T0321434

Tumor Cell Differentiation
Biology and Pharmacology

Experimental Biology and Medicine

Tumor Cell Differentiation

Biology and Pharmacology

Edited by

Jarle Aarbakke, Peter K. Chiang, and H. Phillip Koeffler

Humana Press • Clifton, New Jersey

Library of Congress Cataloging-in-Publication Data:

Tumor cell differentiation.

     (Experimental biology and medicine)
     Contains the proceedings of an International Symposium on the Biology and
Pharmacology of Tumor Cell Differentiation, held on June 29–July 1, 1986, at the University
of Tromsö, Norway.
     Includes index.
     1. Cancer cells—Congresses.
2. Cell differentiation—Congresses.
3. Cell transformation—Congresses.
I. Aarbakke, Jarle II. Chiang, Peter K. III. Koeffler, H. Phillip. IV. International Symposium
on the Biology and Pharmacology of Tumor Cell Differentiation (1986: University of Tromsö)
V. Series: Experimental biology and medicine (Clifton, NJ)
[DNLM: 1. Cell transformation, Neoplastic—congresses. QZ 202 T9216 1986]

RC268.5.T86 1987   616.99'4071   87-17012
ISBN 0-89603-134-9

Preface

This volume contains the proceedings of an International Symposium on the Biology and Pharmacology of Tumor Cell Differentiation-held on June 29–July 1, 1986 at the University of Tromsö, Norway.

The objective of this meeting was to bring together scientists from various disciplines to discuss recent advances in the understanding of tumor cell differentiation and to bridge the gap between experimental findings and clinical application of new knowledge. Thus the information will be of value not only to basic scientists involved in molecular and cell biology, but also to pharmacologists and clinicians trying to develop the concept of tumor cell differentiation as a therapeutic modality. Each plenary speaker and selected poster presenters were requested to submit a comprehensive, up-to-date review of recent contributions to their disciplines related to differentiation and: hematopoietic factors and leukemic cells in culture; vitamin derivatives and polyamines; nucleosides and methylation; and cell interactions.

Jarle Aarbakke
Peter K. Chiang
H. Phillip Koeffler

Acknowledgments

The organizers gratefully acknowledge the financial support provided by the following firms and organizations:

The University of Tromsö
The Norwegian Cancer Society   *Main Sponsors*

Apothekernes Laboratorioum A/S
Bayer Kjemi A/S
Bristol Meyers A/S
Norsk Hydro A/S, Department of Biotechnology
Nycomed A/S
Mack Bryggeri A/S
Roche, Norway
SAS, Tromsö
The Erna and Olav Aakre Foundation for Cancer Research
The Norwegian Society for Science and the Humanities (NAVF)
The Wellcome Foundation Ltd
Tromsbanken/Bergen Bank
Weiders Farmasoytiske A/S

Contents

Hematopoietic Factors, Leukemic Cells in Culture, and Differentiation

Vitamin Derivatives, Polyamines, and Differentiation

Nucleosides, Methylation, and Differentiation

Cell Interactions and Differentiation

Contributors

J. Aarbakke • Department of Pharmacology, Institute of Medical Biology, University of Tromsö, Tromsö, Norway

J. P. Abita • INSERM Hôpital Saint Louis, Paris, Fance

Ateeq Ahmad • Department of Applied Biochemistry, Division of Biochemistry, Walter Reed Army Institute of Research, Washington, DC

Berit E. Bang • Department of Pharmacology, Institute of Medical Biology, University of Tromsö, Tromsö, Norway

Edward J. Benz, Jr. • Department of Internal Medicine, and Human Genetics, Yale University School of Medicine, New Haven, Connecticut

Atle Bessensen • Institute of Medical Biology, University of Tromsö, Tromsö, Norway

R. Bjerkvig • Department of Pathology, The Gade Institute, Haukeland Hospital, University of Bergen, Bergen, Norway

Magnus Björkholm • Department of Medicine, Danderyd Hospital, Danderyd, Sweden

Nesbitt D. Brown • Department of Applied Biochemistry, Walter Reed Army Institute of Research, Washington, DC

Sara Chaffee • Duke University Medical Center, Durham, North Carolina

Peter K. Chiang • Department of Applied Biochemistry, Walter Reed Army Institute of Research, Washington, DC

Ruud Delwel • The Dr. Daniel den Hoed Cancer Center, Rotterdam, The Netherlands

Rune Djurhuus • Clinical Pharmacological Unit, Department of Pharmacology, University of Bergen, Bergen, Norway

Walter Doerfler • Institute of Genetics, University of Cologne, Cologne, Germany

xi

John A. Duerre • *Department of Microbiology and Immunology, Ireland Research Laboratory, University of North Dakota Medical School, Grand Forks, ND*

Stefan Einhorn • *Department of Medicine, Karolinska Hospital, Stockholm, Sweden*

A. Faille • *INSERM Hôpital Saint Louis, Paris, France*

Gösta Gahrton • *Department of Medicine, Huddinge University Hospital, Huddinge, Sweden*

B. Geny • *INSERM Hopital Saint Louis, Paris, France*

Richard K. Gordon • *Department of Applied Biochemistry, Walter Reed Army Institute of Research, Washington, DC*

Michael L. Greenberg • *Duke University Medical Center, Durham, North Carolina*

Gunnar Grimfors • *Department of Medicine, Danderyd Hospital, Danderyd, Sweden*

U. Gullberg • *Division of Hematology, Department of Medicine, University of Lund, Lund, Sweden*

Barton F. Haynes • *Duke University Medical Center, Durham, North Carolina*

Svein Helland • *Clinical Pharmacological Unit, Department of Pharmacology, University of Bergen, Bergen, Norway*

Eva Hellström • *Department of Medicine, Huddinge University Hospital, Huddinge, Sweden*

Michael S. Hershfield • *Duke University Medical Center, Durham, North Carolina*

Katherine A. High • *Department of Medicine, and Human Genetics, Yale University School of Medicine, New Haven, Connecticut*

Arnd Hoeveler • *Institute of Genetics, University of Cologne, Cologne, Germany*

Monica Hollstein • *International Agency for Research on Cancer, Lyon, France*

Andreas Killander • *Department of Medicine, University Hospital, Uppsala, Sweden*

Dagmar Knebel • *Institute of Genetics, University of Cologne, Cologne, Germany*

H. P. Koeffler • *University of California, Los Angeles, California*

I. Krawice • *INSERM Hôpital Saint Louis, Paris, France*

Joanne Kurtzberg • *Duke University Medical Center, Durham, North Carolina*

A. Ladoux • INSERM Hôpital Saint Louis, Paris, France

O. D. Laerum • Department of Pathology, The Gade Institute, Haukeland Hospital, University of Bergen, Bergen,Norway

Beverly Lange • The Wistar Institute of Anatomy and Biology and the Department of Oncology, The Children's Hospital of Philadelphia, Philadelphia, Pennsylvania

Klaus-Dieter Langner • Institute of Genetics, University of Cologne, Cologne, Germany

Ursula Lichtenberg • Institute of Genetics, University of Cologne, Cologne, Germany

Christina Lindemalm • Department of Medicine, Karolinska Hospital, Stockholm, Sweden

Sverre O. Lie • Pediatric Institute, Rikshospitalet, Oslo, Norway

Karen Lomax • Department of Internal Medicine, and Human Genetics, Yale University School of Medicine, New Haven, Connecticut

Bob Lowenberg • The Dr. Daniel den Hoed Cancer Center, Rotterdam, The Netherlands

Hakan Mellstedt • Department of Medicine, Karolinska Hospital, Stockholm, Sweden

Robert W. Mercer • Department of Internal Medicine, and Human Genetics, Yale University School of Medicine, New Haven, Connecticut

Malcolm A. S. Moore • Memorial Sloan-Kettering Cancer Center, New York, New York

Lee D. Nelson • Walter Reed Army Institute of Research, Washington, DC

Bo Nilsson • Department of Medicine, Helsingborg Hospital, Helsingborg, Sweden

A. Norman • University of California, Riverside, California

I. Olsson • Division of Hematology, Department of Medicine, University of Lund, Lund, Sweden

Ake Öst • Department of Medicine, Southern Hospital, Stockholm, Sweden

Felipe N. Padilla • Walter Reed Army Institute of Research, Washington, DC

J. B. Paukovits • Institute for Tumor Biology / Cancer Research, University of Vienna, Austria

W. R. Paukovits • Institute for Tumor Biology / Cancer Research, Universtiy of Vienna, Austria

Mona Pederson • Department of Pharmacology, Institute of Medical Biology, University of Tromsö, Tromsö, Norway

O. Poirier • INSERM Hôpital Saint Louis, Paris ,France

Per S. Prytz • Institute of Medical Biology, University of Tromsö, Tromsö, Norway

Thomas A. Rado • Department of Internal Medicine, and Human Genetics, Yale University School of Medicine, New Haven, Connecticut

Helga Refsum • Clinical Pharmacological Unit, Department of Pharmacology, University of Bergen, Bergen , Norway

H. Reichel • University of California, Riverside, California

Doris Renz • Institute of Genetics, University of Cologne, Cologne, Germany

Karl-Henrik Robert• Department of Medicine, Huddinge University Hospital, Huddinge, Sweden

Giovanni Rovera • The Wistar Institute of Anatomy and Biology and the Department of Oncology, The Children's Hospital of Philadelphia, Philadelphia, Pennsylvania

Leo Sachs • Department of Genetics, Weizmann Institute of Science, Rehovot, Israel

Georg Sager • Department of Pharmacology, Institute of Medical Biology, University of Tromsö, Tromsö, Norway

Jan Samuelsson • Department of Medicine, Southern Hospital, Stockholm , Sweden

Joel Schindler • Department of Anatomy and Cell Biology, University of Cincinnati College of Medicine, Cincinnati, Ohio

Jay W. Schneider • Department of Internal Medicine, and Human Genetics, Yale University School of Medicine, New Haven, Connecticut

Eric J. Stanbridge • Microbiology and Molecular Genetics, University of California, Irvine, California

S. K. Steinsvaag • Department of Pathology, The Gade Institute, Haukeland Hospital, University of Bergen, Norway

Catherine Stolle • Department of Internal Medicine, and Human Genetics, Yale University School of Medicine, New Haven, Connecticut

Asbjörn M. Svardal • Clinical Pharmacological Unit, Department of Pharmacology, University of Bergen, Bergen Norway

A. Tobler • University of California, Los Angeles, California

Ann-Mari Uden • Department of Medicine, Southern Hospital, Stockholm, Sweden

Per M. Ueland • Clinical Pharmacological Unit, Department of Pharmacology, University of Bergen, Bergen, Norway

William P. Wiesmann • Walter Reed Army Institute of Research, Washington, DC

Bernd Weisshaar • Institute of Genetics, University of Cologne, Cologne, Germany

Ingemar Winqvist • Department of Medicine, Lund Hospital, Lund, Sweden

Hiroshi Yamasaki • International Agency for Research on Cancer, Lyon, France

Hematopoietic Factors, Leukemic Cells in Culture, and Differentiation

HEMATOPOIETIC GROWTH AND DIFFERENTIATION FACTORS AND THE REVERSAL OF MALIGNANCY

Leo Sachs

Department of Genetics, Weizmann Institute of Science, Rehovot 76100, Israel

ABSTRACT

"The described cultures thus seem to offer a useful system for a quantitative kinetic approach to hematopoietic cell formation and for experimental studies on the mechanism and regulation of hematopoietic cell differentiation" (1). Our development of systems for the in vitro cloning and clonal differentiation of normal hematopoietic cells made it possible to identify A. The factors that regulate growth and differentiation of these normal cells. B. The changes in the normal development program that result in leukemia, and C. How to reverse malignancy in leukemic cells. I have mainly used myeloid cells as a model system. Normal hematopoietic cells require different proteins to induce growth (growth factors) and differentiation (differentiation factors). There is a multigene family for these factors. Identification of these factors and their interaction has shown how growth and differentiation can be normally coupled. The development of leukemia involves uncoupling of growth and differentiation. This can occur by changing the requirement for growth without blocking cell response to the normal inducers of differentiation. Addition of normal differentiation factors to these malignant

cells still induces their normal differentiation,
and the mature cells are then no longer malignant. Genetic changes which inhibit differentiation by normal differentiation factors can occur
in the progression of leukemia. But even these
leukemic cells may still be induced to differentiate by other compounds, including low doses of
compounds now being used in cancer therapy, that
can induce differentiation by alternative pathways. The differentiation of leukemic to mature
cells results in the reversion of malignancy by
by-passing genetic changes that produce the
malignant phenotype. We have obtained this differentiation of leukemic cells <u>in vitro</u> and <u>in vivo</u>
and by-passing genetic defects by inducing differentiation can be a useful approach to therapy.

INTRODUCTION

The multiplication and differentiation of normal
cells is controlled by different regulatory molecules. These regulators have to interact to
achieve the correct balance between cell multiplication and differentiation during embryogenesis and during the normal functioning of the
adult individual. The origin and further progression of malignancy results from genetic changes
that uncouple the normal balance between multiplication and differentiation so that there are
too many growing cells. This uncoupling can occur
in various ways (2-6). What changes in the normal
development program produce cells with different
degrees of malignancy? When cells have become
malignant, can malignancy again be suppressed so
as to revert malignant back to non-malignant
cells? Malignant cells can have different abnormalities in the controls for multiplication and
differentiation. Do all the abnormalities have
to be corrected, or can they be by-passed in
order to suppress malignancy? I will discuss our
results obtained with normal and leukemic myeloid
hematopoietic cells, and also some results with
sarcomas, as model systems that can be used to
try and answer these questions.

NORMAL HEMATOPOIETIC GROWTH FACTORS AND DIFFERENTIATION FACTORS

An understanding of the mechanisms that control multiplication (growth) and differentiation in normal cells would seem to be an essential requirement to elucidate the origin and reversibility of malignancy. The development of appropriate cell culture systems (Table 1) has made it possible to identify the normal regulators of growth (growth factors) for various types of cells, and also in some cell types the normal regulators of differentiation (differentiation factors). This approach has been particularly fruitful in identifying the normal growth factors for all the different types of hematopoietic cells, first for myeloid cells (1,7-10) and then for other cell types, including T lymphocytes (11) and B lymphocytes (12). The growth and differentiation factors for hematopoietic cells are different proteins that can be secreted by the cells that produce them. The normal differentiation factors but not the growth factors for myeloid cells are DNA binding proteins (13,14). It will be interesting to determine how far this applies to normal differentiation factors for other cell types.

Table 1.
History of cloning and clonal differentiation of normal hematopoietic cells in culture

---

1963.	Cloning and clonal differentiation in liquid medium (1).
1965.	Cloning and differentiation in agar (7).
1965.	Factors for growth and differentiation secreted by cells (7).
1966.	Factors in conditioned medium from cells (8,9).
1966.	Cloning and differentiation in methylcellulose (9).
1966.	Confirmation of cloning and differentiation in agar (10).

In cells of the myeloid series four different growth-inducing proteins have been identified. These have been given various names and are now called macrophage and granulocyte inducers-types 1 (MGI-1), or colony stimulating factors (CSF) (2,3,15,16). Of the four growth factors, one protein (M) induces the development of clones with macrophages, another (G) clones with granulocytes, the third (GM) clones with both macrophages and granulocytes, and the fourth (also called Interleukin-3, IL-3), clones with macrophages, granulocytes, eosinophils, mast cells, erythroid cells, or megakaryocytes (Table 2, Fig. 2). Cloning of the genes for the IL-3 (17,18) GM (19), M (20) and G (21) growth factors has shown that these genes are unrelated in their nucleotide sequence. This multigene family represents a hierarchy of growth factors for different stages of hematopoietic cell development as the precursor cells become more restricted in their developmental program. It can be assumed that in the normal development program IL-3 functions as a growth factor at an early stage when the precursors have the potential to develop into 6 cell types, GM at a later stage when the precursors have a more limited potential and can develop into 2 cell types, and that G and M are growth factors when the developmental potential is still more restricted to produce only one cell type (Fig. 1). There is presumably also such a hierarchy of growth factors in the developmental program of other types of cells.

How do normal myeloid precursor cells induced to multiply by these growth factors develop into clones that contain mature differentiated cells that stop multiplying when they terminally differentiate? It appears unlikely that a growth factor which induces cell multiplication is also a differentiation factor whose action includes the stopping of cell multiplication in mature cells. Proteins that act as myeloid cell differentiation factors have been identified and these have been called MGI-2 or differentiation factors (DF) (2,3,15,22-24). Experiments with normal myeloid cell precursors have shown that in these

HIERARCHY OF GROWTH FACTORS IN DEVELOPMENT

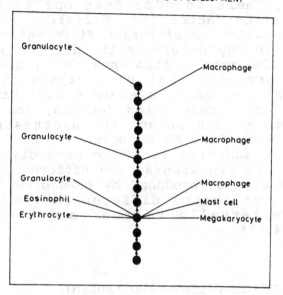

Fig.1. Myeloid precursors can be induced to grow by 4 different growth factors (Table 1). One (IL-3) induces growth in precursors that have the potential to develop into 6 cell types, the second (GM) when the precursors can develop into 2 cell types, and the third (M) and fourth (G) when the precursors produce one cell type.

cells the growth factors induce cell viability and cell multiplication and also production of different factors (2,3,25,26). The myeloid differentiation factors induce differntiation directly, whereas the growth factors induce differentiation indirectly by inducing the production of differentiation factors (Table 2). This induction of differentiation factor by growth factor thus ensures the normal coupling of growth and differentiation, a coupling mechanism that may also apply to other cell types. Diffe-

rences in the time of the switch-on of the differentiation factor would produce differences in
the amount of cell multiplication before differentiation. There is more than one type of
differentiation factor (5). Different growth
factors may switch on different differentiation
factors which may determine the differentiated
cell type. The results thus show that there are
different proteins that participate in the
developmental program of myeloid cells, growth
factors and differentiation factors, and that
growth factors can induce the synthesis of
differentiation factors in normal myeloid precursors. In addition to their production by
normal myeloid precursors, the differentiation
factors can also be produced by some other cell
types and can induce differentiation when
supplied externally to the target cells
(2,3,5,22-24,27).

GROWTH FACTORS AND LEUKEMIA

Identification of these normal growth and differentiation factors and the cells that produce
them, has made it possible to identify the different types of changes in the production or
response to these normal regulators that occur in
leukemia. The normal myeloid growth factors can
be produced by various cell types. However, these
growth factors are not made by the normal myeloid
precursors (25,26), so that the normal precursors
require an external source of growth factor for
cell viability and growth. Cells that become
malignant have escaped some normal control, which
can be associated with changes from an induced to
a constitutive expression of certain genes
(2,28,29). In myeloid leukemic cells different
clones of malignant cells have been identified
which have shown the various types of changes
that can occur in the normal response to growth
factors (2,3,5,30). There are different leukemic
clones that A. Need less or have become independent of normal growth factor for growth. B.
Constitutively produce their own growth factor,

and C. Are blocked in the ability of growth
factor to induce production of differentiation
factor. The cells blocked in the ability of
growth factor to induce production of differentiation factor include some cell lines in culture
which require an external source of growth factor
for growth (25,26), and in some leukemic cells
which constitutively produce their own growth
factor, changes in specific components of the
culture medium can restore the ability of growth
factor to induce differentiation factor (15,31).

Growth factors induce cell viability and cell
multiplication (25,26,32). Independence from
normal growth factor or constitutive production
of their own growth factor, can also explain the
survival and growth of metastasizing malignant
cells in places in the body where the growth
factor required for the survival of normal cells
is not present. In cells that are malignant and
may still need some growth factor, the organ pre-
ference of metastasis could be due to production
of the required growth factor in the organ where
the metastasis occurs. Normal macrophages and
granulocytes, and other cell types, move in
certain directions in response to various chemotactic stimuli (33). But the myeloid leukemic
cells which metastasize did not respond to these
chemotactic stimuli (34). A decrease or lack of
response to chemotactic stimuli which are
presumably produced in certain organs could also
explain the ability of metastatic, and non-
metastatic tumor cells, to move in a more dis-
organized manner than normal cells.

The transformation of normal into malignant cells
can involve different genetic changes including
changes in gene dosage (27), gene mutations, de-
letions and gene rearrangements (see 35,36). The
genes involved in the expression of malignancy
are now called oncogenes (see 36-39), and the
changes of normal genes to oncogenes are in all
cases associated with changes in the structure
or regulation of the normal genes (see 36-39).
Some oncogene products are related to a growth
factor or a receptor for growth factor.

The sis oncogene is derived from one of the normal genes for platelet derived growth factor (40,41), the erb B oncogene from the gene for the receptor for epidermal growth factor (42), and the fms proto- oncogene is related (43) to the receptor for one of the hematopoietic growth factors, CSF-1 = MGI-1M = M-CSF (Table 2). These results are thus providing further information on the genetic differences that result in changes in the normal production or response to growth factors that occur in malignancy.

DIFFERENTIATION FACTORS IN LEUKEMIA

The different types of myeloid leukemic cells include clones that have changed their normal requirement for growth factor and in which growth factor no longer switches on production of differentiation factor, but which can still be induced to differentiate to mature non-dividing cells by a normal differentiation factor. These clones, which are called D$^+$ clones (D for differentiation) can be induced to differentiate normally to mature macrophages and granulocytes via the normal sequence of gene expression that occurs during differentiation by incubating the cells with normal differentiation factor (see 2,3,27). The mature cells, which can be formed from all the cells of a leukemic clone, then stop multiplying like normal mature cells and are no longer malignant. Experiments carried out in animals have shown that normal differentiation of these myeloid leukemic cells to mature non-dividing cells can be induced not only in culture but also in the body (44-49). These leukemias therefore grow progressively when there are too many leukemic cells for the normal amount of differentiation factor in the body. The development of leukemia can be inhibited in mice with these leukemic cells by increasing the normal amount of differentiation factor either by injecting it, or by injecting a compound that increases production of differentiation factor by cells in the body (45,46).

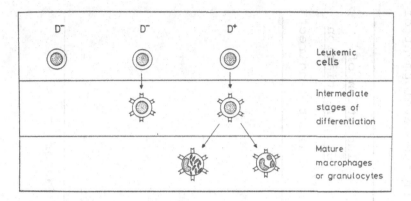

Fig. 2. Classification of different types of clones of myeloid leukemic cells according to their ability to be induced to differentiate by normal differentiation factors. Some differentiation-defective (D⁻) clones can be induced by normal differentiation factors to intermediate stages by differentiation, whereas other D⁻ clones were not induced to differentiate by these factors even to an intermediate stage.

The culture of different clones of myeloid leukemic cells in the presence of differentiation factor has shown that in addition to D⁺ clones there are also differentiation-defective clones (called D⁻ clones). Some of these clones were induced to an intermediate stage of differentiation which then slows down the growth of the cells, and others could not be induced to differentiation even to this intermediate stage (see 3,27,30,50) (Fig. 2). Since normal differentiation factor can induce differentiation to mature non-dividing cells in the D⁺ clones, it can be suggested that D⁺ clones are the early stages of leukemia and that the formation of different types of D⁻ clones may be later stages in the further progression of malignancy. Does this progression include complete loss of the genes for differentiation in D⁻ clones?

Table 2. Growth factors and differentiation factors in the development of myeloid hematopoietic cells

Nomenclature	Differentiated cell type	Induction of differentiation	
		Direct	Indirect*
Growth factors			
MGI-1M = M-CSF = CSF-1	Macrophages	–	+
MGI-1G = G-CSF	Granulocytes	–	+
MGI-1GM = GM-CSF	Macrophages and granulocytes	–	+
IL-3	Macrophages, granulocytes and others	–	+
Differentiation factors			
MGI-2 = DF	Macrophages and granulocytes	+	–

*Growth factor induces production of differentiation factor

To answer this, experiments were carried out to determine whether compounds other than normal differentiation factor can induce differentiation in myeloid leukemic cells.

Studies with a variety of chemicals other than normal differentiation-inducing protein have shown that many compounds can induce differentiation in D^+ clones of myeloid leukemic cells. These include certain steroid hormones, chemicals such as cytosine arabinoside, adriamycin, methotrexate and other chemicals that are used to-day in cancer chemotherapy, and also x-irradiation (Table 3). At high doses these compounds used in cancer chemotherapy and x-irradiation kill cells, whereas at low doses they can induce differentiation. Not all these compounds are equally active on the same leukemic clone. A variety of chemicals can also induce differentiation in clones that are not induced to differentiate by normal differentiation factor, and in some clones induction of differentiation requires combined treatment with different compounds (see 3,5,30). The results show that although the response for induction of differentiation by differentiation factor has been altered, the D^- clones have not lost all the genes for differentiation.

Table 3.
Compounds used to-day in cancer therapy that can induce differentiation in clones of myeloid leukemic cells at low doses

Adriamycin, cytosine arabinoside daunomycin, hydroxyrea, methotrexate, mitomycin C, prednisolone, X-irradiation

In addition to certain steroids and chemicals used to-day in chemotherapy and irradiation, other compounds that can induce differentiation in myeloid leukemic cells include insulin, bacterial lipopolysaccharide, certain plant lectins and phorbol esters, together with or without differentiation factor (see 5,30). It is probable that all myeloid leukemic cells no longer susceptible to the normal differentiation factor by it self can be induced to differentiate by choosing the appropriate combination of compounds.

The ability of a variety of compounds to induce differentiation in malignant cells is not restricted to myeloid leukemic cells. Erythro-leukemic cells can be induced to differentiate by various chemicals (51,52). Erythropoietin, a normal protein that induces the production of hemoglobin in normal erythrocytes, did not induce hemoglobin in these erythroleukemias. These erythroleukemias are thus like D^- myeloid leukemias that are not induced to differentiate by the normal myeloid differentiation factor. It has also been shown that some of the compounds that induce differentiation in leukemic cells can induce differentiation in tumors derived from other types of cells (52).

Studies on the way in which different compounds act in myeloid leukemic cells have shown that there are different ways of inducing differen-tiation. Some compounds induce differentiation by inducing the production of differentiation-inducing protein (differentiation factor) in the D^+ leukemic cells, whereas others such as the steroid hormones induce differentiation without inducing this protein. Various compounds can also induce differentiation in D^- clones that are not induced to differentiate by normal differen-tiation factor, not all clones respond to the same compound, and in some clones differentiation requires combined treatment with more than one compound. Not all compounds act in the same way and in cases of combined treatment each compound induces changes not induced by the other.

The combined treatment then produces, by comple-
mentation, the appropriate gene expression that
is required for differentiation (see 3,5).

Further evidence that there are different ways of
inducing differentiation in leukemic cells was
obtained from studies on changes in the synthesis
of cellular proteins in normal myeloid precursors
and different types of myeloid leukemic cells
(2,28,29). These experiments have shown that
there are protein changes that have to be induced
in normal cells and are constitutive in leukemic
cells. The leukemic cells were found to be
constitutive for changes in the synthesis of a
group of proteins that were only induced in
normal cells after the addition of growth factor.
These protein changes, which include the appearance of some proteins and disappearance of
others, where constitutive in all the leukemic
clones studied derived from different leukemias.
They have been called C_{leuk}, for constitutive in
leukemia. D^+ leukemic cells can be induced to
differentiate to mature cells by normal differentiation factor. This showed that the differentiation program induced by differentiation factor
can proceed normally, even when the protein
changes induced in normal cells by growth factor
have become constitutive. There were other
protein changes that were induced by differentiation factor in normal and D^+ leukemic clones but
were constitutive in the differentiation-
defective D^- leukemic clones. With this group of
proteins, the most differentiation-defective
clones showed the highest number of constitutive
protein changes. These protein changes have been
called C_{def}, for constitutive in differentiation
defective (2,28) (Fig. 3).

The protein changes during differentiation of
normal myeloid precursors are induced as a series
of parallel multiple pathways of gene expression.
It can be assumed that normal differentiation
requires synchronous initiation and progression
of these multiple parallel pathways. The
presence of constitutive instead of induced gene
expression for some pathways can be expected to

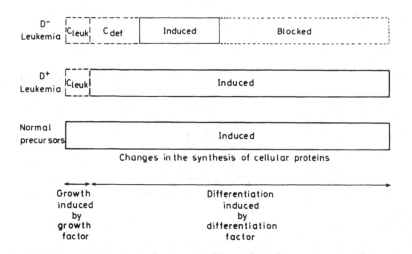

Fig. 3. Schematic summary of changes in the synthesis of cellular proteins associated with growth and differentiation. C_{leuk}, constitutive expression of changes in all the clones of myeloid leukemic cells compared to normal myeloblasts. C_{def}, constitutive expression of changes in differentiation-defective (D⁻) clones of leukemic cells compared to differentiation-competent (D⁺) leukemic clones and normal myeloblasts. The most differentiation-defective D⁻ clones (Fig. 5) showed the highest number of C_{def} constitutive protein changes (28).

produce asynchrony in the co-ordination required for differentiation. Depending on the pathways involved, this asynchrony can then produce blocks in the induction and termination of the differentiation program (2,28,29). D⁻ leukemic cells can be treated so as to induce the reversion of C_{def} proteins from the constitutive to the induced state. This reversion was associated with restoration of inducibility for differentiation by the normal differentiation factor. Reversion from constitutive to the induced state in these cells thus restored the synchrony of

gene expression that is required for differentiation (53).

The study of different mutants of myeloid
leukemic cells has shown that in addition to the
existence of constitutive protein changes that
inhibit differentiation of myeloid leukemic cells
by normal differentiation factor, there are also
constitutive protein changes that inhibit differentiation by the steroid hormone dexamethasone. The constitutive changes that inhibit
differentiation by dexamethasone are different
form those that inhibit differentiation by normal
differentiation factor (29). These experiments
have thus identified different pathways of gene
expression for inducing differentiation, and have
also shown that genetic changes which inhibit
differentiation by one compound need not affect
differentiation by another compound that uses
alternative pathways. Since the normal differentiation factor for myeloid cells has been
identified and leukemic clones have been found
that respond to this normal differentiation
factor, it was possible to compare the ability of
clones of myeloid leukemic cells to be induced to
differentiation by the normal inducer and by
other compounds. Even though the normal differentiation factors or many other cell types have
not yet been identified, it seems likely that the
conclusion on the different pathways of inducing
differentiation derived from studies with myeloid
leukemic cells will also apply to other types of
tumors.

ONCOGENE SUPPRESSORS AND BY-PASSING OF GENETIC DEFECTS IN THE REVERSAL OF MALIGNANCY

Evidence has been obtained with various types of
tumors including sarcomas (27), myeloid leukemias
(27,30) and teratocarcimomas (54) that malignant
cells have not lost the genes that control normal
growth and differentiation. This was first shown
in sarcomas by the finding that it was possible
to reverse the malignant to a non-malignant
phenotype with a high frequency in cloned sarcoma

cells whose malignancy had been induced by
chemical carcinogens, x-irradiation, or by a
tumor-inducing virus (27,55,56). In sarcomas
induced after transformation of normal
fibroblasts in culture with chemical carcinogens
(57,58) or x-irradiation, (59,60) this reversibility of malignancy included reversion to the
limited life-span found with normal fibroblasts
(61).

Chromosome studies on normal fibroblasts,
sarcomas, revertants from sarcomas which had
regained a non-malignant phenotype, and re-
revertants, showed that the difference between
these malignant and non-malignant cells is
controlled by the balance between genes for
expression (E) and suppression (S) of malignancy
(27,56,62-65). When there is enough S to
neutralize E malignancy is suppressed, and when
the amount of S is not sufficient to neutralize E
malignancy is expressed. These early experiments
have shown (4,27,56,62-65) that in addition to
genes for expression of malignancy (E)
(oncogenes), there are other genes, S genes (that
have now been called soncogenes (4), or anti-
oncogenes (66), that can suppress the action of
oncogenes. Suppression of the action of the Ki-
ras oncogene in revertants (66,67), is presumably
due to such suppressor genes. The balance between
oncogenes and their suppressors also seems to
determine malignancy in other tumors including
human retinoblastomas (68).

In the mechanism found with sarcomas (see 4,27)
reversion was obtained by chromosome segregation,
resulting in a change in gene dosage due a change
in the balance of specific chromosome. This
suppression of malignancy by chromosome segregation, with a return to the gene balance
required for expression of the non-malignant
phenotype, occurred without hybridization between
different types of cells. The non-malignant
cells were thus derived form the malignant ones
by genetic segregation. Suppression of malignancy
associated with chromosome changes including
changes in gene balance have also been found

after hybridization between different types of cells (35,69-73). These studies on cell hybrids have led to similar conclusion to those obtained from the reversal of malignancy in sarcomas without hybridisation between different cell types.

In addition to this reversion of malignancy by chromosome segregation another mechanism of reversion was found in myeloid leukemia. These leukemic cells also have an abnormal chromosome composition (74). In this second mechanism reversion to a non-malignant phenotype was also obtained in certain clones with a high frequency, but this reversion was not associated with chromosome segregation. Phenotypic reversion of malignancy in these leukemic cells was obtained by induction of the normal sequence of cell differentiation by the normal differentiation factor (2,3,27,30). In this reversion of the malignant phenotype, the stopping of cell multiplication by inducing differentiation to mature cells by-passes genetic changes in the requirement for the normal growth factor, and the block in the ability of growth factor to induce differentiation factor, that produced the malignant phenotype. Genetic changes which make cells defective in their ability to be induced to differentiate by the normal differentiation factor occur in the evolution of myeloid leukemia. But even these cells can be induced to differentiate by other compounds, either singly or in combination, that can induce the diffe-rentiation program by other pathways. (2,5,30) Also in these cases the stopping of cell multi-plication by inducing differentiation by these alternative pathways by-passes the genetic changes that inhibit response to the normal differentiation factor. This by-passing of genetic defects is presumably also the mechanism for the suppression of malignancy by inducing differentiation in other types of tumors such as erythroleukemias (51,52) and neuroblastomas.

There is also the possibility that all the oncogenes are lost (75), or that the changes of normal genes into oncogenes are actually reversed. Chromosome changes can also change malignant ceells from D⁻ to D+ (74) so that the cells can then be induced to differentiate when exposed to normal differentiation factors.

It can, therefore, be concluded that the changes of normal genes into oncogenes that result in the expression of malignancy does not mean that this expression of malignancy can not again be suppressed. The results on the reversibility of malignancy have shown that there are different ways of suppressing malignancy (Fig.4), that reversion does not have to restore all the normal controls and that the stopping of cell multiplication by inducing differentiation can by-pass genetic defects that give rise to malignancy.

HEMATOPOIETIC GROWTH AND DIFFERENTIATION FACTORS IN THERAPY

I have suggested from these results that the reversibility of malignancy provides new possibilities for therapy (27,30). This is an alternative approach to therapy based on the use of cytotoxic agents which with the agents used so far kills many normal cells as well as tumor cells. The reversion of malignancy by correcting genetic abnormalities may be of therapeutic value in the future. However, the therapeutic possibilities of reverting malignancy by inducing differentiation and thus by-passing the genetic abnormalities are already now testable. Results showing that the development of myeloid leukemia can be inhibited in mice with D+ leukemic cells by injecting a normal differentiation factor, or injecting a compound that increases the production of differentiation factor in the body (45,46), indicate a therapeutic potential for normal differentiation factors. The induction of growth of normal myeloid precursors by myeloid growth factors and their differentiation to macrophages and granulocytes by the differentiation factors, also indicates (45,46) that

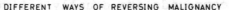

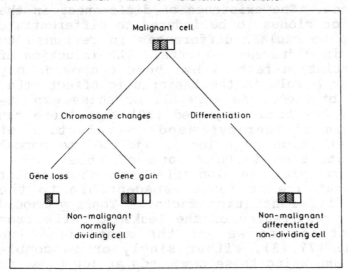

Fig. 4. Malignancy can be suppressed in different ways. <u>A</u>. By chromosome changes that change the balance between genes for the expression of malignancy (oncogenes) and genes that suppress oncogenes, or <u>B</u>. The stopping of cell multiplication by inducing differentiation to mature cells can by-pass genetic changes that produce the malignant phenotype. Chromosome changes can also change malignant cells from D⁻ to D⁺ so that the cells can then be induced to differentiate when exposed to normal differentiation factors.

injection of these factors and the use of compounds that increase their production in the body can be of value in restoring the normal macrophage and granulocyte population after cytotoxic therapy. The use of these factors may also be of value for treating non-malignant macrophage and granulocyte defects (30). Chemicals and irradiation used to-day in cancer therapy at high doses to kill cells can induce differentiation in leukemic cells at low doses.

not all these compounds are equally active on the
same clone. The existence of differences in the
ability of clones to be induced to differentiate
may help to explain differences in response to
therapy in different patients. The induction of
differentiation factors by these compounds may
also play a role in the therapeutic effects that
can be obtained. As a result of these experiments it has been suggested (30) that there can
be a form of therapy based on induction of
differentiation by using in addition to normal
differentiation factors some of these other
compounds, which can also affect mutant malignant
cells that are no longer susceptible to the
normal differentiation factor. Therapy should
include prescreening of the leukemic cells from
each patient to select the most effective
compound (77,78), either singly or in combination, and using these compounds at low doses to
induce differentiation. Differentiation therapy
could also in some cases be combined with cytotoxic therapy to reduce the number of malignant
cells. Based on these suggestions some
encouraging clinical results with myeloid
leukemia have been obtained with low doses of
cytosine arabinoside (79-87) which is one of the
compounds that can induce differentiation in
myeloid leukemic cells (30,50). Differentiation
therapy should also be applicable to tumors
derived from other types of cells whose growth
and differentiation are controlled by other
normal factors.

ACKNOWLEDGMENTS

This research is now supported by the Albert and
Victoria Ebner Foundation for Leukemia Research
the National Foundation of Cancer Research,
Bethesda, and the Jerome A. and Estelle R. Newman
Assistance Fund.

REFERENCES

1. Ginsburg H. and Sachs L. (1963) J Natl Cancer Inst **31**, 1-40.
2. Sachs L. (1980) Proc Natl Acad Sci, U.S.A. **77**, 6152-6156.
3. Sachs L. (1982) Cancer Surveys **1**, 321-342.
4. Sachs L. (1984) Cancer Surveys **3**, 219-228.
5. Sachs L. (1985) In Molecular Biology of Tumor Cells,pp. 257-280, Nobel conference, Stockholm, New York, Raven Press
6. Sachs L. (1986) Scientific American **254**, 40-47.
7. Pluznik D.H. and Sachs L. (1965) J Cell Comp Physiol **66**, 319-324.
8. Pluznik D.H. and Sachs L. (1966) Exper Cell Res **43**, 553-563.
9. Ichikawa Y., Pluznik D.H. and Sachs L. (1966) Proc Natl Acad Sci, U.S.A. **56**, 488-495.
10. Bradley T.R. and Metcalf D. (1966) Aust J Exp Biol Med Sci **44**, 287-300.
11. Mier J.W. and Gallo R.C. (1980) Proc Natl Acad Sci, U.S.A. **77**, 6134-6138.
12. Möller G (ed) (1984) Immunol Rev 78
13. Weisinger G. and Sachs L. (1983) EMBO J **2**, 2103-2107.
14. Weisinger G., Korn A.P. and Sachs L. (1985) Europ J Cell Biol **37**, 196-202.
15. Sachs L. and Lotem J. (1984) Nature **312**, 407
16. Metcalf D. (1985) Science **299**, 16-22.
17. Fung M.C., Hapel S.J., Ymer S., Cohen D.R., Johnson R.M., Campbell H.D. and Young I.G. (1984) Nature **307**, 233-237.
18. Yokota T., Lee F., Rennick D, Hall C. Arai N., Mosmann T., Nabel G., Cantor H. and Arai K-I. (1984) Proc Natn Acad Sci, U.S.A. **81**, 1070-1074.
19. Gough N.M. Gough J. Metcalf D., Kelso A., Grail D., Nicola N.A., Burgess A.W. and Dunn A.R. (1984) Nature **309**, 763-767.
20. Kawasaki E.S., Ladner M.B:, Wang A.M., Van Arsdell J., Kim Warren M., Coyne M.Y., Schweickart V.L., Lee M-T., Wilson K.J., Boosman A., Stanley E.R., Ralph P. and Mark D.F. (1985) Science **230**, 291-296.

21. Nagata S., Tsuchiya M., Asano S., Kaziro Y., Yamazaki T.,Yamamoto O., Hirata Y., Kubota N., Oheda M., Nomura H. and Ono M. (1986) Nature **319**, 415-418.
22. Ichikawa Y., Maeda N. and Horiuchi M. (1976) Int J cancer **17**, 789-797.
23. Tomida M., Yamamoto-Kamaguchi Y. and Hozumi M. (1984) J Biol Chem **259**, 10978-10982.
24. Olsson I., Sarngadharan M.G., Breitman T.R. and Gallo R.C. (1984) Blood **63**, 510-517.
25. Lotem J. and Sachs L. (1982) Proc Natl Acad Sci, U.S.A. **79**, 4347-4351.
26. Lotem J. and Sachs L. (1983) Int J Cancer **32**, 127-134.
27. Sachs L. (1974) Harvey Lectures. Vol. 68 pp. 1-35. New York, Academic Press (1974)
28. Liebermann D., Hoffman-Liebermann B. and Sachs L. (1980) Develop Biol **79**, 46-63.
29. Cohen L. and Sachs L. (1981) Proc Natl Acad Sci, U.S.A. **78**, 353-357.
30. Sachs L. (1978) Nature **274**, 535-539.
31. Symonds G. and Sachs L. (1982) EMBO J **1**, 1343-1346.
32. Tushinski R.J., Oliver I.T., Guilbert L.J., Tynan P.W., Warner J.R. and Stanley E.R. (1982) Cell **28**, 71-81.
33. Wilkinson P.C. (1974) Chemotaxis and inflammation, London Churchill Livingstone.
34. Symonds G. and Sachs L. (1979) Somat Cell Genet **5**, 931-944.
35. Klein G. (1981) Nature **194**, 313-318.
36. Land H., Parada L.F. and Weinberg R.A. (1983) Science **222**, 771-778.
37. Bishop J.M. (1983) Ann Rev Biochem **52**, 301-354.
38. Cooper G.M. (1982) Science **218**, 801-806.
39. Temin M. and Miller K. (1984) Cancer Surveys **3**, 229-246.
40. Waterfield M.D., Scrace G.T., Whittle N., Stroobant P., Johnsson A., Wasteson A., Westermark B., Heldin C.H., Huang J.S. and Deuel T.F. (1983) Nature **304**, 35-39.

41. Doolittle R.F., Hunkapiller M.W., Hood L.E., Devare S.G., Robbins K.C., Aaronson S.A. and Antoniades H.N. (1983) Science **221**, 275-277.
42. Downward J., Yarden Y., Mayers E., Scrace G., Totty N., Stockwell P., Ulrich A., Schlessinger J. and Waterfield M.D. (1984) Nature **307**, 521-527.
43. Sherr C.J., Rettenmier C.W., Sacca R., Roussel M.F., Look A.T. and Stanley E.R. (1985) Cell **41**, 665-676.
44. Lotem J. and Sachs L. (1978) Proc Natl Acad Sci, U.S.A. **75**, 3781-3785.
45. Lotem J. and Sachs L. (1981) Int J Cancer **28**, 375-386.
46. Lotem J. and Sachs L. (1984) Int J Cancer **33**, 147-154.
47. Lotem J. and Sachs L. (1985) Leukemia Res **9**, 249-258.
48. Gootwine E., Webb C.G. and Sachs L. (1982) Nature **299**, 63-65.
49. Webb C.G., Gootwine E. and Sachs L. (1984) Develop Biol **101**, 221-224.
50. Lotem J. and Sachs L. (1974) Proc Natl Acad Sci, U,S.A. **71**, 3507-2511.
51. Friend C. (1978) Harvey Lectures. Vol 72, pp. 253-281, New York, Academic Press.
52. Marks P. and Rifkind R.A. (1978) Ann Rev Biochem **47**, 419-448.
53. Symonds G. and Sachs L. (1983) EMBO J **2**, 663-667.
54. Stewart T.A. and Mintz B. (1981) Proc Natl Acad Sci, U.S.A. **78**, 6314-6318.
55. Rabinowitz Z. and Sachs L. (1968) Nature **220**, 1203-1206.
56. Rabinowitz Z. and Sachs L. (1970) Nature **225**, 136-139.
57. Berwald Y. and Sachs L. (1963) Nature **200**, 1182-1184.
58. Berwald Y. and Sachs L. (1965) J Natl Cancer Inst **35**, 641-661.
59. Borek C. and Sachs L. (1966) Nature **210**, 276-278.
60. Borek C. and Sachs L. (1967) Proc Natn Acad Sci, U.S.A. **57**, 1522-1527.

61. Rabinowitz Z. and Sachs L. (1970) Int J Cancer **6**, 388-398.
62. Hitotsumachi S., Rabinowitz Z. and Sachs L. Nature **231**, 511-514.
63. Yamamoto T., Rabinowitz Z. and Sachs L. (1973) Nature New Biol **243**, 247-250.
64. Bloch-Shtacher N. and Sachs L. (1976) J Cell Physiol **87**, 89-100.
65. Bloch-Shtacher N. and Sachs L. (1977) J Cell Physiol **93**, 205-212.
66. Craig R.W. and Sager R. (1985) Proc Natl Acad Sci, U.S.A. **82**, 2062-2066.
67. Noda M., Selinger Z., Scolnick E.M. and Bassin R.H. (1983) Proc Natl Acad Sci, U.S.A. **80**, 5602-5606.
68. Murphree A.L. and Benedict W.P. (1984) Science **223**, 1028-1033.
69. Ringertz N.R. and Savage R.E. (1976) Cell Hybrids New York, Academic Press.
70. Stanbridge E.J., Der C.J., Doersen C-J, Nishimi R.Y., Peehl D.M., Weissman B.E. and Wilkinson J.E. (1982) Science **215**, 252-259.
71. Evans E.P., Burtenshaw M.D., Brown B.B., Hennion R. and Harris H. (1982) J Cell Sci **56**, 113-130.
72. Kitchin R.M., Gadi I.K., Smith B.L. and Sager R. (1982) Somat Cell Genet **89**, 677-689.
73. Benedict W.F., Weissman B.E., Mark C. and Standbridge E.J. (1984) Cancer Res **44**, 3471-3479.
74. Azumi J. and Sachs L. (1977) Proc Natn Acad Sci, U.S.A. **74**, 253-257.
75. Frankel A.E., Haapala D.K., Newbouer R.L. and Fischinger P.J. (1976) Science **191**, 1264-1266.
76. Fibach E., Landau T. and Sachs L. (1972) Nature New Biol **237**, 276-278.
77. Lotem J. and Sachs L. (1980) Int J Cancer **25**, 561-564.
78. Lotem J., Berrebi A. and Sachs L. (1985) Leukemia Res **9**, 249-258.
79. Castaigne S., Daniel M.T., Tilly H., Gerait P. and Degos L. (1983) Blood **62**, 85-86.
80. Wischz J.S., Griffin J.D. and Kufe D.W. (1983) New Engl J Med **309**, 1599-1602.

81. Manoharan A. (1983) New Engl J Med **309**, 1652-1653.
82. Mufti G.J., Oscier D.G., Hamblin T.J. and Bell A.J. (1983) New Engl J Med **309**, 1563-1564.
83. Michalewicz R., Lotem J. and Sachs L. (1984) Leuk Res **8**, 783-790.
84. Ishikura H., Sawada H., Okazaki T., Mochizuki T., Izumi Y., Yamagishi M. and Uchino H. (1984) Brit J Haemat **58**, 9-18.
85. Tilly H., Castaigne S., Bordessoule D., Sigaux F., Daniel M-T., Monconduit M. and Degos L. (1985) Cancer **55**, 1633-1636.
86. Jensen M.K. and Ahlbom G. (1985) Scand J Haematol **34**, 261-263.
87. Shtalrid M., Lotem J., Sachs L. and Berrebi A. (1986) Scand J Haematol in press.

G-CSF AS A DIFFERENTIATION-INDUCING AGENT IN NORMAL AND LEUKEMIC MYELOPOIESIS.

MALCOLM A.S. MOORE.

MEMORIAL SLOAN-KETTERING CANCER CENTER

NEW YORK, NEW YORK.

The "reversal of malignancy" in leukemia, while an attractive goal, is one that is rarely attainable in its entirety in clinical or experimental systems. What is more feasible and has proved attainable, is removal of the maturation block in the leukemic lineage with resulting development of varying but incomplete functional and phenotypic features of lineage-specific differentiation.

Post-deterministic differentiation of normal hematopoietic progenitors is under the control of lineage-specific growth factors and lineage fidelity is the norm. The last five years have seen accelerated progress in the characterization and purification of murine and human hematopoietic growth factors, culminating in the current availability of recombinant material in sufficient quantities for extensive in vitro and in vivo testing. Hematopoietic growth factors can be considered in three categories. Type A mediate terminal differentiation by action on a specific lineage restricted progenitor; Type B have more extensive action where there is mediation of differentiation in one or two lineages by action on specific lineage-restricted progenitors and a survival promoting and proliferation-inducing action on earlier progenitors of other lineages without induction of differentiation. Type C factors would be pluripotent,

supporting proliferation, self-renewal and differentiation of pluripotent stem cells with multiple differentiation potential and self-renewal capacity. The
class C pluripotent factors have proved the hardest to
characterize because their action may be considered
permissive for survival or proliferation of cells whose
commitment to any lineage is the result of stochastic
events rather than deterministic ones. Furthermore,
terminal expression of differentiation may invariably
require synergistic interaction with class A growth
factors.

It has recently become clear that human myeloid leukemias retain responsiveness to hematopoietic growth
factors which they can produce themselves (autocrine)
or that are provided from an exogenous source. As with
normal hematopoietic progenitors, proliferative and
differentiation changes may be induced and current
strategy is designed to accentuate differentiation at
the expense of leukemic stem cell self-renewal. In
contrast to the high degree of fidelity seen in normal
hematopoiesis, a high degree of lineage infidelity in
leukemic blast cell populations has been reported in
some studies. This controversial observation suggests
that the differentiation program of leukemic cells is
constructed abnormally relative to the programmatic
components of normal lineages.

It remains to be seen whether lineage-specific growth
factors, or other differentiation-inducing agents,
while not being deterministic may nevertheless impact
on, or maintain the fidelity of expression of, differentiation in terminal stages of leukemic cell maturation.

A major goal of current therapy in leukemia is the
selective inhibition of leukemic cell proliferation
relative to the proliferation of normal stem cells.
Decades of chemotherapy research have defined some
clinically effective agents but in general the "toxic
window" has proved too narrow for highly selective
erradication of leukemic stem cells without damage,
frequently irreversible, to the normal stem cell
compartment. Differentiation-inducing agents, while
falling short in their ability to "reverse" malignancy,

can nevertheless prove highly effective in suppressing leukemic stem cell self-renewal capacity by inducing "death" by differentiation to a post-mitotic stage. Reduction or elimination of leukemic stem cell self-renewal, together with restoration of responsiveness to homeostatic control, may prove to be the most effective therapeutic strategy in myeloid leukemia since the leukemic cells would lose their competitive advantage over normal stem cells and would no longer clonally dominate hematopoiesis.

In designing strategies to test some of the above hypotheses, various differentiation inducible leukemic cell lines have been utilized. Much of the history of the development of an effective chemotherapy for leukemia was based on the availability of cell lines, or transplantable leukemias, with sensitivity to cell cycle specific agents. The development of biological response modification therapy and the recognition of leukemic cell differentiation as an obtainable goal led to the use of leukemic cell lines capable of terminal maturation. The human cell lines HL-60 and U937 and the murine lines WEHI-3 and Ml are examples. HL-60 was isolated from the peripheral blood of a patient with acute promyelocytic leukemia. U937 originated from the pleural fluid of a patient with diffuse histiocytic lymphoma. At present these lines are cloned, readily maintainable in culture and, most important, exist in an arrested yet differentiation inducible phenotype. These lines in the uninduced state resemble blast cells of their lineage and are believed to be the neoplastic equivalents of committed progenitors of granulocytes and/or monocytes and the histochemistry and morphology of these cell lines typify them as immature cells of myelomonocytic lineages.

Recognition that physiological inducers of differentiation of normal hematopoietic cells could also influence proliferation and differentiation of leukemic cell lines, led to a series of studies over the last decade involving characterization of hematopoietic growth factors, in many cases using leukemic cell lines as sources of growth factor and/or as targets for growth factors in various bioassays. In order to consider the role of a specific growth factor - G-CSF- as a

physiological inducer of myeloid leukemic
differentiation and to understand the nature and extent
of uncoupling of growth factor proliferation and
differentiation responses in leukemic transformation,
the properties of existing growth factors will be
reviewed. In doing so, the problem of nomenclature
arises and while no true logic exists in this area,
Table 1 provides the most current, and hopefully to be
agreed upon, nomenclature of growth factors influencing
hematopoiesis.

TABLE 1.

NOMENCLATURE OF HEMATOPOIETIC GROWTH FACTORS

INTERLEUKIN-2 (IL-2):	T cell growth factor. TCGF.
INTERLEUKIN-3 (IL-3):	Multi-CSF, PSF, Mast cell growth factor, HCGF, BPA, Hemopoietin-2 etc.
INTERLEUKIN-4 (IL-4):	MCGFII/TCGFII, BCGF-I, BSF, IgG-induction factor.
INTERLEUKIN-5 (IL-5):	Eosinophil differentiation factor (EDF), Eo-CSF, TRF, BCGFII, Interleukin-4.
GRANULOCYTE-MACROPHAGE CSF (GM-CSF):	CSFα, MGI-IGM, CSF-2, NIF-T, Pluripoietin α.
GRANULOCYTE CSF (G-CSF):	Pluripoietin, CSFβ, MGI-1G, GM-DF.
MACROPHAGE CSF (M-CSF):	CSF-1, MGI-1M.
ERYTHROPOIETIN (Epo):	Ep, ESF.
HEMOPOIETIN-1 (H-1):	Synergistic Factor.

In general, terminology imposed by hematologists has
reflected function as defined by the assay, for example, a colony stimulating assay, or by a growth
(-poietic) response, both further modified by a lineage
specificity. Immunological terminology favours nomenclature based upon cell network concepts defining
producer and target cells, thus, interleukins numbered
chronologically in order of first publication of the

full sequence of the molecule. A further defining
feature of Interleukins 2 to 5 is that they appear to
be products of T cells, in contrast to G-CSF, M-CSF,
Epo and H-1, which are products of macrophages, endothelial cells, fibroblasts, uroepithelium, etc., but
not T cells. GM-CSF is certainly a T cell product, but
is also an inducible product of endothelial cells and
fibroblasts, but possibly not of macrophages.

MOLECULAR AND BIOLOGICAL CHARACTERISTICS OF HEMATO-
POIETIC GROWTH FACTORS.

Recent progress in the cloning of hematopoietic growth
factor and lymphokine genes and the availability of
recombinant factors for research has led to an escalating interest in the therapeutic potential of these
agents. Table 2 is a summary of the currently characterized factors that influence hematopoietic cell
differentiation. All the native factors are heavily
N-glycosylated, or in the case of G-CSF, O-glycosylated, and all are active in vitro in a nonglycosyla-
ted state. Where tested for in vivo activity (CSF-1,
IL-3, GM-CSF, G-CSF, Epo.) non-glycosylated E.coli
recombinant material is active, with the exception of
Erythropoietin, where glycosylation appears necessary
for in vivo stabilization. In almost every case, both
murine and human gene products are available which is
important in the case of factors whose action is
species restricted (IL-3, IL-4, GM-CSF). No significant sequence homology exists between the different
factors arguing against their evolution from a common
primordial gene. Between species, considerable structural conservation at the nucleotide and amino acid
level is seen when murine and human are compared, with
G-CSF and CSF-1 being the most conserved and IL-3 being
the least conserved. All the molecules are in the
range of 120-178 amino acids with the exception of
CSF-1 whose gene codes for 224 amino acids. However,
its active form is much smaller, coding for a subunit
of 14,500 MW., presumably resulting from cleavage.

The spectrum of biological activity of the factors is
summarized in Table 3. IL-3 is capable of stimulating
proliferation of all classes of myeloid progenitors
including a subset of late pluripotential stem cells

TABLE 2.
RECOMBINANT HEMATOPOIETIC GROWTH FACTORS

NAME	m/h	MOL.WEIGHT** Gly.	Non-Gly.	AMINO ACIDS Total	%Homol	FIRST PURIFIED	FIRST CLONED
IL-3	m	28,000	15,000	134		Ihl et al 1982(1)	Fung et al 1984(2)
	h	25,000	14,600	133	29%		Yang et al 1986(3)
IL-4	m	20,000	14,000	120			Lee et al 1986(4) / Noma et al 1986(5)
	h	20,000	15,000	129	50%		Yokota et al 1986(6)
IL-5	m	18,000	12,300	133	?	Sanderson et al 1986(7)	Kinashi et al 1986(8)
M-CSF	m	66,000	14,500	?		Stanley & Heard 1977(9)	
	h	45,000	14,500	224	80%	Das & Stanley 1982(10)	Kawasaki et al 1985(11)
G-CSF	m	25,000	19,000	178		Nicola et al 1983(12)	Tsuchiya et al 1986(13)
	h	19,600	18,000	174	69%	Welte et al 1985(14)	Souza et al 1986(15) / Nagata et al 1986(16)
GM-CSF	m	23,000	14,100	124		Burgess et al 1977(17)	Gough et al 1984(18)
	h	22,000	14,500	127	54%	Gasson et al 1984(19)	Wong et al 1985(20)
Epo.	h	34,000	18,400	166	?	Miyake et al 1977(21)	Jacobs et al 1985(22)

* m/h mouse or human.
** estimated Mr of fully glycosylated or non-glycosylated molecule.

TABLE 3.

SITES OF ACTION OF INTERLEUKINS AND HEMATOPOIETIC GROWTH FACTORS

CYTOKINE	S.C.*	ERYTH.	MEGA.	NEUT.	Eo.	BAS-MAST.	MONO-MAC.	B	T
IL-2	–	–	–	–	–	–	–	±	++
IL-3	+	+	+	+	+	+	+	–	–
IL-4	–	(+)	(+)	(+)	(+)	++	–	+	+
IL-5	–	–	–	–	++	–	–	+	–
GM-CSF	+	+	+	+	–	–	+	–	–
G-CSF	(+)	(+)	(+)	++	–	–	+	–	–
M-CSF	–	–	–	±	–	–	++	–	–
Epo.	–	++	–	–	–	–	–	–	–
H-1	+	(+)	(+)	(+)	(+)	–	(+)	?	–

* Hematopoietic stem cells (CFU-s CFU-GEMM)

** Parentheses indicate indirect action via accessory cells or synergism with other obligatory growth factor.

that form mixed colonies of neutrophils, monocytes, eosinophils, megakaryocytes and - with the addition of erythropoietin - erythrocytes (12). Despite earlier confusion, there is no evidence of direct action of IL-3 on B or T lineage cells, however, IL-3 is a major growth factor for the mast cell lineage.

Interestingly, inappropriate production of IL-3 by the myelomonocytic leukemia WEHI-3, together with ability of the factor to cause leukemic cell proliferation, but not differentiation, implicates this factor in an autocrine model of leukemogenesis. IL-4 is a lympho-kine that is intimately involved in the allergic response, stimulating mast cell growth and differen-tiation, inducing IgE receptors, promoting B cell proliferation and Ig secretion and acting as a T cell growth factor (4,5,6). IL-5 is a lymphokine pre-dominantly involved in the eosinophil response, acting as a CSF for eosinophil-restricted progenitors and as a functional activator of the mature eosinophil (7,8). In addition, it acts as a growth factor for pre-activated B cells and is a T cell replacing factor in certain antibody responses. The conventional CSF's include GM-CSF that in humans is capable of stimulating colonies of neutrophils, eosinophils and monocytes and appears to have megakaryocyte and erythroid (with erythropoietin) colony stimulating activity (17,20). Its action on myeloid leukemic cells is as a prolif-eration-inducing agent with uncoupling of differen-tiation, however, some differentiation of HL-60 cells can be induced by GM-CSF (34). Like IL-3, autocrine production of GM-CSF by human leukemic cells may be a critical component of malignant tranformation in certain myeloid leukemias. CSF-1 is a monocyte-macrophage proliferation and differentiation inducing agent with the potential for activating monocyte-macrophage production of a variety of monokines (TNF, interferon, GM-CSF prostaglandin E, plasminogen acti-vator, Interleukin-1) (9-11). The identity of the fms protooncogene and the CSF-1 receptor has raised con-siderable interest in the factor and in its role in malignant transformation in certain hematopoietic and fibroblast systems. The CSF-1 receptor may be up-regulated on early hematopoietic stem cells by brief exposure of such cells to a partially purified factor

termed synergistic activity or hemopoietin-1 (36)
originally identified in human spleen of placental
conditioned medium and subsequently purified from the
bladder carcinoma line 5637(36). Hemopoietin-1 has no
direct colony stimulating activity but synergises with
other hematopoietic growth factors.

MURINE G-CSF.

The existence of a regulatory factor specific for
neutrophils was unclear for a long time, due to confusion with the activities of pluripotential IL-3 and
oligopotential GM-CSF. It is now clear that a specific
G-CSF does exist in mouse and man. It was first recognized that a number of active tissue sources of murine
GM-CSF contained an additional structurally and functionally distinct CSF species capable of stimulating
exclusively neutrophil colony formation and neutrophil
differentiation of WEHI-3 myelomonocytic leukemic cells
(12,23). This G-CSF-Dif activity was reported in mouse
post-endotoxin serum (24) and could be distinguished
from GM-CSF by Con-A sepharose binding capacity and
lack of immuno cross reactivity with GM-CSF antisera.
The first purification of mouse G-CSF from endotoxin-
treated mouse lung conditioned medium was reported by
Nicola et al. (12). The differentiating activity
against WEHI-3 cells was purified $x10^5$ fold using
salting out chromatography, phenylsepharose hydrophobic
chromatography, gel filtration and RP-HPLC on phenyl
silica columns and HPLC on gel filtration columns. In
the first two purification steps the Dif. activity
separated from GM-CSF but at all later stages it
co-purified with a distinct neutrophil-specific CSF.
The common identity of the two activities was further
suggested by their localization in a single protein
band on SDS PAGE. The murine factor is a 25,000 Mr.
glycoprotein of considerable hydrophobicity containing
internal disulfide bonds essential for maintaining
structural integrity and biological activity.

Purification of a factor distinct from GM-CSF and also
capable of Dif. activity against M1 mouse leukemic
cells has been reported by the Israel group (25) and
has been termed MGI-2 to distinguish it from MGI-1
which stimulates normal marrow granulocyte-macrophage

colony formation. The hypothesis of this research group is that MGI-2 is a molecule uniquely active in causing leukemic differentiation to granulocytes and macrophages, whereas MGI-1 is the regulator of normal granulocyte-macrophage proliferation and differentiation, being capable of inducing normal or leukemic cells to produce MGI-2. This conflicts with the view that MGI-2 is G-CSF and the Israel group have identified a separate MGI-1G and MGI-1M stimulating proliferation and differentiation of normal progenitors to neutrophil or macrophage suggesting G-CSF is MGI-1G and CSF-1 is MGI-1M (25).

G-CSF interacts with specific high-affinity receptors present in relatively low numbers on mature human and mouse PMN and on all neutrophil lineage progenitors. The receptors are lacking in eosinophil, monocytes, macrophages, erythroid or lymphoid tissue and appear to be specific for neutrophil G-CSF since there is no competition for binding with other CSF-species. Receptors have been purified from the WEHI-3 differentiation-inducible line, but they appear to be lacking on the D non-inducible line (26). Interestingly, but anomalously, the murine macrophage leukemic line, alone among macrophage leukemias tested, possessed high affinity G-CSF receptors and it is this line that was used for isolation of the specific CSF-1 receptor. Conflicting reports exist as to the capacity of mouse G-CSF to stimulate human normal granulocyte progenitor cell differentiation (26) although a differentiation action on human HL-60 or fresh leukemic cells is well established. The most current studies, using highly enriched FACS separated human marrow showed the same degree of colony formation with mouse G-CSF and human CSF-beta with colonies being small, appearing early and degenerating after 7 days of culture (26). The concentration of G-CSF influenced the morphology of colonies since at high concentration, mixed neutrophil-macrophage (but never pure macrophage or eosinophil) colony formation was seen in addition to pure neutrophil colonies, whereas at low concentrations only neutrophil colonies were seen. This differentiation downgrading phenomena is the reverse of that reported for GM-CSF (24).

Some action of G-CSF on the survival and initial proliferation of pluripotent progenitors is seen, for in
delayed addition colony transfer experiments, clones
initiated with GM- or G-CSF for the first few divisions
could be transferred to secondary cultures containing
only IL-3 and colonies of mixed erythroid, megakaryocyte and myeloid cells developed (27).

HUMAN G-CSF.

The association of neutrophil leukocytosis with a
variety of neoplasias in man has in certain cases been
attributed to inappropriate production of hematopoietic
growth factors by tumor tissue. In a patient with
squamous carcinoma of the oral cavity and in a case of
squamous cell carcinoma of the lung and in a pancreatic
carcinoma (28-30) associated with leukocytosis, transplantation of tumor tissue in nude mice provoked a
leukocytosis in recipient animals (28-30) which was
tumor mass dependent and reversed upon excision of the
tumor (30). The neutrophil leukocytosis in nude mice
induced by a transplanted lung tumor was associated
with marked splenomegaly and an increase in myeloid,
erythroid and megakaryocytic progenitor cells and
pluripotential stem cells detected by the CFU-s assay
(31-32). Freshly isolated tumor cells and cell lines
established from leukocytosis-inducing tumors have also
been shown to produce CSF active in human marrow
culture and tumor cell production of CSF is not un-
common since nine of 67 tumors screened were found to
be positive in one survey and nearly 50% of lung,
pancreas and urinary bladder carcinomas were found to
produce CSF (33). The human hepatoma cell line Hep-1
and the bladder carcinoma cell line 5637 are both
constitutive producers of high levels of both G- and
GM-CSF (14,34) Interleukin-1 (35 and Moore MAS.,
unpublished observation) and 5637 produces a synergistic factor, Hemopoietin-1 (36). Whether CSF production by the preceding tumor types reflects aberrant
gene expression associated with malignant transformation, or is a true reflection of the functional
capacity of the normal tissue from which the tumor
arose, is unclear. Certainly in man, fibroblasts,
endothelial cells, trophoblasts, monocyte-macrophage
and activated T cells are the only normal sources of

CSF that have been clearly defined and recently it has been reported that normal human prostate and uretral epithelia, cultured or freshly isolated, have the capacity to produce CSF that is active on both human and murine bone marrow (33). The cross species activity of human tumor-derived CSF and its ability to induce a neutrophil leukocytosis in nude mice, clearly points to the active CSF species being C-GSF since it acts across species barriers, while human GM-CSF does not and M-CSF is only weakly active as a colony stimulus in man and its action is predominantly to induce monocyte-macrophage production.

CSF activity in the conditioned medium of the human bladder carcinoma cell line 5637 was purified by sequential ammonium sulfate precipitation, anion-exchange chromatography, and gel filtration (14). In the final purification step on RP-HPLC human CSF activity and a differentiating (GM-DF) activity for both HL-60 and WEHI-3B (D+) leukemic cells eluted together at a propanol concentration of 42%. An additional peak of GM-DF activity eluted at a lower propanol concentration and fractions from this peak were highly active in inducing differentiation of HL-60 cells, but were inactive on WEHI-3 cells and in the human GM-CSF colony assay at day 7. The least hydrophobic activity called CSF-alpha (26) or pluripoietin alpha (34) is structurally and functionally homologous to murine GM-CSF (although not species cross reactive) and the hydrophobic species called CSF-beta (26) or pluripoietin (14) is the human analogue of murine G-CSF, since these two CSF's exhibit similar activities on murine and human cells and are fully cross-reactive with each others specific cellular receptors (14,15,26). This latter CSF species was purified to homogeneity and was shown to be O-glycosylated and to have a molecular weight of 19,600 (14). The gene encoding this pluripotent human G-CSF was subsequently cloned and expressed in E.coli (15,16). The E-coli rh-G-CSF was comprised of 174 amino acids with a deduced molecular weight of 18,700 and it had no significant homology with any other previously sequenced growth factors. Recently, the cDNA sequence coding for murine G-CSF has been isolated from a cDNA library prepared with mRNA derived from murine fibrosarcoma NFSA cells, which

produce G-CSF constitutively (13). The nucleotide
sequence and the deduced amino acid sequence of murine
G-CSF cDNA were 69% and 73% homologous, respectively,
to the corresponding sequences of human G-CSF cDNA.

Native and recombinant G-CSF had comparable biological
activity, stimulating neutrophil granulocyte colonies
of mouse and man with a specific activity of 1×10^8
units per milligram of pure protein (15).

The action of hG-CSF on mature hematopoietic cells
appears to be confined to an action on neutrophils
involving increased expression of chemotactic receptors, and enhanced phagocytic ability, cellular metabolism associated with the respiratory burst, antibody-
dependent cell killing and the expression of function-
associated cell surface antigens (37,38). Our earlier
observation with purified G-CSF showing that at high
concentrations, the factor stimulated BFU-E and CFU-
GEMM in methylcellulose cultures of adherent and T cell
depleted human marrow (14) were confirmed using rh-G-
CSF (15). More recent studies in our laboratory (14)
using highly enriched hematopoietic progenitor cells
failed to demonstrate a direct effect of human G-CSF on
BFU-E and CFU-GEMM, suggesting that the earlier observations may have been the consequence of an indirect
mechanism involving non-T accessory cells (39). We
have documented that G-CSF can stimulate the generation
of new CFU-GM in suspension culture of accessory cell
depleted human marrow, suggesting a recruitment action
on some pre-CFU-GM populations and/or enhanced self
renewal of pre-existing CFU-GM capable of responding to
both G-CSF and GM-CSF (40). This observation provides
evidence for a stimulatory action of G-CSF on a progenitor population with a differentiation potential more
extensive than that of neutrophil lineage-restricted
CFU-G. The CFU-GM generated in suspension cultures with
G-CSF responded to GM-CSF in colony assay by a normal
pattern of differentiation into eosinophils and macrophages as well as neutrophils.

In vivo, administration of G-CSF by the intraperitoneal
route led to sustained serum levels of bioactive G-CSF
comparable to those found 3-6 hrs. post injection of
endotoxin in endotoxin responsive strains of mice (40).

The use of highly purified recombinant G-CSF, absence
of significant contamination of our G-CSF with endotoxin and the use of C3H/HeJ mice, allowed us to
conclude that the in vivo responses seen were due to
the action of G-CSF, rather than any contaminant, acting directly or synergistically on neutrophil production. The predominant response involved elevation of
peripheral blood neutrophils by 6-9 fold in C3H/HeJ
mice, which was somewhat lower than we have observed in
other strains, since up to a 20 fold increase in blood
neutrophils can be obtained in Balb/c mice. Studies in
hamsters also indicated a specific action on the
neutrophil lineage with an increase of 3-6 fold in
peripheral blood neutrophils (41), and in monkeys
receiving 10ug/kg/days of rh-G-CSF, neutrophil counts
rose five fold and up to 12 fold with 100/ug/kg/day
(42). In mice, demand for increased hematopoiesis
following such insults as endotoxin treatment, irradiation or cytotoxic drug treatment is met by a marked
expansion of splenic hematopoiesis with little absolute
change in marrow cellularity. Thus it was not surprising that the major expansion of neutrophil production
elicited by chronic G-CSF treatment was met by a rapid
onset of extensive splenic myelopoiesis. What was
surprising was that the splenic phase of hematopoiesis
was associated with increased erythropoiesis, megaka-
ryocytopoiesis, and elevated numbers of pluripotential
stem cells and progenitors of all hematopoietic lineages. Indeed, the splenic increase led to an absolute
total body expansion of production of these cell
populations, although only neutrophils and to a lesser
extent monocytes, but not red cells, platelets and
eosinophils increased in the circulation. It is
possible that G-CSF acts directly to activate pluripotential stem cells detected by the day 12 CFU-s assay
leading to their enhanced proliferation, mobilization,
migration to the spleen and subsequent expansion. In
this scenario, progenitors for lineages other than
neutrophil, could be generated in increased numbers as
a result of stochastic mechanisms believed to operate
at the level of pluripotential stem cell self-renewal
and differentiation. Alternatively, indirect mechanisms may operate whereby G-CSF-induced differentiation
depletes a population of neutrophil progenitors which
in turn triggers activation of the pluripotential stem

cell pool and expansion of the marrow microenvironment. A third possibility is that G-CSF acts in vivo upon an accessory cell population to induce release of other hematopoietic growth factors known to influence multiple hematopoietic lineages.

G-CSF AND LEUKEMIC CELLS.

The action of G-CSF on leukemic cells is receptor mediated and competitive binding studies with ^{125}I-labeled hG-CSF (15) or murine G-CSF (26) revealed receptors on fresh human leukemic marrow cells classified as M2,M3 and M4, on murine WEHI-3 and human HL-60 and U937 leukemic cell lines. Furthermore, these leukemic cell lines and receptor positive human leukemic cells were induced by recombinant G-CSF to undergo terminal differentiation to macrophages and granulocytes (15).

HL-60 and WEHI-3 cells were differentially sensitive to native human G-CSF in the colony assay measuring conversion of leukemic colonies from compact undifferentiated to diffuse, differentiated, with HL-60 cells requiring approximately five times more G-CSF for comparable effect. Morphological and cytochemical analysis of HL-60 colonies with cytochemical analysis of colony morphology revealed that up to 75% of HL-60 colonies were induced to contain significant numbers (>10%) of polymorphonuclear neutrophils and there was increased intensity of alpha-napthyl acetate esterase staining (37).

Many endogenous cytokines and lymphokines appear capable of inducing both neutrophil and monocytoid maturational changes in HL-60 cells and of mature monocyte and macrophage functional features in the U937 monocytic leukemic cell line. Since functional neutrophil and macrophage maturation involves changes in lysosomal enzyme activity, in cytoskeletal protein, glycolipid profiles and altered expression of cell surface receptors in a coordinated temporal sequence, no single criterion of differentiation can establish the exact developmental state of induced cells. For this reason, we elected to characterize leukemic cell differentiation, using a panel of markers characteristic of mature granulocytes and macrophages and applied to leukemic cells cultured for 206 days in simple sus- pension culture in the presence of various sources of cytokine/lymphokine differentiation inducers (42, 44). Table 4 shows the various parameters of differentiation monitored in U937 and HL-60 cultures exposed for varying intervals to unseparated conditioned media, partially purified fractions of inducer activity and pure natural or recombinant cytokines and lymphokines.

TUMOR NECROSIS FACTOR AND G-CSF.

The ability of endotoxin to elicit production of G-CSF can account for most reports of the leukemia- differentiation action of post-endotoxin serum in mouse and man (45), however, the elevation of bioactive G-CSF in post-endotoxin serum is partially masked at high serum concentrations by an inhibitory activity which is particularly evident in post-endotoxin sera of mice primed with BCG or C.parvum ()45. This hematopoietic or colony inhibitory activity was shown to be directed at both normal CFU-GM and myeloid leukemic cells. Bio- chemical characterization showed that it co-purified with an activity with both in vitro L cell cytotoxicity and in vivo tumor necrosis action. Subsequent studies distinguished between the antiproliferative effects of tumor necrosis factor on CFU-GM and myeloid leukemic cells and the proliferation and differentiation induc- ing action of the G-CSF co-induced with similar kinet- ics in the serum of C. parvum-endotoxin treated mice (45). With the availability of recombinant human TNF alpha (18) it was possible to demonstrate that human CFU-GM, BFU-E and CFU-GEMM were inhibited by relatively low concentrations of TNF (<100 Units/ml) and that the inhibition was potentiated by addition of gamma inter- feron (46). We have explored the antagonism between CSF species and TNF alpha in both short-term clonogenic assays and long-term bone marrow cultures(40). The stimulation of increased granulopoiesis persists as long as G-CSF is administered in vivo although the duration of studies to date have been limited to 4-5 wks. In long-term marrow culture much longer periods, up to 4 months, with sustained high levels of G-CSF have been obtained, with persisting elevation of

TABLE 4.

G-CSF INDUCIBLE FEATURES OF HL-60 AND U937.

1. Neutrophil/macrophage or macrophage morphology.

2. Adherence.

3. Activation of lysozomal enzymes (myeloperoxidase, α-naptha esterase, alkaline and acid phosphatase, lysozyme, lactoferrin).

4. Reactive oxygen production, NBT reduction.

5. Enhanced expression of the Fc, C3 and fMLP chemotactic receptors.

6. Enhanced phagocytosis and bacteriacidal capacity.

7. Antibody-dependent cell-mediated tumor cell killing.

8. Induction of monocyte-related antigens OKM1 and Leu M2.

9. Stimulation of ConA-induced release of Prostaglandin E_2, 6-keto $PGE_{1\alpha}$ and Thromboxane B_2.

10. Enhanced glucosamine uptake and glycoconjugate synthesis.

11. Conversion of compact, undifferentiated leukemic colonies to diffuse differentiated.

12. Reduced recloning capacity of leukemic colonies.

neutrophil production relative to control cultures and no evidence was obtained for premature exhaustion of stem cells or accelerated depletion of cultures.

The ability of low concentrations (100μ/ml) of TNF alpha to counteract the proliferative action of G-CSF in vitro in clonal assay and long-term bone marrow cultures (40) suggests a physiological role for TNF as a natural inhibitor of neutrophil granulopoiesis. The co-ordinate inducibility of G-CSF and TNF alpha following endotoxin-activation of macrophages may provide a mechanism self-limiting the chronic generation of neutrophils from marrow progenitors following bacterial infection. Alternatively, the relative resistance to TNF inhibition of myeloid progenitors stimulated by GM-CSF may provide an alternate pathway for generating neutrophils in the face of elevated TNF levels. The interrelationship of TNF and CSF in the production and function of neutrophils is further emphasised by the observation that TNF can enhance both the phagocytic ability and the antibody-dependent cytotoxicity of neutrophils, increase their superoxide anion production and stimulate their adherence to endothelial cells (47). In addition, TNF has been shown to stimulate growth factor production by endothelial cells, due in part to activation of transcription of the GM-CSF gene (48).

REFERENCES

1. Ihle,J.N.,Keller,J.,Henderson L.,Klein.,F.,
   and Palaszinski,E.(1982)J.Immunol.129,
   2431-2435
2. Fung,M.C.,Hapel,A.J.,Ymer,S.,Cohan,D.R.,
   Johnson,R.M.,Campbell,H.D.,and Young,I.G.
   (1984)Nature(Lond)307,233-237.
3. Yang,Y.C.,Ciarletta,A.B.,Temple,P.A.,Chung,
   M.P.,and Kovacic,S.(1986)Cell 47,3-10.
4. Lee, F.,Yokota,T.,Otsuka,T.,Meyerson,P.,
   Villaret,D.,Coffman,R.,Mosmann,T.,Rennick,
   D.,Roehm,N.,Smith,C.,Zlotnik,A.,and Arai,
   K-I.(1986)Proc.Natl.Acad.Sci.USA.83,
   2061-2065.
5. Noma,Y.,Sideras,P.,Naito,T.,Bergstedt-
   Lindquist,S.,Azuma,C.,Severinson,E.,Tanabe,T.,
   Kinashi,T.,Matsuda,F.,Yaoita,Y.,and Honjo,T.
   (1986)Nature 319,640-646.
6. Yokota,T.,Otsuka,T.,Mosmann,T.,Banchereau,J.,
   DeFrance,T.,Blanchard,D.,DeVries,J.E.,Lee,F.
   and Arai,K-I.(1986)Proc.Natl.Acad.Sci.USA.
   83,5894-5898.
7. Sanderson,C.J.,O'Garra,A.,Warren,D.J.,and
   Klaus,G.G.B.(1986)Proc.Natl.Acad.Sci.USA.
   83,437-440.
8. Kinashi,T.,Harada,N.,Severinson,E.,Tanabe,T.,
   Sideras,P.,Konishi,M.,Azuma,C.,Tominaga,A.,
   Bergstedt-Lindquist,S.,Takahashi,M.,Matsuda,
   F.,Yaoita,Y.,Takatsu,K.,and Honjo,T.(1986)
   Nature 324,70-73.
9. Stanley,E.R.,and Heard,P.M.(1977)J.Biol.Chem.
   252,4045-4052.
10. Das,S.K.,and Stanley,E.R.(1982)J.Biol.Chem.
    256,13679-13684.
11. Kawasaki,E.S.,Ladner,M.B.,Wang,A.M.,VanArsdell,J.,
    Warren,M.K.,Coyne,M.Y.,Schweickart,V.L.,Lee,M-T.,
    Wilson,K.J.,Boosman,A.,Stanley,E.R.,Ralph,P.,
    and Mark,D.F.(1985)Science 230,291-230.
12. Nicola,N.A.,Metcalf,D.,Matsumoto,M.and Johnson
    G.R.(1983)J.Biol.Chem.258,9017-9021.
13. Tsuchiya,M.,Shigetaka,A.,Kaziro,Y.,and Shigekazu
    N.(1986)Proc.Natl.Acad.Sci.USA.83,7633-7637.
14. Welte,K.,Platzer,E.,Lu,L.,Gabrilove,J.L.,Levi,E.,
    Mertelsmann,R. and Moore,M.A.S.(1985)Proc.Natl.

Acad.Sci.USA.82,1526-1530.

15. Souza,L.M.,Boone,T.C.,Gabrilove,J.,Lai,P.H.,Zsebo,
     K.M.,Murdock,D.C.,Chazin,V.R.,Bruszewski,J.,
     Lu,H.,Chen,K.K.,Barendt,J.,Platzer,E.,Moore,
     M.A.S.,Mertelsmann,R.,and Welte,K.(1986)Science
     232,61-65.

16. Nagata,S.,Tsuchiya,M.,Asano,S.,Kaziro,Y.,Yamazaki,
     T.,Yamamoto,O.,Hirata,Y.,Kubota,N.,Oheda,M.,
     Nomura,H.and Ono,M.(1986)Nature 319,415-418.

17. Burgess,A.W.,Camakaris,J.,and Metcalf,D.(1977)
     J.Biol.Chem.252,1998-2003.

18. Gough,N.M.,Gough,J.,Metcalf,D.,Kelso,A.,Grail,D.,
     Nicola,N.A.,Burgess,A.W.,and Dunn,A.R.(1984)
     Nature(London)309,763-767.

19. Gasson,J.C.,Weisbart,R.H.,Kaufman,S.E.,Clark,S.C.,
     Hewick,R.,Wong,G.G.,and Golde,D.W.(1984)Science
     226,1339.

20. Wong,G.G.,Witek,J.S.,Temple,P.A.,Wilkens,K.M.,
     Leary,A.C.,Luxenberg,D.P.,Jones,S.S.,Brown,E.L.,
     Kay,R.M.,Orr,E.C.,Shoemaker,C.,Golde,D.W.,
     Kaufman,R.J.Hewick,R.M.,Wang,E.A.,and Clark,S.C.
     (1985)Science 228,810-815.

21. Miyake,T.,Kung,C.K-H.,and Goldwasser,E.(1977)J.
     Biol.Chem.252,5558-5564.

22. Jacobs,K.,Shoemaker,C.,Rudersdorf,R.,Neill,S.D.,
     Kaufman,R.J.,Mufson,A.,Seehra,J.,Jones,S.S.,
     Hewick,R.,Fritsch,E.F.,Kawakita,M.,Shimizu,T.,
     and Miyake,T.(1985)Nature 313,806-810.

23. Nicola,N.A.,and Metcalf,D.(1981)J.Cell Physiol.
     109,253-264.

24. Burgess,A.W.,and Metcalf,D.(1980)Blood 56,947-958.

25. Lotem,J.,Lipton,J.H.,and Sachs,L.(1980)Int.J.
     Cancer 25,763-771.

26. Nicola,N.A.,Begley,C.G.and Metcalf,D.(1985)Nature
     316,625-628.

27. Metcalf,D.,and Nicola,N.A.(1983)J.Cell Physiol.
     116,198-206.

28. Asano,S.,Urabe,A.,Okabe,T.,Sato,N.,Kondo,Y.,
     Ueyama,Y.,Chiba,S.,Ohsawa,S.,and Kosaka,K.(1977)
     Blood 49,845-852.

29. Sato,N.(1979)Cancer 43,605-609.

30. Yunis,A.A.,Jimenez,J.J.,Wu,M-C.,and Andreotti,P.E.
     (1984)Exp.Hematol.12,838-843.

31. Motoyoshi,K.,Suda,T.,Takaku,F.,and Miura,Y.(1983)
     Blood 62,980-987.

32. Mizoguchi,H.,Suda,T.,Miura,Y.,Kubota,K.,and
     Takaku,F.(1982)Exp.Hemat.10,874-880.
33. Zinzar,S.N.,Svet-Moldavsky,G.J.,Fogh,J.,Mann,P.E.,
     Arlin,Z.,Iliescu,K.,and Holland J.F.(1985)Exp.
     Hematol.13,574-580.
34. Gabrilove,J.,.Welte,K.,Harris,P.,Platzer,E.,Lu,L.,
     Levi,E.,Mertelsmann,R.and Moore,M.A.S.(1986)Proc.
     Natl.Acad.Sci.USA.83,2478.
35. Doyle,M.V.,Brindley,L.,Kawasaki,E.,and Larrick,J.
     (1985)Biochem.and Biophys.Res.Comm.130,768-773.
36. Jubinsky,P.T.,and Stanley,E.R.(1985)Proc.Natl.
     Acad.Sci.82,2764-2768.
37. Platzer,E.,Welte,K.,Gabrilove,J.L.,Lu,L.,Harris,
     P.,Mertelsmann,R.,and Moore,M.A.S.(1985)J.Exp.
     Med.162,1788-1801.
38. Metcalf,D.(1986)Blood 67,257-267.
39. Ottmann,O.G.,Welte,K.,Souza,L.M.,and Moore,M.A.S.
     (1987)Blut (in press).
40. Moore,M.A.S.,Welte,K.,Gabrilove,J.,and Souza,L.M.
     (1987)Blut (in press).
41. Zsebo,K.M.,Cohen,A.M.,Murdock,D.C.,Boone,T.C.,
     Inoue,H.,Chazin,V.R.,Hines,D.,and Souza,L.M.
     (1987)Immunobiol.(in press).
42. Welte,K.,Bonilla,M.A.,Gillio,A.P.,Boone,T.C.,
     Potter,G.K.,Gabrilove,J.L.,Moore,M.A.S.,
     O'Reilly,R.J.,and Souza,L.M.(1987)J.Exp.Med.
     (in press).
43. Harris,P.,Ralph,P.,Litkofski,P.,and Moore, M.A.S.
     (1985)Cancer Res.45,9-13.
44. Harris,P.,Ralph,P.,Gabrilove,J.,Welte,K.,Karmali,
     R.,andMoore,M.A.S.(1985)CancerRes.45,3090-3095.
45. Moore,M.A.S.(1982)J.Cell.Physiol.Suppl.1,53-64.
46. Broxmeyer,H.E.,Williams,D.E.,Lu.L.,Cooper,S.,
     Anderson,S.L.,Beyer,G.S.,Hoffman,R.,and
     Rubin,B.Y.(1986)J.Immunol.136,4487-4496.
47. Shalaby,M.R.,Pennica,D.,and Palladino,M.A.,(1986)
     Springer Seminars in Immunopathol.9,34-43.
48. Broudy,V.C.,Kaushansky,K.,Segal,G.M.,Harlan,J.M.,
     and Adamson,J.W.(1986)Proc.Natl.Acad.Sci.U.S.A.
     83,7467-7472.

INDUCTION OF DIFFERENTIATION IN MYELOID LEUKEMIC CELLS AND THE DIFFERENTIATION INDUCING FACTOR (DIF)

U Gullberg and I Olsson

Division of Hematology, Department of Medicine,
University of Lund, S-221 85 Lund, Sweden

ABSTRACT

Results from work on immortalised cell lines indicate that the maturation arrest of leukemic cells can be reversed. Mitogen-stimulated lymphocytes and some T-lymphocyte lines produce a polypeptide called differentiation-inducing factor (DIF), which gives maturation of promyelocytic HL-60 cells into macrophage-like cells. DIF also mediates a primary growth inhibition of some myeloid leukemic cell lines as well as of fresh clonogenic cells from patients with acute myeloid leukemia and normal granulocyte-macrophage progenitors. Also the Tumor Necrosis Factor, which is not identical with DIF, displayed differentiation effects and growth inhibitory effects, which were similar to those of DIF. Our data indicate that there are a number of ways to induce differentiation in leukemia but that final common pathways may exist. That complementary, synergistic differentiation effects were found between some agents may be of clinical utility.

INTRODUCTION

The stemcells constitute the basis for the hematopoiesis. A stemcell shows two major capabilities: one is to produce identical copies of itself by cell proliferation (self renewal) and the other is to yield daughter cells which are committed to differentiation. The capacity for differentiation is restricted by the determination of the stemcell. The mature phenotype is the visible result of stemcell determination. Hematopoietic stemcells are likely targets for leukemia inducing agents and as a result a transformed cell is produced from which leukemia manifests itself by clonal expansion.

Proliferation and differentiation are normally coupled processes i.e. daughter cells which are committed to diffe-rentiation along a hematopoietic lineage also passes seve-ral cellcycles during this maturation to reach terminal differentiation where proliferation no longer can occur. In leukemia the processes of proliferation and differentia-tion are uncoupled (1) with a very low probability for differentiation. This leads to an expanding clone of proli-ferating immature leukemic cells. However, a stemcell rela-tionship is maintained so far that usually a minority of the cells are clonogenic in vitro. This minor population is responsible for maintenance of the leukemic growth and is most important from a therapeutic point of view.

Human leukemic clonogenic cells are not independent of physiological growth factors (2). Thus it seems unlikely that the leukemic cells produce endogenous growth factors that are of importance for stimulating growth in an auto-crine fashion. For stationary cells it is suggested that autonomous growth of transformed cells might be due to a constitutive expression of any of the controlling elements along the normal mitogenic pathway, (3). Hematopoietic cells are not stationary and normally depend on a continuous supply of adequate physiological growth factors. Therefore, transformed hematopoietic cells are not under pressure to develop independency of growth factors which are supplied by the environment. On the other hand, immortalised leukemic cell lines may produce their own growth factor or develop an independency of growth factors (1).

Induction of Differentiation

Is the differentiation block in leukemia reversible? An extensive work on both animal models and on leukemic cell lines suggests that the normal maturation may be reestab-lished, (4-11). Injection of mouse myeloid leukemic cells into embryos resulted in the appeerence of mature leukocytes in the adult mice partially derived from the leukemic clone

(10) indicating that the malignant cells responded to normal differentiation control in the embryo. Many studies on differentiation induction in leukemia have been performed on cell lines. In these the immortalising genes, which normally can be induced or repressed, have become constitutively expressed or amplified. Sachs and coworkers showed that some leukemia clones were induced to mature macrophages or granulocytes by a physiological inducer called MGI (macrophage and granulocyte inducer) (11). Such clones did not require MGI as a proliferation stimulus because they multiplied in its absence. In spite of this, they were still induced to mature by the addition of this physiological inducer of differentiation. Similarly, G-CSF has been reported to have a differentiation effect on myeloid leukemic cells (12).

The human promyelocytic HL-60 (5) and the monoblast-like U-937 (6) lines have been widely used in a search for differentiation agents, some of which are listed in Table I. HL-60 cells are bipotent and mature into granulocyte-like cells. Incubation with interferon-γ lead to the development of markers of myelo-monocytic cells on U-937 (13).

Inducer	Conc.(M)	Cell product
Dimethyl sulfoxide (DMSO)	10^{-1}	granulocyte
Hypoxanthin	10^{-3}	macrophage
Thioguanine	$10^{-6}-10^{-5}$	granulocyte
dbcAMP	10^{-4}	macrophage
Prostaglandin E	$10^{-7}-10^{-6}$	macrophage
Phorbol diesters	$10^{-9}-10^{-8}$	macrophage
Retinoic acid	$10^{-7}-10^{-6}$	granulocyte
1,25(OH)$_2$ vitamin D$_3$	$10^{-10}-10^{-9}$	macrophage
Polypeptides: Differentiation inducing factor (DIF)	10^{-11}	macrophage
Tumor necrosis factor (TNF)	10^{-10}	macrophage

TABLE I
dbcAMP: dibutyryl cyclic adenosine monophosphate

The differentiation-inducing factor (DIF)

In our work we demonstrated that mitogen-stimulated human mononuclear blood cells released polypeptide factors, which produced mature monocyte-like HL-60 cells (14). These polypeptides are called differentiation-inducing factors (DIFs). Mononuclear blood cells released one or two species of DIF depending on which type of mitogen was used; apparent molecular weights were 40,000 and 25,000. At least the 40,000 mw species of DIF was distinct from colony-stimulating factor. It was shown that the T-lymphocyte cell-line HUT-102 produced DIF constitutively (15). Others have also demonstrated that mitogen-stimulated blood cells produced differentiation inducing factors (16, 17). As the parameter of maturation in HL-60 we have used nitroblue tetrazolium (NBT) reduction as well as phagocytic capacity, cell-surface antigen expression detected with monoclonal antibodies, non-specific esterase, and composition of cytoplasmic granules.

We have attempted large scale purification of DIF using the HUT-102 cell line as the producer (15). Batches of HUT-102 supernatant are prepared and after processing including concentration by ultrafiltration, DEAEcellulose chromatography and high-resolution ion-exchange chromatography on MonoQ, a 50,000-fold purification is achieved. Final purification in µg quantities is obtained by SDS-PAGE. On the basis of partial amino acid sequence determinations, corresponding oligonucleotides can be synthesised and used as probes for screening a cDNA-library established from HUT-102 cells. Subsequent production of recombinant DIF may be of clinical utility in leukemia.

High-resolution ion-exchange chromatography showed a considerable charge heterogeneity also demonstrated by chromatofocusing, revealing isoelectric points in the pH range 5.4-5.9. DIF is a relatively heat-stable protein destroyed by proteases. It is not inactivated by periodate oxidation indicating that carbohydrate moieties are unimportant for biological activity. DIF does not have colony-stimulating activity; thus it is distinct from G-CSF. The DIF-effect is likely to be mediated through binding to a cell-surface receptor. The second messenger is unlikely to be cAMP as no increase in cAMP was observed after addition of DIF. A synergistic inducing effect between DIF and retinoic acid (15) was expressed in the production of granulocyte-like cells.

DIF induces maturation of "wild" type HL-60 along the monocyte pathway leading to a secondary inhibition of growth.
However, we have also showed that DIF, at a ten-fold lower
concentration (1 pM), inhibited proliferation of subclones
of both HL-60 and U-937 (18). This effect was displayed
without visible differentiation. Therefore the antiproliferative effect was unlikely to be secondary to differentiation in this case. Thus there are different actions on clones from the same cell line and target cells that are resistant to a direct antiproliferative effect of DIF, may respond with differentiation (and secondary growth inhibition)
at higher concentrations. The final result will be inhibition of self-renewal in both cases. Differentiation and
antiproliferative effects are expressed by the same polypeptide as both activities cochromatographed during all purification steps.

The antiproliferative effect of DIF was not exclusive
for myeloid cell lines but also clonogenic cells from bone
marrow of patients with acute myeloid leukemia were growth
inhibited (18). Our findings demonstrated that normal hemopoietic stem cells (CFU-GM and BFU-E) are inhibited too. It
is therefore possible that DIF may be involved in a physiological regulation of hemopoiesis perhaps as a link in a
feedback regulation involving T-lymphocytes. DIF may be of
utility in the treatment of leukemia only if normal multipotent stem cells are resistant, which is not yet demonstrated.

An identity between DIF and interferon-γ was ruled out
based on the use of a neutralising antibody against interferon-γ that did not affect the DIF-effect (18).

The tumor necrosis factor (TNF)

As DIF caused a primary growth inhibition of both leukemic and normal hemopoietic cells, we investigated if the
cytostatic and cytotoxic factor TNF had similar properties.
TNF is produced by macrophages (19) and has been purified
and cloned (20-23). Recombinant TNF produced by Genentech,
Inc. and supplied by Boehringer-Ingelheim was used in our
studies. A factor called cachectin, which is released from
macrophages and which specifically suppressed the enzyme
lipoprotein lipase is identical with TNF (24) and may play
a role in the development of the cachexia of chronic inflammatory disease.

Neutralizing antibodies against TNF did not neutralize the effect of DIF and biochemical characteristics are not identical, but we found very striking effects of TNF reminiscent of the DIF effects (25). Thus TNF displayed a profound growth inhibitory effect on some myeloid leukemia cell lines at 1-10 pM concentration. However, the susceptibility for TNF varied among different clones of HL-60. Some of these were highly susceptible to growth inhibition except for wild type HL-60, which was induced to differentiate into monocyte-like cells at 100 pM TNF. Thus TNF showed different actions on clones from the same cell line and target cells that are resistant to the antiproliferative effect at low concentrations may respond with differentiation at higher concentrations of TNF.

The clonogenic growth of fresh acute myeloid leukemia cells was inhibited with 50% at approximately 15 pM TNF. The sensitivity to TNF was not specific for transformed cells as the growth of normal granulocyte-macrophage progenitors (CFU-GM) was also inhibited as was the growth of erythroid progenitors (25). A synergistic antiproliferative effect was demonstrated between TNF and recombinant interferon-γ . By use of radioiodinated TNF 1,500-2,100 cell surface receptors were detected on myeloid cell lines at 4^0 C with K_d of approximately 300 pM. A very high affinity binding observed at elevated temperature may be an expression of a temperature sensitive class of receptors or result from ligand internalization (25). At 20^0C internalization occurred of bound ligand into receptosomes, but without transfer to lysosomes and degradation. At 37^0 bound ligand was transferred to lysosomes and after 2 hours degradation was visible. No correlation was observed between the number of binding sites or affinity and antiproliferative or differentiation resppponse to the addition of TNF. No differences in pattern of internalization of the receptor-ligand complex were observed between sensitive and resistant clones. Most likely differences in post. receptor events are responsible for different responses among cell lines to TNF and not differences in binding to the receptor.

A relationship between DIF and lymphotoxin (LT)?

Also lymphotoxin produced by B-cell lines is active in the classical tumor necrosis assay (26). The sequence comparison revealed extensive homologies between TNF and LT (20).

One neutralizing antibody against LT neutralized all DIF
effects but some monoclonal antibodies against LT did not
bind to DIF (27). Biochemical characteristics also seem to
differ between DIF and LT. The data may however, indicate
a structural relationship between DIF and LT. A comparison
of aminoterminal sequence data for DIF with the sequence
for LT will resolve this question.

       Mechanisms for induction of differentiation
       - a common pathways?

     If mechanisms by which agents act to induce differen-
tiation are defined this may lead to an understanding of
the maturation arrest in leukemia. We found a synergistic
effect between retinoic acid and cAMP agents (28) and that
cells could be "primed" for differentiation by preincubation
with low concentrations of retinoic acid followed by exposure to low concentrations of DIF. Priming was independent of
the normal rate of protein synthesis suggesting that an
initial decrease in synthesis of some protein(s) favored
differentiation. Short-time incubation with $1,\alpha25$-dihydoxy-
cholecalciferol $(1,25(OH)_2D_3)$ "primed" for the maturation
effect of cAMP agents (29). It was noticed that the "priming" did not depend on the normal rate of RNA or protein
synthesis. We also demonstrated that U-937 were "primed"
for differentiation by preincubation with $1,25(OH)_2D_3$ followed by exposure to interferon-γ (13). This priming did not
depend on the normal rate of RNA synthesis. All the data
reviewed suggest that an initial step in differentiation
induction is independent of RNA and/or protein synthesis
and that the maturation arrest may therefore be due to the
production, or overproduction, of a polypeptide and that
maturation is facilitated when the production of this inhibitor is decreased.

     Different agents obviously act by different mechanisms
to induce the production of more or less identical maturation products. This diversity indicates that there are a
number of ways to induce differentiation but there are final
common pathways. Proliferation and differentiation may be
regulated by a network which spans the cell from the plasma
membrane to the nucleus. The network may be touched at specific points to change the balance so that the maturation block
is released. A network theory explains complementary maturation effects between different agents; the network being

touched at different points simultaneously to give a synergistically amplified effect.

Cellular oncogenes most likely play a role in hemopoietic growth regulation. There is also evidence for the existence of a family of genes called anti-oncogenes (30), which could have a suppressive effect on oncogene products. Maturation arrest in leukemic cells may result both from constitutive expression of oncogenes or lack of expression of anti-oncogenes. Expression of anti-oncogenes may be directly linked to terminal differentiation.

ACKNOWLEDGEMENTS

This work was supported by the Swedish Cancer Society, the John and Augusta Persson Foundation and the Medical Faculty of Lund.

REFERENCES

1. Sachs L. (1981) Blood Cells 7, 31-44.
2. Moore MAS, Williams N, Metcalf D, (1973) J Natn Cancer Inst 50, 603-623.
3. Heldin C-H, Westermark B. (1984) Cell 37, 9-20.
4. Sachs L. (1978) Nature 274, 535-539.
5. Collins SJ, Gallo RC, Gallagher RE. (1977) Nature (Lond) 270, 347-349.
6. Sundström C, Nilsson K. (1976) Int J Cancer 7, 565-577.
7. Lozzio CB, Lozzio BB. (1975) Blood 45, 321-324.
8. Koeffler HP, Golde DW (1978) Science 200, 1153-1156.
9. Ischikawa Y. (1969) J Cell Physiol 74:3, 223-234.
10. Gootwine E, Webb C, Sachs L. (1962) Nature 299, 63-66.
11. Lotem J, Sachs L. (1981) Int J Cancer 28, 375-386.
12. Metcalf D. (1982) Int J Cancer 30, 203-210.
13. Gullberg U, Nilsson E, Einhorn S, Olsson I.(1985) Exp Hematol 13, 675-679.
14. Olsson I, Olofsson T, Mauritzon N. (1981) J Natn Cancer Inst 67, 1225-1230.
15. Olsson I, Sarngadharan MC, Breitman TR, Gallo RC. (1984) Blood 63, 510-517.
16. Chiao JW, Freitag WF, Steinmetz JC, Andreff M. (1981) Leukemia Res 5, 477-489.
17. Leung K, Chiao JW. (1985) Proc Natl Acad Sci USA 82, 1209-1213.

18. Gullberg U, Nilsson E, Sarngadharan MG, Olsson I. Blood, in press.
19. Carswell EA, Old LJ, Kasssel S, Green S, Fiore N, Williamson B. (1975) Proc Natl Acad Sci USA 72, 3666-3670.
20. Pennica D, Nedwin GE, Hayflick JS, Seeburg PH, Derynck R, Palladino MA, Kohr WJ, Aggarwal BB, Goeddel DV. (1984) Nature (Lond) 312, 724-729.
21. Wang AM, Creasey AA, Ladner MB, Lin LS, Stickler J, van Arsdell JN, Yamoto R, Mark DF. (1985) Science 228, 149-151
22. Marmenout A, Fransen L, Taverenier J, van der Heyden J, Tizard R, Kawashima E, Shaw A, Johnson M-J, Semon D, Muller R, Ruysschaert M-R, van Vliet A, Fiers W. (1985) Eur J Biochem 152, 515-522.
23. Fransen L, Muller R, Marmenout A, Tavernier J, van der Heyden J, Kawashima E, Tizard R, van Heuverswyn H, van Vliet A, Ruysschaert M-R, Fiers W. (1985) Nucleic Acid Res 13, 4417-4429.
24. Beutler S, Greenwald D, Hulmes JD, Chang M, Pan Y-C, Mathison J, Ulevitch R, Cerami A. (1985) Nature 316, 552-554.
25. Peetre C, Gullberg U, Nilsson E, Olsson I. J Clin Invest, in press.
26. Williamson BD, Carswell EA, Rubin BY, Prendergast JS, Old LJ. (1983) Proc Natl Acad Sci USA 80, 5397-5401.
27. Gullberg U, Peetre C, Nilsson E, Olsson I. Submitted
28. Olsson I, Greitman TR, Gallo RC. (1982) Cancer Res 42, 3928-3933.
29. Olsson I, Gullberg U, Ivhed I, Nilsson K (1983) Cancer Res 53, 5862-5867.
30. Knudson AG. (1985) Cancer Res 45, 1437-1443.

PROLIFERATION AND DIFFERENTIATION OF HUMAN LEUKEMIC CELLS IN CULTURE

Giovanni Rovera and Beverly Lange

The Wistar Institute of Anatomy and Biology and the
Dept. of Oncology, The Children's Hospital of Philadelphia

3601 Spruce Street, Philadelphia, PA 19104
and 34th & Civic Center Blvd.

The human leukemic population is an heterogeneous
collection of cells arising from a malignant clone of
undifferentiated progenitor cells analogous in some
respects to the normal hemopoietic cells (1-3). These
leukemic progenitors are capable both of self-renewal and
differentiation that very often is highly abnormal. The
differentiation level (most immature stem cell or intermediate progenitor cell) at which the leukemic transformation occurs has been defined in lymphocytic leukemia,
where marker events involving progressive rearrangement of
specific genes (immunoglobulin genes for B-ALL and and T
cell receptor genes for T-ALL) leave irreversible foot-
prints in the DNA (32,33). In the case of acute undifferentiated leukemias (AUL) or acute myelogenous leukemias
(AML) gene rearrangements during progression of differentiation do not occur, or at least they have not been identified and the differentiation stage of the progenitor
cells that are targets for the various types of AML is
still largely undefined. Genetic evidence (4) indicates
that chronic myelogenous leukemias arise from the malignant
transformation of a very early pluripotent stem cell
(although the expression of the malignancy usually occurs
at the level of the myelomonocytic lineage); in other types
of myeloid leukemia the issue is less clear.

G6PD isoenzyme analysis of the hemopoietic population
in 4 cases of AML showed that clonal proliferation was
limited to progenitor cells with potential for granulocytic

and monocytic differentiation in two young patients and to
involve cells with potential for erythroid as well as
myeloid differentiation in two older patients (5).

The problem of identifying the leukemic progenitor
cells has been approached by studying those leukemic cells
which proliferate in vitro either in semisolid media or in
suspension culture and by investigating the specific factors that allow leukemic progenitor cells to proliferate.
Studies aimed at defining the phenotype of leukemic cells
able to form colonies in vitro (CFU-L) support the concept
of multipotent progenitor or stem cell origin for AML.
Colony-forming cells in ten cases of acute myeloid leukemia
(AML) were studied in our laboratory with six cytotoxic
monoclonal antibodies that react with antigens expressed at
discrete stages of differentiation of normal and leukemic
precursors (6-7) and the reactivity of the entire leukemic
population was measured by indirect immunofluorescence. The
phenotype and the reactivity of the colony-forming cells
was established by complement-mediated cytotoxicity and by
fluorescence activated cell sorting. Comparison of the
immunofluorescent reactivity with cytotoxicity and cell
sorting showed that colony-forming cells were contained
within a fraction of the leukemic subpopulation that
expresses these differentiation antigens. The implication
of this result is that immunofluorescent reactivity of the
total leukemic population does not necessarily predict the
phenotype of the clonogenic cells, but reflects the differentiative heterogeneity of the leukemic population (8).
When the surface phenotype of the CFU-L was compared to the
phenotype previously established for normal marrow hemopoietic clonogenic cells, three patterns were seen: (a) the
clonogenic cells expressed a phenotype similar to that of
relatively mature normal granulocyte-macrophage colony-
forming cells (late CFU-GM) in 4 cases; (b) in two cases,
the phenotype resembled the less mature colony-forming
cells (early CFU-GM or CFU-GEMM), and (c) in four cases a
composite phenotype of early and late CFU-GM (9). Thus, the
level of impairment of differentiation in AML and the hemopoietic progenitor cell target for transformation may vary
from case to case. Essentially, similar studies using
monoclonal antibodies and AML cells were also reported by
Griffin and Lowenberg (10,11). All these studies suggest
that in the majority of AML the cell that is target of
malignant transformation is a cell that is more immature

than the cell that has the potential to generate only monocytes and granulocytes (CFU-GM).

How much more immature is the target progenitor cell
for AML?

A limitation of these studies, is that the leukemic
clonogenic cell (CFU-L) phenotype is established by cloning
the cells using sources of growth factors that, we know,
allow formation of colonies derived only from relatively
late progenitor cells. Unless in vitro clonogenic cells are
self-maintaining, like the in vivo leukemic stem cells,
they may not represent the type of cells from which the
leukemic cells have originated in vivo, but simply an
intermediate population, making it impossible to pinpoint
the target cell for malignant transformation.

The CFU-L studies, therefore, may indicate which are
the more differentiated targets for leukemic transformation,
but, at the present time, they are unable to indicate which
are the most undifferentiated targets.

We have more recently attempted to identify the self-
maintaining population in various cases of leukemia by
identifying those conditions that permit the leukemic cells
to proliferate indefinitely in vitro in suspension cultures.

Presently, accumulating evidence indicates the existence
of a hierarchy of growth factors that control differentiation and proliferation of normal human hemopoietic cells
(35). Pluripotent growth factors have been identified and
characterized (36) although, there is no evidence at the
present time that these factors may support the growth of
the most immature cells. Rather than using monoclonal
antibodies probes and clonogenic assays to identify the
most immature leukemic cells with proliferative potential,
we have attempted to probe the response of leukemic cells
with growth factors with the objective of obtaining self-
maintaining leukemic population of cells and to determine
their differentiation state by immunophenotypic characterization.

It is generally believed that leukemic cells remain
dependent on the same growth factors that control proliferation and differentiation of normal hemopoietic cells.

Factor-independent growth may occur in vivo and in vitro, due possibly to the effect of some oncogenes on the signal-transmission pathway of growth factors (25-27). However, this is probably not the most common event occurring in vivo during progression of human acute leukemia because the cells, in the great majority of cases, seem to maintain, after multiple relapses, the same factor dependence that they had initially.

The dependence of leukemic cells on specific growth factors has been documented in a few cases. Well-differentiated or partially differentiated human T leukemia cells grow in long-term cultures in media supplemented with interleukin-2 (IL2) (12), a molecule required for proliferation of antigen-activated mature T cells (13). However, highly undifferentiated leukemic T cells do not respond to IL2 or any known growth factors. Several types of immature murine leukemia of the B cell and myeloid lineages can be maintained in cultures supplemented with interleukin-3 (IL3) (14), a growth factor that induces proliferation and differentiation of early hemopoietic and lymphoid stem cells (15). Well-differentiated B cell leukemias (hairy cell leukemias) can be grown in long-term cultures using medium supplemented with BCGF (16), a factor that stimulates proliferation of normal mature B cells (17).

In the case of human acute myelogenous leukemia (AML) and most pre-B and early T cell leukemia, the conditions under which progenitor cells can be grown routinely in the presence of growth factors have not yet been defined. Only a small fraction of AML cells can form colonies in semisolid media supplemented with conditioned media containing colony-stimulating activity for normal myeloid cells (18-21). The leukemic colonies often undergo terminal differentiation, and repeated subculturing is not possible. The long-term tissue culture system for normal myeloid and erythroid precursor cells first described by Dexter et al. (22) is inadequate for human leukemia cells since it tends to select for growth of normal rather than malignant clones (23). Recently, Nara and McCulloch (24) have reported success in establishing cultures that grew for more than 7 days and up to 2 months, in 9 out of 17 cases of AML using medium conditioned by phytohemagglutinin (PHA)-stimulated lymphocytes. However, the specific factors responsible for leukemic growth remain to be identified, and only certain subclasses of myelogenous leukemias were responsive.

The long-term culture may be a more relevant test
system than colony formation to assess the efficacy of
potential chemotherapeutic agents in vitro. The identification of those factors that stimulate growth of leukemic
cells would help to establish their relationship to the
well-characterized factors that stimulate growth of normal
myeloid progenitor cells and their relationship with potential oncogenes. In addition, the question of whether
autocrine stimulation (28) plays a role in maintaining
leukemic growth at any stage during leukemic progression
can be addressed. Finally, long-term culture of leukemia
cells would allow analysis of the nature of the leukemic
stem cell and of any functional similarities to normal
hemopoietic precursor cells.

We have examined 50 consecutive cases of childhood
leukemias in order to determine the frequency of leukemias
that are already growth factor independent; to determine
whether conditioned media from 3 cell lines (Mo, JLB-1 and
5637) known to produce a variety of hemopoietic growth factors could increase the survival in vitro of the cells that
were not growth factor independent; to establish whether
any particular leukemic lineage was more responsive to
these factors and to identify any activity present in the
conditioned medium of these cell lines that could favor the
growth and the establishment of leukemic cell lines (29).

The fifty consecutive cases of childhood acute leukemia
included 30 pre-B, 7 T, and 13 ANLL. Five of the 50 cases
(3 pre-B, 1 T, and 1 ANLL) did not require any conditioned
medium factors to grow in vitro and form established cell
lines. This suggest that for any type of lymphoid and
myeloid leukemia, 10% of the cases are growth factor
independent.

In 28/50 cases conditioned medium from three human cell
lines (Mo, JLB-1 and 5637) was able to maintain prolonged
proliferation, from 4 to 12 weeks. A comparison of the conditioned media for their overall growth stimulating activities indicated that the Mo-CM was slightly more efficient
than the JLB-1 and 5637 conditioned medium, but as a general
rule, in every case there was a proliferative response all
three conditioned media were found to be effective,
suggesting that the three conditioned media contained factors with relatively similar activities on leukemic cells.

Although the cultures usually ended in terminally differentiated cells, three cases developed into cell lines in the
presence of conditioned media. Two of the cell lines became
independent after 6 weeks and 6 months; the third required
conditioned medium more then 1 year after establishment.

Utilizing blocking antisera and replacing the conditioned media with recombinant growth factors the growth
factor required to establish the three lines was shown to
be GM-CSF. Unexpectedly, however, the lines requiring this
factor were not all myeloid, but an undifferentiated T, a
biphenotypic B-myelomonocytic and a myelomonocytic. Probing
for the proliferative response of the five cell lines that
did not require at all growth factors indicated that some
clearly could be further stimulated with GM-CSF.

The GM-CSF growth factor dependent TALL-101 cell line
was studied in more detail (30). The cells are genotypi-
cally of the T cell lineage since they have a translocation
t(8;14) involving chromosome 14 in region q1.1, a region
where the gene for the alpha-T cell receptor is localized
(31) and that often is involved in translocations in T cell
leukemia.

The TALL-101 cells also have a rearrangement of the T-
beta receptor. Although the leukemic population was originally positive for TdT and for the T11 pan T surface
antigen, the established line is negative for both markers.
The TALL-101 cells have, however, on the surface the IL2
receptor that can be detected by the anti-Tac monoclonal
antibody and IL2 potentiates GM-CSF in supporting the proliferation of such cells.

TALL-101 cells can grow in synthetic medium only in the
presence of 10 ug/ml of GM-CSF, however, high serum concentration decrease the requirement for GMCSF.

Phenotypically, the TALL-101 population has no lineage
specific markers. However, the majority of the cells carry
on the surface a carbohydrate antigen recognized by monoclonal antibody S4.7 (32). This antigen is abundant on the
surface of cells of the myelomonocytic lineage.

These studies suggest that in some cases acute leukemias may arise from cells that are highly immature, e.g.,
at the level of precursors of both the T and the myeloid
lineage.

Since it has been shown that GM-CSF is a factor that
acts on pluripotent cells (34) it is, however, surprising
that the majority of AMLs cannot be maintained in vitro in
its presence, and it is not yet clear what differentiates
these cases, which have prolonged growth in vitro from those
that die or differentiate almost immediately. In some cases
(M4 and M5 most commonly) terminal differentiation occurs.
In other cases (M1 and M2 cells), rapidly die. This suggest that the target cell is probably different from the
various subtypes of leukemias and that most of AML may be
even more immature than one would expect or alternatively
that leukemic transformation, alters the distribution of
growth factor receptors. In any case, the issue remains
open: what are the factors that in vivo maintain the self-
replication of AML cells? Is human IL3 going to be the
answer? Or will we have to identify those factors that
support the proliferation of pluripotent stem cells in
order to be able to support leukemic growth?

Acknowledgement

This work was support by grants CA 10815 and CA 21124
from the National Cancer Institute and grant CH-279 from
the American Cancer Society.

References

1. Steel, G.G. (1977) Growth Kinetics of Tumors. Oxford,
   Claredon, 205-232.
2. Lajtha, L.F. (1982) Stem cells: Properties and
   Malfunctions. London. Leukemia Research Fund.
3. McCulloch, E.A. and Till, J.E. (1981) Blood Cells 7,
   63-68.
4. Fialkow, P.J. (1982) J. Cell Phys. 131, Suppl. 1 37-43.
5. Fialkow, P.J., Gartler, S.M., Yoshida, A. (1967) Proc.
   Natl. Acad. Sci. USA 58, 1468-1471.
6. Ferrero, D., Pagliardi, G.L., Broxmeyer, H.E., Venuta,
   S., Lange, B., Pessano, S. and Rovera, G. (1983) Proc.
   Natl. Acad. Sci. USA 80, 4114-4118.
7. Ferrero, D., Gabbianelli, M., Peschle, C., Lange, B.
   and Rovera, G. (1985) Blood 66, 496-502.

8. Pessano, S., Palumbo, A., Ferrero, D., Pagliardi, G.L.,
    Bottero, L., Lai, S.K., Meo, P., Carter, C., Hubbell,
    H., Lange, B. and Rovera, G. (1984) Blood 64, 275-281.
9. Lange, B., Ferrero, D., Pessano, S., Palumbo, A.,
    Faust, J., Meo, P. and Rovera, G. (1984) Blood 64, 693-
    700.
10. Sabbath, K.D., Ball, E., Larcom, P., Davis, R.B. and
    Griffin, J. (1985) J. Clin. Invest. 75, 746-753.
11. Lowenberg, B. and Baumann, J.G.J. (1985) Blood 66,
    1225-1232.
12. Poiesz, B.J., Ruscetti, F.W., Mier, J.W., Woods, A.M.
    and Gallo, R. (1980) Proc. Natl. Acad. Sci. USA 77,
    6815-6819.
13. Smith, K.A. (1980) Immunol. Rev. 51, 337-357.
14. Oliff, A., Oliff, I., Schmidt, B. and Famulari, H.
    (1984) Proc. Natl. Acad. Sci. USA 81, 5464-5467.
15. Ihle, J.N. (1985) Contemp. Top. Mol. Immunol. 10,
    93-119.
16. Ford, R.J., Yoshimura, L., Morgan, J., Quesada, J.,
    Montagna, R. and Maizel, A. (1985) J. Exp. Med. 162,
    1093-1098.
17. Ford, R.J., Metha, S.R., Franzini, D., Montagna, R.,
    Lachman, L. and Maizel, A.L. (1981) Nature 294, 261-263.
18. Broxmeyer, H.E. and Moore, M.A.S. (1978) Biochem.
    Biophys Acta. 516, 129-166.
19. Buck, R.N., Till, J.E. and McCulloch, E.A. (1977)
    Lancet 1, 862-868.
20. Moore, M.A.S., Williams, N. and Metcalf, D. (1973)
    J. Natl. Cancer Inst. 50, 603-623.
21. Metcalf, D. et al. (1974) Blood 43, 847-859.
22. Dexter, T.M., Allen, T.D. and Lajtha, L. (1977) J. Cell.
    Physiol. 91, 335-344.
23. Coulombel, L., Kalousek, D.K., Eaves, C.J., Gupta, C.M.
    and Eaves, A.C. (1983) N. Engl. J. Med. 308, 1493-1498.
24. Nara N. and McCulloch, E.A. (1985) Blood 65, 1484-1493.
25. Pierce, J.H., Di Fiore, P.R., Aaronson, S.A., Potter,
    M., Pumphrey, J., Scott, A. and Ihle, J.N. (1985) Cell
    41, 685-693.
26. Ihle, J.N., Keller, J, Rein, A., Cleveland, J. and
    Rapp, U. (1985) Cancer Cells 3, 211-219.
27. Oliff, A., Agranovsky, O., McKinney, M.D., Murty,
    V.V.S., Bauchwitz, R. (1985) Proc. Natl. Acad. Sci.
    USA 82, 3306-3310.
28. Sporn, M.B. and Roberts, A.B. (1985) Nature 313, 745-
    747.

29. Lange, B., Valtieri, M., Caracciolo, D., Mavilio, F., Griffin, C., Emanuel, B., Finan, J., Nowell, P. and Rovera, G. (1986) submitted.
30. Valtieri, M., Caracciolo, D., Altmann, S., Santoli, D., Tweardy, D.J., Lange, B. and Rovera, G. (1986) submitted.
31. Croce, C.M., Isobe, M.I., Palumbo, A., Puck, J., Ming, J., Tweardy, D., Erikson, J., Davis, M. and Rovera, G. (1985) Science 227, 1044-1047.
32. Korsmeyer, S.J., Bieter, P.A., Ravetch, J.V., Poplack, D.G., Waldmann, T.A. and Leder, P. (1981) Proc. Natl. Acad. Sci. USA 78, 7096-7100.
33. Minden, M.D. and Mak, T.W. (1986) Blood 68, 327-336.
34. Emerson, S.G., Sieff, C.A., Wang, E.A., Wong, G.G., Clark, S.C. and Nathan, D.G. (1985) J. Clin. Invest. 76, 1286-1290.
35. Walker, F., Nicola, N.A., Metcalf, D. and Burgess, A.W. (1985) Cell 43, 269-275.
36. Metcalf, D., Johnson, G.R. and Mandel, T.E. (1979) J. Cell Physiol. 98, 401-412.

INFREQUENT PHENOTYPES OF CLONOGENIC CELLS IN AML: EVIDENCE
FOR ABNORMAL DIFFERENTIATION AND POSSIBILITIES FOR DETECTING
MINIMAL DISEASE?

BOB LÖWENBERG AND RUUD DELWEL
The Dr Daniel den Hoed Cancer Center,
P.O. Box 5201, 3008 AE Rotterdam,
The Netherlands.

INTRODUCTION

Efforts to detect minimal numbers of AML clonogenic
cells (AML-CFU) in the marrow during complete remission
depend on phenotypic properties which distinguish AML-CFU
from normal marrow stem and progenitor cells.
We and others have previously shown that AML-CFU represent a
minority population among the total leukemic blast pool
(1,2,3). Among the phenotypically heterogeneous AML cells,
the AML-CFU are typically the most immature subset of cells
which give rise to maturing progeny during proliferation in
vitro (3,4,5). Earlier studies have established that the
phenotypes of AML-CFU differ but the differences correlate
with the heterogeneous classes of normal progenitors as a
function of maturity (14). Although AML-CFU phenotypes show
considerable variability when different cases of AML are
compared, it is noteworthy that surface markers to
distinguish AML-CFU from their normal counterparts have not
been reported as yet.
We wished to investigate whether abnormal surface markers
are expressed on the subset of clonogenic cells of AML and
whether these differences provide clues for the diagnosis of
minimal numbers of AML cells among normal marrow. In a
systematic search for identifying discriminative markers
between AML-CFU and normal hematopoietic precursor cells, we
selected a combination of surface markers (i.e., three MCA
and a fucose binding lectin), which are expressed as a
consistent phenotype on early as well as late hematopoietic
progenitors. These investigations were conducted with

71

fluorescence activated cell sorting (FACS) of colony forming cells. We assessed the membrane marker expression not only by presence or absence of the marker but also by relative fluorescence intensity to measure the antigen density on the cell surface.

MATERIALS AND METHODS

The collection and processing of marrow and blood from patients with AML and from normal individuals (3), the colony assay for AML-CFU (6,7,8) and for normal myeloid progenitors (CFU-GM) (8), the use of indirect immunofluor-escence (3,4), fluorescence activated cell sorting (9) and the application of the fucose binding lectin UEA (Ulex Europaeus Agglutinin) coupled to the fluorescent label FITC (9) have been described in detail.
Vim-2 is a murine MCA (IgM) which recognizes an antigen expressed on granulocytic cells (from myeloblasts to polymorphonuclear cells) and monocytes (10). The mouse MCA My-10 (IgG1) is expressed on immature human marrow cells, including normal hematopoietic in vitro colony forming cells (11). The MCA, RFB-1 (IgG1), reacts with immature progenitor cells of the granulocytic-monocytic cells, including colony forming units and terminal deoxynucleotidyl transferase-positive (TdT$^+$) cells in the marrow and thymus (12).

RESULTS

Characterization Of CFU-GM In Normal Marrow With Four Surface Markers.

We have previously reported that a varying proportion of Ficoll separated normal bone marrow cells are UEA positive. Normal CFU-GM are UEA negative or only weakly positive, i.e., they express receptors for the lectin UEA at only low density on the cell surface (9). Normal marrow shows a bimodal Vim-2 fluorescence profile indicative of distinct Vim-2 positive and Vim-2 negative populations. CFU-GM are almost entirely recovered among the Vim-2 negative cells. The My10 fluorescence histogram reveals a minor (approximately 5%) subset of highly reactive cells from which fairly all CFU-GM are recoverable. Finally, normal marrow contains 20-50% RFB-1 positive cells and all CFU-GM are RFB-1 strongly positive. Thus, in summary, CFU-GM

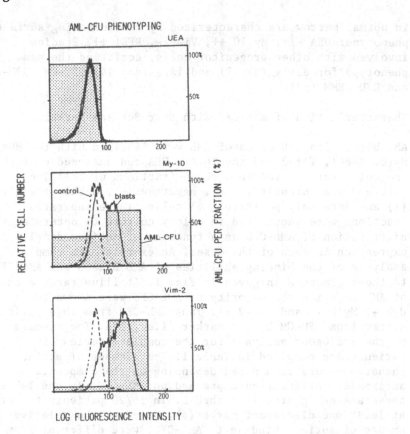

LOG FLUORESCENCE INTENSITY

Fig. 1 - Legend.
The surface marker profile was established in the individual
patients with FACS using the lectin UEA-FITC and three
monoclonal antibodies (My-10, Vim-2, RFB-1) as illustrated
in the example of Fig. 1. Negative -; weakly positive +;
strongly positive ++.
1) Reference data for normal hematopoietic precursor cells
CFU-GM, BFU-e and CFU-GEMM.
2) 45-50% of normal precursors are UEA negative, 50% are UEA
+, and less than 10% UEA ++.
3) Between 90-100% of normal progenitors.
4) Between 90-100% of normal progenitors.
5) 100% of normal progenitors.

in normal marrow are characterized by the following surface phenotype: UEA -/+, My 10 ++, Vim-2-, RFB1 ++. Studies involved with other progenitor cells, confirmed the same phenotype for early (day 7) and late (day 14) CFU-GM, BFU-e and CFU-GEMM (13).

Characterization of AML-CFU With Four Surface Markers.

AML blasts from 20 cases of AML were labelled with the MCA My10, RFB-1, Vim-2 and the lectin UEA and analyzed by FACS. The cells were sorted into three fractions of relative fluorescence intensity, i.e., negative (-), weakly positive (+) and intensely positive (++) cells. These separated fractions were inoculated in colony culture to determine the distribution of AML-CFU as a function of antigen density expression in each of the cases. An example of a complete analysis of the binding abilities of AML blasts and AML-CFU to these reagents is geven in Fig. 1. It illustrates a case of AML in which the majority of AML-CFU were shown to be UEA -, My10 ++ and Vim-2 ++. Thus AML-CFU from this patient differ from CFU-GM by one marker, i.e., UEA. The results of the analogous analyses for the complete series of patients are compiled in Table 1. Ten classes of surface phenotypes were recognized depending on the composite antigenic configuration expressed on AML-CFU. In the Table these are designated as A thru L. In 16/20 patients two or at least one discrepant marker(s), based on the relative amount of surface binding to AML-CFU, were different from normal CFU-GM. This refers to the surface categories A through K. In contrast, in the four patients 17, 18, 19 and 20, AML-CFU phenotypes (profile L) were indistinguisable from their normal counterparts.

TABLE 1. Surface phenotypes of AML-CFU in 20 patients with AML.

pat	FAB	reactivity with surface markers				patterns of reactivity	number of markers different from normal
		UEA	My-10	Vim-2	RFB-1		
1	M2	++	++	-	++	A	2
2	M4	++	++	+	++		
3	M4	++	++	+	++	B	2
4	M4	++	++	+	++		
5	M4	++	++	++	++	C	2
6	M2	+	++	++	++	D	1
7	M1	-	++	++	++		
8	M1	-	++	++	++	E	1
9	M1	-	++	++	++		
10	M2	-	++	++	++		
11	M1	-	++	++	+	F	2
12	M4	-	+	++	++	G	2
13	M5	-	-	++	++	H	2
14	M2	-	-	++	++		
15	M1	-	+	++	++	K	2
16	M4	-	-	+	++		
17	M1	-	++	-	++	L	0
18	M2	-	++	-	++		
19	M2	-	++	-	++		
20	M2	-	++	-	++		
normal[1]		-/+[2]	++[3]	-[4]	++[5]	L	

CONCLUSION

No unique AML associated surface markers have been
reported. AML-cells share differentiation antigens with
normal marrow cells. In the present study we have phenotyped
the clonogenic cells in 20 cases of human AML (AML-CFU) with
three MCA (monoclonal antibodies), My-10, Vim-2 and RFB1 and
the fucose binding lectin UEA. Using fluorescence activated
cell sorting and colony culture of subpopulations with
different fluorescence intensities, we did not only the
determine the abnormal presence or absence of these surface
markers on AML-CFU but also whether the expression was
apparent at an abnormal (i.e., increased or decreased)
density on the cell surface. Based on this approach, the
surface profile was established in each of the individual
cases of AML.
We demonstrate that AML-CFU phenotypes are highly variable
and 10 combinations of phenotypes were distinguished. In 16
of these 20 cases, we were able to differentiate AML-CFU
from the majority of the normal hematopoietic precursors,
i.e., CFU-GEMM, early (day 14) and late (day 7) CFU-GM and
BFU-e. Only, in 4 cases AML-CFU phenotypes were identical to
the normal counterparts as far as these four markers are
concerned. Other studies involving monoclonal antibodies
have previously indicated discrepancies as regards their
reactivity with AML-CFU and CFU-GM. However, these
approaches have usually been based on complement mediated
lysis so that more subtle distinctions founded on relative
binding abilities were not made.
We have defined a reference phenotype, which included 4
heterogeneous classes of normal precursors. The frequent
discrepancies between the AML and normal precursors are
striking. The fact that AML-CFU phenotypes were so diverse
and so frequently dissimilar to the standard surface pattern
of each of the types of normal progenitors, suggests that
these polymorphic phenotypes of AML-CFU reflect
abnormalities of differentiation. At the present time we can
not distinguish between the two possibilities to explain
this bizarre marker expression: i.e., AML-CFU present
altered phenotypes as the result of malignant transformation
or they correlate with expansions of precursors with
essentially normal but unfrequent phenotypes.
The problem of the identification of minimal numbers of AML
clonogenic cells in a remission bone marrow aspirate relates
not only to the unfavourable quantitative ratio of AML
versus normal cells, but also to the cross reactivity of the

surface reagents with AML cells and diverse normal cell types. The experiments presented utilizing FACS allow for differentiating AML-CFU from the normal hematopoietic precursors by fluorescence intensity and thus open new possibilities for detecting minimal leukemia. These possibilities increase when surface markers are selected which indicate a stable phenotype for the different categories of normal hematopoietic precursors and which permit the identification of a high frequency of deviations in AML.

In order to successfully detect minimal numbers of AML cells, the marrow cell suspension needs to be processed so that a fraction is obtained from which contaminant normal precursors are removed and which is highly enriched for AML precursors. It is conceivable that this goal can be reached if advantage is taken of the disordered differentiation which characterizes most cases of AML as demonstrated in our studies. Attempts at detection can for instance be made by sorting My10 positive cells in a first separation step, so that 95% of contaminant non leukemic marrow is removed. In a second step utilizing a discriminative marker the AML-CFU can be recovered and CFU-GM removed. This may result in the ultimate concentration of AML-CFU by 30-100 fold.

Preliminary data (not shown) indicate possibilities for detection of AML cells when they make up only 0.1-1% of a mixed normal marrow and AML cell preparation.

ACKNOWLEDGEMENTS

This work was supported by the Netherlands Cancer Society "Queen Wilhelmina Fund". The monoclonal antibodies My-10, Vim-2 and RFB-1 were kindly provided by Dr. C.I. Civin (Baltimore), Dr. W. Knapp (Vienna) and Dr. M.P. Bodger (London), respectively.

REFERENCES

1. Lange, B., Ferrero, D., Pessano, S., Palumbo, A., Faust, J., Meo, P., Rovera, G. (1984) Blood 64, 693.

2. Sabbath, K.D., Ball, E.D., Larcom, P., Davis, R.B., Griffin, J.D. (1985) J.Clin.Invest. 75, 746.

3. Löwenberg, B., Bauman, J.G.J. (1985) Blood 66, 1225.

4. Wouters, R., Löwenberg, B. (1984) Blood 63, 684.

5. Touw, I.P., Löwenberg, B. (1985) Brit.J.Haemat. 59, 37.

6. Löwenberg, B., Swart, K., Hagemeijer, A. (1980)
   Leuk.Res. 4, 143.

7. Löwenberg, B., Hagemeijer, A., Swart, K. (1982) Blood
   59, 641.

8. Swart, K., Hagemeijer, A., Löwenberg, B. (1982) Blood
   59, 816.

9. Delwel, H.R., Touw, I.P., Löwenberg, B. (1985) Blood 68,
   41.

10. Majdic, O., Bettelheim, P., Stockinger, H., Aberer, W.,
    Liszka, K., Lutz, D. and Knapp, W. (1984) Int.J. Cancer
    33, 617.

11. Civin, C.I., Strauss, L.C., Brovall, C., Fackler, M.J.,
    Schwartz, J.F., Shaper, J.H. (1984) J.Immunol. 133, 157.

12. Bodger, M.P., Francis, G.E., Delia, D., Granger, S.M.
    and Janossy, G. (1981) J.Immunol. 127, 2269.

13. Delwel, R., Bot, F., Touw, I.P. and Löwenberg, B.
    Exceptional phenotypes of progenitors in acute
    myelocytic leukemia (AML-CFU): possibilities for
    separating AML-CFU from normal marrow progenitors.
    (1986) Blood submitted.

14. Griffin, J.D. and Löwenberg, B. (1986) Blood in press.

Studies of Gene Expression During Granulocyte Maturation

Edward J. Benz, Jr., Katherine A. High, Karen Lomax,
Catherine Stolle, Thomas A. Rado, Jay W. Schneider and
Robert W. Mercer

Departments of Internal Medicine
and Human Genetics
Yale University School of Medicine
New Haven, Connecticut 06510

Introduction

Hematopoiesis is the process by which a pluripotent stem cell gives rise to the formed elements (recognizable differentiated cells) of the blood. These include red cells, platelets, lymphocytes, and cells of the granulocyte monocyte series (neutrophils, eosinophils, basophils, and monocyte-macrophages). The cellular biology and biochemistry of hematopoiesis have been intensively studied because the hematopoietic system is of fundamental scientific and clinical importance. As a biological phenomenon, hematopoiesis represents the most striking and readily examined example of differentiation by a single parent stem cell along several alternate cellular pathways. At the clinical level, hematopoiesis represents the means by which the body is supplied with cells needed for oxygen transport, infection resistance, and hemostasis. Disorders of hematopoiesis, such as the aplastic anemias, myeloproliferative syndromes, leukemias, and lymphomas, represent a major cause of morbidity and mortality for which increasingly effective but incomplete treatments have become available.

Abundant evidence, reviewed elsewhere (cf, for example, references 1,2), has established the existence of a single stem cell which gives rise to all of the formed elements of the blood. Very little is known about

the morphologic or biochemical features of stem cells.
However, much has been inferred about their capacity to
generate mature blood cells by use of clonal colony
assays. These measure the ability of stem cells to
generate unique subsets of red cell, white cell, or
platelet precursors under defined culture conditions.
This information has permitted useful generalizations to
be postulated about the development of each of the
mature blood cell types.

Hematopoiesis can be considered to consist of two
distinct phases: <u>differentiation</u>, during which the
potential of the pluripotent stem cell to develop along
several lines becomes restricted; and <u>maturation</u>, during
which the committed stem cell acquires the actual
phenotype found in the mature of that lineage.

The pluripotent stem cell begins to differentiate
by forming "committed stem cells", which have more
restricted potential to form blood elements. For
example, a committed erythroid stem cell has the
capacity to form only red cells, while a committed
granulocyte-monocyte stem cell can give rise only to
those particular cell types. These stem cells do not
express the actual phenotypic features of the line to
which they are committed. Rather, during the
"differentiation" phase, the genetic program of
pluripotent stem cells simply becomes restricted with
respect to the array of genes they potentially express.
Actual execution of the genetic program is delayed until
the "maturation" phase during which the committed stem
cell pool, now expanded and further restricted by virtue
of several "differentiating" cell divisions, begins to
express, during a period of three to seven days, the
recognizable, distinctive phenotypes of the particular
cell line to which the parent stem cells were committed.
During this phase the maturing progenitor cells usually
undergo only three to six cell divisions and
progressively develop the characteristics of the cell
lineage, from the earliest recognizable precursor stage
(e.g. erythroblasts or myeloblasts) to the release of
the fully mature cell into the circulation.

Relatively little is known about the biochemistry
of the differentiation phase. The biochemical markers of
the maturation phase seem to be controlled by mechanisms
determined during the silent or cryptic portion of
hematopoiesis. At the present time, maturation is the
phase that can be better studied biochemically, even

though this stage represents only the manifestation and execution of the genetic program determined in early stem cells during the differentiation phase. In this manuscript, we summarize some of our efforts to analyze the expression of selected genes during the maturation phase of granulopoiesis.

Maturation of blood cell lines clearly involves the enhanced expression of a few genes whose products characterize the mature cell, concomitant with orderly repression of the vast majority of the genome. For example, granulocyte maturation is characterized by selective expression of the genes encoding the structures of secondary granules and their contents, lactoferrin and vitamin B12 binding proteins (cf reference 3); conversely expression of globin and glycophorin genes, (cf reference 4) is a hallmark of maturing erythroid cells. Repression of the majority of the genome can readily be appreciated by morphologic criteria, such as the progressive condensation of chromatin as progenitors acquire more mature characteristics (1,2). In order to examine more closely the processes governing gene activation and inactivation during cellular differentiation, we have studied changes in gene expression in normal and leukemic human granulocytes, and in a human leukemia cell line (HL60) that can, when exposed to inducing agents, undergo terminal maturation.

Characteristics of Maturing Neutrophils.

As shown in figure 1, the earliest recognizable neutrophil progenitor is the myeloblast, which exhibits features typical of immature blood cell precursors, including open chromatin, multiple nucleoli, and highly basophilic, scant cytoplasm; these features correlate with active cell division and protein synthesis. Blasts may still have some capacity to pursue an alternative maturation pathway into monocytes, as may the next maturation stage, the promyelocyte. Promyelocytes exhibit some of the earliest features of specialization, including azurophilic (primary, or "non-specific") granules, and production of characteristic enzymes, such as neutrophil myeloperoxidase. Actual restriction or "commitment" to granulocytic maturation with loss of proliferation potential appears to occur during the transition from promyelocyte to myelocyte stage, a process that is also accompanied by the acquisition of the neutrophilic or "specific" granules containing

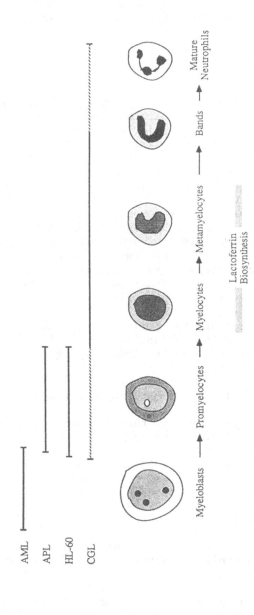

FIGURE 1 - Neutrophil Maturation. The bars above the cells show the maturation stages at which acute myelogenous leukemia (AML), acute promyelocytic (APL) and HL60 cells are fixed.

lactoferrin and vitamin B12 binding protein (cf reference 3). Subsequent stages (metamyelocyte, band and mature polymorphonuclear leukocytes) are characterized by progressive dominance of neutrophilic granules, condensation of chromatin, loss of protein synthesizing capacity, and lobulation of the nucleus.

Granulocyte maturation stages are largely preserved in chronic myelogenous leukemia, even though the total number of granulocytic progenitors is abnormally high, and there is a "shift to the left" toward dominance of more immature precursors in both bone marrow and peripheral blood (5). Patients in the chronic phase of this disorder thus provide a valuable source of circulating myelocytes and metamyelocytes, cells active in the biosynthesis of the more mature components of the neutrophils; in normal patients, only bands and mature neutrophils circulate. These exhibit very little protein biosynthetic activity. For this reason, studies of protein biosynthesis in normal maturing granulocytes have been relatively limited in the past.

Attempts to investigate neutrophil maturation have been greatly enhanced in recent years by the discovery and characterization of the HL60 cell line by Gallo and co-workers (6,7). HL60 cells are a permanent cell line derived from a patient with acute promyelocytic leukemia. These cells undergo maturation along other granulocytic pathways (following induction with compounds such as dimethyl sulfoxide or retinoic acid) or a macrophage-monocyte pathway (following induction with phorbol esters) [6-8]. Upon induction, HL60 cells acquire many of the features of mature granulocytes, including phagocytosis, staining with specific histochemical markers, motility, and acquisition of characteristic morphology. However, even maximal inducing conditions, do not cause HL60 cells to produce specific granules or to express proteins contained in these granules, such as lactoferrin (9,10). Although these facts limit the utility of the HL60 cell line as a complete model for granulocyte maturation, the cell remains useful for a number of important studies, particularly those that examine on the early commitment of immature progenitors to terminal maturation along this pathway. The HL60 line appears, even after induction, to be "locked" or "frozen" at an early myelocyte stage of differentiation.

Our attempts to examine some aspects of granulocyte

maturation at the genetic level have focused on two genes: The lactoferrin gene, whose expression appears to occur only in late progenitors, and the c-myc oncogene, which, as discussed below, is expressed actively in HL60 cells before induction but is strongly repressed upon addition of inducers. We chose these genes as potentially illuminating examples which might reveal interesting aspects of the processes by which the majority of genes are repressed during maturation while a few are selectively expressed.

Lactoferrin and c-myc Proto-oncogene Expression in Maturing Neutrophil Precursors.

Lactoferrin is an iron binding protein with a molecular weight of approximately 79,000 daltons that is known to be present among hematopoietic cell types only in neutrophilic secondary granules (11-13). Lactoferrin has been implicated as an important protein in bacteriostasis and as an agent required for optimal neutrophil function during phagocytosis (14-16); lactoferrin deficient patients have abnormal secondary granules, functional neutrophil abnormalities, and increased susceptibility to infection (16,17). Some investigators (cf 18,19) have suggested that lactoferrin is also a participant in the servoregulation of granulocyte mass. We chose lactoferrin for further study because its onset of accumulation in late progenitors identifies it as a potentially interesting marker for study of the commitment to terminal phases of maturation.

The c-myc proto-oncogene is a cellular DNA sequence homologous to the transforming DNA sequence of MC-29 avian myelocytomatosis virus (20). The oncogenic activity of c-myc remains mysterious, but it does appear to be a nuclear DNA binding protein expressed in a cell cycle specific manner (cf reference 1). Gallo and co-workers (21) have previously reported that expression of c-myc is abundant in uninduced HL60, but declines upon induction to terminal maturation. The gene is amplified 16-32 fold in HL60 cells (22). We chose to analyze c-myc expression as a potential model for shut down of the bulk of genomic DNA during the induction of HL60 cells. The abundant expression of c-myc in a continuous cell line also provided an opportunity to study expression of a specific gene in a system providing sufficient material for detailed analysis of mRNA and gene configuration in chromatin.

Analysis of Lactoferrin Biosynthesis During Granulocytopoiesis.

Figure 2 summarizes the methods we utilized to study lactoferrin biosynthesis in granulocytic cells (cf also reference 3). Briefly intact cells were incubated with ^{35}S methionine. The radiolabelled protein was extracted by mild detergent lysis of the cells and removal of nuclei and mitochondria by centrifugation. The lysates were then incubated with specific antilactoferrin antibody (we tried several sources from our own and other laboratories, but found commercially available preparations to be equally suitable). Immune complexes were immunoprecipitated by exposure to killed Staphylococcal cell bearing the "Staph A" protein. The immunoprecipitated proteins were analyzed by polyacrylamide gel electrophoresis and autoradiography. As indicated in the figure, biosynthesis of lactoferrin is readily detected by the presence of a radiolabelled band at the appropriate molecular weight from lysates immunoprecipitated with specific antiserum, whereas no such band is seen when pre-immune serum was used instead. The results shown in figure were obtained using a sample of peripheral blood from a patient with chronic myelogenous leukemia who exhibited abundant myelocytes and metamyelocytes in peripheral blood.

We applied this method to they study of lactoferrin biosynthesis in peripheral blood and bone marrow specimens from patients with a variety of hematologic abnormalities, as well as uninduced and DMSO induced HL60 cells. These data have been presented previously (3), and are summarized in table 1. These results can be summarized as follows: The presence, and approximate amount, of lactoferrin biosynthesis always correlated with the presence and cellular content of myelocytes, metamyelocytes, and bands in the specimen. In particular, abundant lactoferrin synthesis was seen only when myelocytes and metamyelocytes were abundant in the specimen. On the basis of these findings, we concluded that lactoferrin biosynthesis was confined to a narrow "window" of granulocyte maturation, beginning with the myelocyte and ending at or just prior to the band stage.

Our studies of de novo lactoferrin biosynthesis correlated well with earlier studies of lactoferrin accumulation using cytochemical and immunochemical techniques (cf reference 3). Moreover, we established

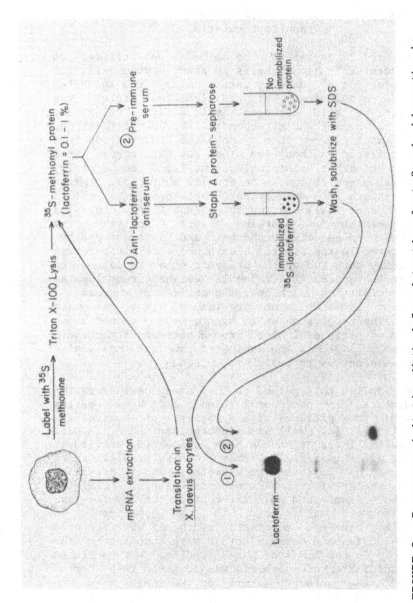

FIGURE 2 - Immunoprecipitation Method for detecting lactoferrin biosynthesis. See text for details.

Table 1.

Synthesis of Lactoferrin in Leukocytes

Source of Cells	Cellular Content of Myelocytes, Metamyelocytes, Bands	Amount of Lactoferrin Biosynthesis
Normal Bone Marrow	Moderate	Moderate
Normal Blood	Bands only	Minimal
CGL[1] Bone Marrow	Very Abundant	Very Abundant
CGL Peripheral Blood	Abundant	Abundant
APL Bone Marrow	Absent	Absent
APL Remission Bone Marrow	Abundant	Abundant
AML Bone Marrow	Absent	Absent
AML Remission Bone Marrow	Moderate	Moderate
HL60 cells (uninduced)	-	Absent
HL60 cells (induced)	-	Absent

Lactoferrin synthesis was analyzed as described in Figure 2. Cellular content of specimens was determined by quantitative differential counting of Wright-Giemsa stained smears. For details concerning these experiments cf reference 3. [1]CGL-chronic Granulocytic Leukemia; APL-Acute Promyelocytic Leukemia; AML-Acute Myelogenous Leukemia. Leukemic and remission specimens were obtained from the same patients before and after treatment. AML and APL specimens contained only myeloblasts and promyelocytes, respectively, before remission; in both conditions patients in remission exhibited the full range of granulocytic precursors in their marrows.

that synthesis of lactoferrin polypeptides was not
adversely affected by inhibitors of glycosylation such
as tunicamycin (3), and, as shown in figure 3, that the
presence or absence of lactoferrin biosynthesis appeared
to correlate with the presence or absence of
translatable mRNA in chronic granulocytic leukemia and
HL60 cells.

More recently, we have characterized the size of
lactoferrin mRNA and analyzed its presence or absence in
different granulocytic cells by direct hybridization
analysis, using Northern blotting methods. As shown in
figure 4, when mRNA from chronic granulocytic leukemia
cells is fractionated according to size by sucrose
gradient centrifugation, the strongest lactoferrin mRNA
translational activity appears in fractions of
approximately 22S in size, corresponding to about 3,000
bases of mRNA length.

We next developed synthetic oligonucleotide probes,
17 bases long, directed against known regions of the
amino acid sequence of lactoferrin. We deduced a mixture
of oligonucleotides that represented all possible codon
choices for these amino acids; the derivation of these
oligonucleotides is discussed elsewhere (3). As shown in
figure 5, these oligonucleotides, when used to probe
Northern blots of RNA from chronic granulocytic leukemia
and HL60 cells, detect a 22S mRNA band that is abundant
in the chronic granulocytic leukemia cells, but absent
in all other cell types, including induced and uninduced
HL60 cells. No combination of inducers we have yet
studied generates any detectable lactoferrin mRNA
(unpublished results).

Our examination of lactoferrin gene expression in
granulocytic progenitors suggests strongly that onset of
lactoferrin biosynthesis occurs at the myelocyte stage
and results from de novo accumulation of a 22S mRNA
species. Failure of induced and uninduced HL60 cells to
produce lactoferrin appears to be related to failure of
these cells to produce this mRNA. Our current studies
focus on determining whether or not these differences in
lactoferrin gene expression result from differences in
transcriptional or post transcriptional events. (We have
recently isolated cDNA clones for lactoferrin and
confirmed the Northern blotting data shown here with
these more specific probes).

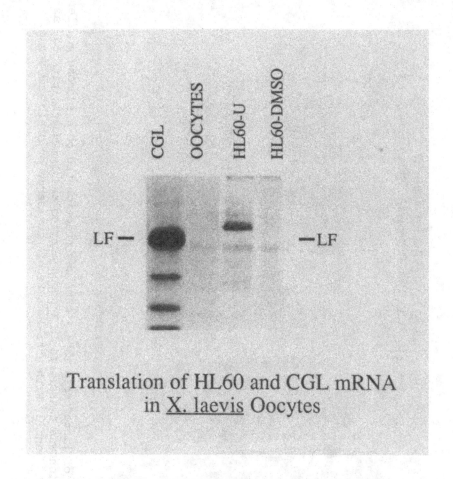

Translation of HL60 and CGL mRNA in X. laevis Oocytes

FIGURE 3 - Translation of lactoferrin mRNA in Xenopus oocytes. Autoradiographs of gel slots loaded with immunoprecipitated ^{35}S proteins synthesized by oocytes injected with mRNA from the indicated cell sources are shown. See text and Figure 2.

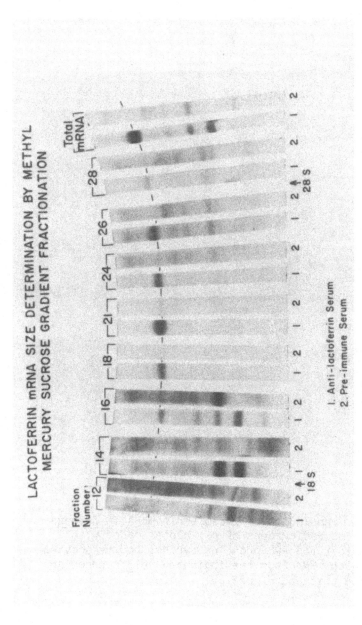

FIGURE 4 – Size of lactoferrin mRNA – mRNA was fractionated on a sucrose gradient. Each mRNA fraction was translated in Xenopus oocytes and immunoprecipitated, as shown in Figures 2 and 3, with anti-lactoferrin antiserum or preimmune serum.

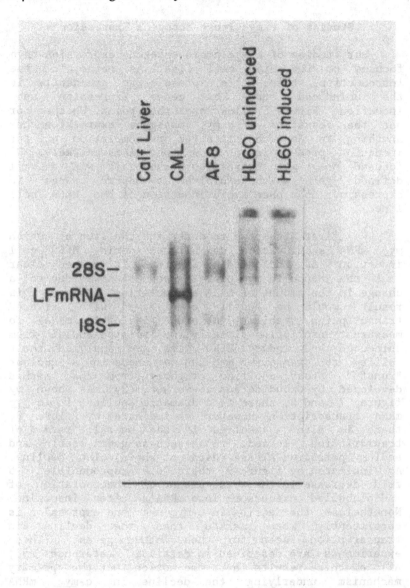

FIGURE 5 - Northern Blot analysis of mRNA. Poly (A)$^+$
mRNA from each cell source was blotted and then hybridized to a 17 oligonucleotide deduced from the amino
acid sequence of a segment of lactoferrin. See text.

Studies of c-myc Proto-oncogene Expression

Our studies of c-myc proto-oncogene expression have focused on the HL60 cell line. As noted in the introduction, these cells express c-myc abundantly in the uninduced state, but cease expression upon induction. Figure 6 illustrates this point. Whether or not the cessation of c-myc oncogene expression has anything to do with initiation or completion of the induction process is not known, but seems unlikely. We focused on c-myc expression because it was a well defined gene which exhibited a marked change in expression upon phenotypic induction of the HL60 cell line.

We first attempted to determine the step at which myc mRNA accumulation was altered during HL60 cell induction. As indicated by figure 6, it seemed clear that the change in myc protein production was due to a change in the amount of mRNA accumulation. However, this result would be equally consistent with altered transcription, stability, or processing of the mRNA. To measure transcription directly, we isolated nuclei from uninduced and induced HL60 cells, and analyzed their ability to transcribe myc RNA sequences in a nuclear "runoff" assay modified slightly from the method developed by Groudine and co-workers (24). As shown by figure 7 and 8, there is a dramatic decline in c-myc mRNA transcription. However, as indicated by figure 9, there is also a decline in the overall rate of transcription. Indeed, genes such as gamma actin and sodium potassium ATPase (data not shown) also decline. As indicated by figure 9, there is a reproducible 3-5 fold decrease in the total amount of incorporation of radiolabelled precursor into mRNA's after induction. Nonetheless, the decline in c-myc oncogene expression is consistently more marked than the decline in transcription seen for these other genes. [These experiments are described in detail in reference 25.] All of these results favor the notion that the primary mechanism underlying the decline in c-myc mRNA expression occurs at the level of transcription. As discussed by us elsewhere (25) several groups, including ours, have documented that c-myc mRNA is a particularly unstable mRNA species with a half life of approximately 20 minutes. Our results (cf 25) suggest that in the HL60 cell line, in contrast to other cell lines, there is no major change in mRNA stability as a result of induction.

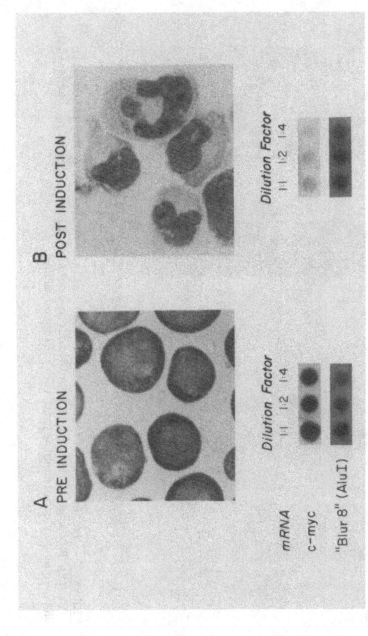

FIGURE 6 - Loss of c-myc mRNA upon induction of HL60 cells with DMSO. The altered cell morphology of induced HL60 is shown as is the loss c-myc mRNA detectable by quantitative dot-blotting of cytoplasmic extracts. The "Blur 8" probe detects a common replated sequence.

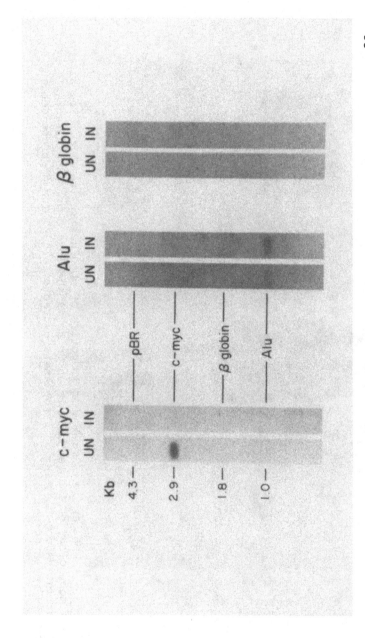

FIGURE 7 - Nuclear run-off analysis of HL60 cells. Nuclei were incubated with ^{32}P-UTP; the RNA was isolated and hybridized to Southern blots containing bands with DNA sequences complementary to the indicated mRNAs.

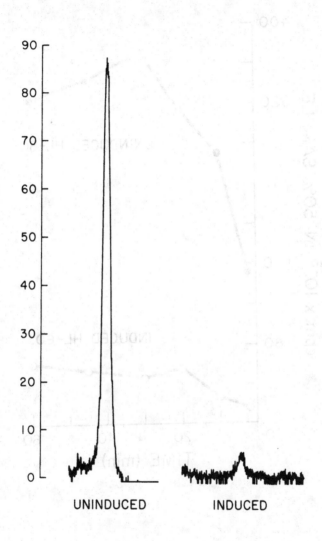

UNINDUCED   INDUCED

<u>FIGURE 8</u> - Densitometry scan of c-myc bands in Figure 7.

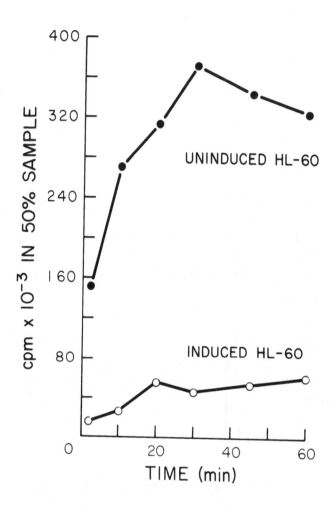

FIGURE 9 - Rates of ³H-UTP uptake into mRNA in induced and uninduced HL60 cells.

Transcriptional activity of the gene often correlates well with the development or loss of DNA'se I hypersensitive sites in the chromatin surrounding the affected gene domains (26,27). These sites can be detected by exposing nuclei to minute amounts of DNA'se I, and then digesting with informative restriction endonucleases, followed by restriction endonuclease mapping by Southern gene blotting techniques (cf reference 25-29 for details). A DNA'se I hypersensitive site is detected by progressive loss of the parent band seen in control DNA and the appearance of smaller sub bands as DNA'se concentrations are progressively increased (cf figure 10). When we performed this analysis on the c-myc loci in uninduced and induced HL60 cells, we found three DNA'se hypersensitive sites. Figure 10 shows a representative analysis illustrating detection of these sites. Precise localization and enumeration of these sites requires multiple restriction endonuclease digestions and analysis of the blots with a variety of probes directed toward various regions of the gene. We have presented these results in detail in reference 25.

Figure 11 summarizes the results of our DNA'se I hypersensitivity mapping of the c-myc proto-oncogenes present in HL60 cells. We identified three definitive DNA'se I hypersensitive sites, but only one (site II) was found to change on induction (25). Appropriately, this site is located within the 5' flanking sequence of the gene, a region frequently implicated as being important in gene regulation. Is is noteworthy that these sites can be detected in HL60 cells despite the fact that the gene is highly amplified. This implies the existence of "trans" acting factors capable of interacting with multiple copies of the c-myc genes.

Summary and Conclusion

Granulocyte maturation is characterized by the selective onset of expression of a few genes and the repression of the bulk of genomic DNA expression. We have begun to analyze expression of two genes, one that increases as neutrophils mature and one that decreases when induction of maturation takes place in a leukemia cell line. We have demonstrated that lactoferrin gene expression appears to be regulated by accumulation of new mRNA molecules, quite possibly at the level of transcription. In any event, its absence, even after induction, in HL60 cells appears to be due to failure to

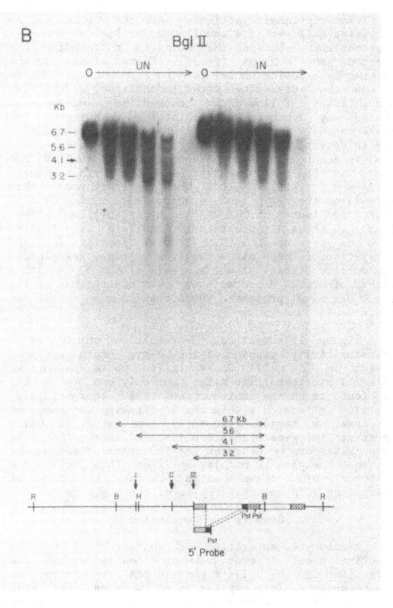

<u>FIGURE 10</u> - DNAse Hypersensitivity Analysis of c-myc
genes in HL60 cells. See text and Reference 25 for
details.

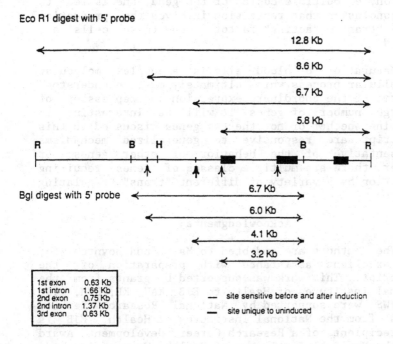

DNA'se Hypersensitive Sites Near
c-myc in HL-60

FIGURE 11 - Map of DNAse Hypersensitive sites in HL60.
See text for details.

accumulate the characteristic 22S mRNA species. c-myc proto-oncogene expression appears to be repressed when HL60 cells are induced to mature by transcriptional mechanisms which appear to act at least in part by altering a DNA'se I hypersensitive site near the transcription start site in the 5' flanking sequences. Furthermore, since this change appears to develop in synchrony on multiple copies of the gene, one is led to the conclusion that repression involves the production of a "trans" "acting" factor when these cells are induced.

Maturation of blood cells is a complex molecular and cellular process which ultimately must be understood in terms of the coordinate expression and repression of a large number of genes. It will be interesting to determine whether or not the two genes discussed in this manuscript are responsive to generalized mechanisms representative of the behavior of other genes, or whether there are multiple classes of genes requiring regulation by a variety of different "trans" regulating factors.

Acknowledgments

The authors are indebted to Ms. Linda Boynton for her excellent assistance with preparation of the manuscript. This work was supported by grants from the National Institutes of Health to EJB. KAH, KL, RWM, TR, and JWS were supported by National Research Service Awards from the National Institutes of Health. EJB is the recipient of a Research Career Development Award from the National Institutes of Health. We are indebted to a large number of investigators who generously provided us with cell lines and molecular hybridization probes.

References

1. Takeshita, K., Benz, E.J., Jr.: Analysis of gene expression during hematopoiesis: present and future applications. CRC Critical Reviews in Oncology/Hematolgy, 4:67-102, 1985.

2. Nienhuis, A.W., Benz, E.J., Jr.: Regulation of hemoglobin synthesis during the development of the red cell, N. Engl. J. Med. 297:1318, 1977.

3. Rado T.A., Bollekens, J., St. Laurent, G., Parker, L., Benz, E.J., Jr.: Lactoferrin biosynthesis during granulocytopoiesis. Blood 64(5):1103-1109, 1984.

4. Tonkonow, B.L., Hoffman, R., Burger, D., Elder, J.T., Mazur, E.M., Murnane, M.J., Benz, E.J., Jr.: Differing responses of globin and glycophorin gene expression to hemin in the human leukemia cell line K562. Blood 59(4):738-746, 1982.

5. Wintrobe, M., Clinical Hematology, 8th Ed., Lea and Fibiger, Philadelphia, 1981.

6. Collins, S.J., Gallo, R.C., Gallagher, R.E.: Continuous in suspension culture. Nature 270:347-349, 1977.

7. Collins, S.J., Ruscett, F.W., Gallagher, R.E., Gallo, R.C.: Terminal differentiation of human promyelocytic leukemia cells induced by dimethyl sulfoxide and other polar compounds. Proc. Nat. Acad. Sci. (USA) 24588-2462, 1978.

8. Haberman, E., Callahan, M.: Induction of terminal differentiation in human promyelocytic leukemia cells by tumor-promoting agents. Proc. Nat. Acad. Sci. (USA) 1293-1297, 1979.

9. Fontana, J.A., Wright D.G., Schiffman, E. Corcoran, B.A., Deisseroth A.B.: Development of chemotactic responsiveness in myeloid precursor cells: Studies with a human cell line. Proc. Nat. Acad. Sci. (USA) 77:3664, 1980.

10. Fibach, E., Peled, T., Treves, A., Kornberg, A., Rachmilewitz, E.: Modulation of the maturation of

human leukemic promyelocytes (HL 60) to
granulocytes or macrophages. Leukemia Res. 6:781,
1982.

11. Mason, D.Y.: Intracellular lysozyme and lactoferrin
    in myeloproliferative disorders. J. Clin. Pathol.
    30:541, 1977.

12. Pryzwansky, K.B., Martin, L.E., Spitznagel, J.K.:
    Immunocytochemical localization of myeloperoxidase,
    lactoferrin, lysozyme, and neutral proteases in
    human monocytes and neutrophilic granulocytes. J.
    Reticuloendothel. Soc. 24:295, 1978.

13. Briggs, R.C., Glass, W.F. II, Montiel, M.M.,
    Hnilica, L.S.: Lactoferrin: Nuclear localization in
    the human neutrophilic granulocyte? J. Histochem.
    Cytochem. 29:1128, 1981.

14. Osease, R., Yang, H-H., Baehner, R.L., Boxer L.A.:
    Lactoferrin: A promoter of polymorphonuclear
    leukocyte adhesiveness. Blood 57:939, 1981.

15. Boxer, L.A., Haak, R.A., Yang, H-H., Wallace, J.B.,
    Whitcomb, J.A., Butterick, C.J., Baehner R.L.:
    Membrane-bound lactoferrin alters the surface
    properties of polymorphonuclear leukocytes. J.
    Clin. Invest. 70:1049, 1982.

16. Breton-Gorius, J., Mason, D.Y., Buriot D., Vilde,
    J-L., Griscelli, C.: Lactoferrin deficiency as a
    consequence of a lack of specific granules in
    neutrophils from a patient with recurrent
    infections. Am. J. Pathol. 99:413, 1980.

17. Boxer, L.A., Coates, T.D., Haak, R.A., Wolach,
    J.B., Hoffstein, S., Baehner, R.L.: Lactoferrin
    deficiency associated with altered granulocyte
    function. N. Engl. J. Med. 307:404, 1982.

18. Broxmeyer, H.E., DeSousa, M., Smithyman, A., Ralph,
    P., Kurland, J.I., Bognacki, J.: Specificity and
    modulation of the action of lactoferrin, a negative
    feedback regulator of myelopoiesis. Blood 55:324,
    1980.

19. Bagby, G.C., Jr., McCall, E., Layman, D.L.:
    Regulation of colony stimulating activity
    production. J. Clin. Invest. 71:340, 1983.

20. Dalla Favera, R., Gelman, E.P., Martinotti, S., Franchini, G., Papas, T.S., Gallo, R.C., Wong-Staal, F.: Cloning and characterization of different human sequences related to the onc gene (v-myc) of avian myelocytomatosis virus (MCP29). Proc. Nat. Acad. Sci. (USA) 6497-6501, 1982.

21. Westin, E.H., Wong-Stall, F., Gelmann, E.P., Della Favera, R., Papas, T.S., Lautenberger, J.A., Alessandra, E., Reddy, E.P., Tronick, S.R., Aaronson, S.A., Gallo, R.C.: Expression of cellular homologues of retroviral onc genes in human hematopoietic cells. Proc. Nat. Acad. Sci. (USA) 2490-2494, 1982.

22. Dalla Favera, R., Wong-Stall, F., Gallo, R.C.: Onc gene amplification in promyelocytic luekemia cell line HL-60 and primary leukaemic cells of the same patient. Nature 299:61-63, 1982.

23. Lomax, K., Rado, T., Benz, E.J., Jr.: Lactoferrin mRNA accumulation in HL-60 and chronic granulocytic leukemia cells.

24. Groudine, M., Peretz, M., Weintraub, H.: Transcriptional regulation of hemoglobin switching in chicken embryos. Molec. Cellular Biol. 1:281-288, 1981.

25. High, K.A., Schneider, J.W., Hu, W., Benz, E.J., Jr.: C-myc gene inactivation during induced maturation of HL-60 cells: Transcriptional repression and loss of a specific DNAse I hypersensitive site. JCI (in press), 1986.

26. Elgin, S.C.R.: Anatomy of hypersensitive sites. Nature 309:213-214, 1984.

27. Weisbrod, S.: Active Chromatin. Nature 297:289-295, 1981.

28. Weintraub, H., Groudine, M.: Chromosomal subunits in active genes have an altered conformation. Science 193:848-853, 1976.

29. Weintraub, H., Larsen, A., Groudine, M.: Alpha-globin gene switching during the development of chicken embryos: Expression and chromosome structure. Cell 24:333-344, 1981.

GRANULOCYTES OBTAINED FROM HL-60 CELLS BY RETINOIC ACID TREATMENT BEHAVE ABNORMALLY IN HEMATOPOIETIC REGULATION - POSSIBLE CONSEQUENCES FOR DIFFERENTIATION INDUCTION TREATMENT OF LEUKEMIA.

W.R. Paukovits, J.B. Paukovits, O.D. Laerum

Institute for Tumor Biology / Cancer Research, University of Vienna, Austria (W.R.P., J.B.P.) and Department of Pathology, The Gade Institute,University of Bergen, Norway (O.D.L.)

INTRODUCTION

Tumor stem cells, both in hematopoietic and solid neoplasms give rise to differentiated or fully maturated end stage cells at a rate significantly below that of corresponding normal tissues (1,2,3). This aspect of malignancy seems not to be completely irreversible. In several experimental systems chemical induction of differentiation has been accomplished in vitro (see compilation in ref. 4). Based on such observations the emerging concept of differentiation induction therapy was tested in in vivo animal systems (5,6,7,8,9). In contrast to cytotoxic drug therapy which can be based on relatively simple concepts of cellular metabolism and proliferation kinetics the development of rational therapeutic strategies to treat malignant diseases as e.g. leukemia by differentiation induction requires a thorough understanding of the regulation of (granulopoietic) proliferation and differentiation at both the cellular and molecular level. In certain types of leukemia this situation seems to be better understood than for most other hematological and nonhematological malignancies. Several in vitro and in vivo models of myeloid leukemia are known for which regulatory phenomena are relatively well understood. Such systems could also be useful test systems for evaluating the therapeutic efficacy of agents capable of inducing differentiation.

Most of these cellular systems seem to be kinetically compartmentalized in a) a relatively small population of (slowly) proliferating self renewing stem cells, b) transitional cells committed to terminal differentiation, with a re-

stricted   proliferative   capacity,   and   c)
non-proliferating   mature   end-stage   cells
(fig.1). Under   steady state   conditions   (in   a
normal   postembryonic   tissue)   the   various
"fluxes" in   such a   system are under regulatory
control such that a well balanced and (on a time
average) constant population size is maintained.
One of the important factors in such a system is
the probability P_{sr} of self renewal in the stem
cell population,   respectively   the   probability
1-P_{sr} that   a stem   cell will   undergo   terminal
differentiation. In   normal   adult   tissues   the
time average of this   factor   is   exactly   0.5,
whereas the   continuous growth of   a   tumor   is
correlated with $P_{sr}>0.5$. However,   even in such
situations the   majority of the tumor mass still
consists   of   transitional   or   end   cells.

There are   several possible   ways to   reduce the
net growth rate respectively   tumor mass. A) to
remove cells   from the   system, either by mechanical means   (surgery)   or   by   killing   them
(chemotherapy, radiotherapy), and b) to make the
differentiation   probability   1-$P_{sr}>0.5$ thus
increasing the   flux into   the terminal compartment from   which cells   will be   "automatically"
removed according to   their   finite   life   span
(half life $t_{1/2}$). Similar cell kinetic conside-
rations have   earlier   been   made   by   workers
discussing the use of non-cytotoxic chalones for
tumor therapy: "To achieve ... regression of the
tumor it   is only   necessary to   slow down   the
growth rate of the   tumor cells strongly enough
to make   it smaller than the spontaneous rate of
cell loss"   (10). It   is easy   to translate this
sentence   into   the   terminology   used   above.

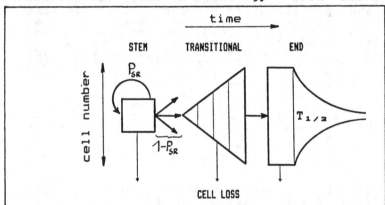

Fig.1: Schematic Presentation of some kinetic
       characteristics of the hemopoietic
       system. P_{sr} is the probability of self
       renewal of the stem cells. $T_{1/2}$ is the
       half life time of the mature end cells.

However real cell growth systems are often much
more complicated than such simplistic reasoning
would imply. Practically all known systems of
this kind are under the control of external
factors, and internal factors, e.g. as in fig.2,
(again oversimplified). The situation in myeloid
leukemia may be discussable in such terms.
Control of stem cell proliferation and
differentiation seems to be exerted by coopera-
ting stimulatory (11,12,13) and inhibitory
(14,15) factors. The situation is often complicated by a strong suppression of the remaining
normal population by the leukemic cells.

One aspect, which may occasionally become important, has been largely neglected by propo-
nents of differentiation induction therapy. The
basic idea assumes that the increase of i-P$_{mr}$
will drive the majority of the leukemic population into the end stage compartment where the
cells have a limited life span. What has been
largely neglected is that the population size in
this compartment will become very high unless
either $t_{1/2}$ is very short, or is shortened by
the treatment. The first is not the case, and
the second is improbable. Physicians will have
to comply with large increases in the number of
end cells. Several aspects may be of
importance here:
a) As schematically indicated in fig.2 these
cells will in one way or another influence the
control circuits in the system;
b) They will be numerous;
c) They will be present in the body for at
least some time;
d) Although non-proliferative they still are of
"malignant" type, possibly resulting in misbe-
haviour of one or another kind.

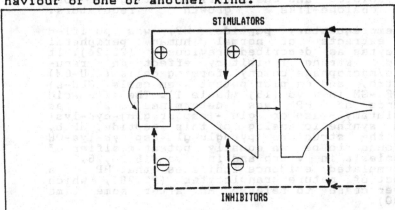

Fig.2: Cell production is often under control of
       well balanced stimulatory and inhibitory
       factors (originating in the system itself
       or elsewhere).

We describe here some experiments concerning the regulatory behaviour of "mature granulocytes" originating from the promyelocytic leukemic cell line HL-60 after treatment with retinoic acid (RA).

MYELOID LEUKEMIA, DIFFERENTIATION, AND HEMOREGULATORY PEPTIDES

Certain types of myeloid leukemia are characterized (among other changes) by a maturation block at a relatively early stage of cellular development. In some cases, however, the leukemic cells retain an inducible capacity to pass this restriction point in response to various kinds of chemicals and biological factors. The HL-60 cell line, derived from a patient with promyelocytic leukemia (16) undergoes such maturational changes when inducers are added to the culture medium. Macrophage-like cells are formed under action of phorbol ester, and dimethyl sulfoxide, retinoic acid, and other compounds (17) induce the development of granulocyte-like cells. Although HL-60 cells grow autonomously in culture, they show some responsiveness to normal regulatoy factors. An autostimulatory mechanism of growth control has been discussed (18), and HL-60 cells, when induced to form macrophages release CSF into their culture medium (19), a necessary growth factor for normal myelopoiesis (20, and Moore, this volume). Under normal conditions cell proliferation in the myeloid lineage has been found to be <u>directly</u> controlled by the interplay of several factors: multi-CSF/IL-3, granulocyte/macrophage CSF, granulocyte CSF (13), and a hemoregulatory peptide (15,21,22,23) which we have isolated and characterized during our work on chalone-like growth regulators.

The hemoregulatory peptide, HP, was purified from extracts of normal human peripheral leukocytes as described previously (22,24). It exerts a strong inhibitory effect on granulocyte/macrophage colony forming cells (CFU-GM) in vitro, and on pluripotent stem cells (CFU-s) and CFU-GM in vivo (15) (table 1). The aminoacid sequence of HP was determined (23) as pyroglutamyl-(asp or glu)-(asp or glu)-cys-lys-OH. A synthetic analog of this peptide, HP5b, with the structure pyroglu-glu-asp-cys-lys-OH was found to be an equally potent modifier of hemopoiesis in vitro and in vivo (15,25,26,27). The cumulated evidence indicates that HP is a product of mature granulocytes (21,28), which however cease to release HP after some time (29,30).

Table 1   EFFECTS OF HEMOREGULATORY PEPTIDE IN VITRO AND IN VIVO.

HP conc. (moles/l)	in vitro[a] CFU-GM (colonies)	in vivo[b] CFU-S (per femur x 10^{-3})	CFU-GM
0	60.5±5.5	3.8±0.7	19.7±2.1
10^{-11}	59.8±2.5		
10^{-10}	21.0±2.4	2.2±0.5	15.5±0.8
10^{-9}	17.2±1.7		
10^{-8}	17		
10^{-7}	21.5±2.5		
10^{-6}	19.0±2.2		
10^{-5}	47.3±4.5		
10^{-4}	49.4±3.1		

a...target: 10^5 mouse bone marrow cells, CSF = mouse lung conditioned medium
b...continuous infusion: 10^{-12} moles/hr for 7 days, total dose: 5.10^{-8} moles. The femoral bone marrow was taken on day 14 for CFU-S and CFU-GM assay.

Table 2:   MORPHOLOGY OF HL-60 CELLS AFTER 6 DAYS TREATMENT WITH 1×10^{-6} M ALL-TRANS-RETINOIC ACID. Functionality was tested by NBT reduction after TPA stimulation.

	promyelo-cytes	myelo-cytes	metamyelo-cytes	granulo-cytes	NBT-positive
control	100	0	0	0	1.3
retinoic	4	36	32	28	51.0

TABLE 3   EFFECTS OF USED HL-60 MEDIA (w/o RA induction) ON CLONAL GROWTH OF HEMOPOIETIC CELLS.

cell type	number of colonies CFU-GM			HL-60	RAJI	Friend
no.cells plated	1 x 10^5			1×10^3	5×10^3	1×10^3
dilution	1:5	1:10	1:50	1:5	1:5	1:5
fresh medium used	65.3±3.8					
HL-60 med.	69.5±6.3	71.0±3.4	70.7±11.1	444±109	9±1	27.8±6.8
used RA-HL-60 med.	27.3±6.1	27.6±5.8	62.0±7.0	77±32	32±4	130±21
percent	39	39	88	17	356	468

HL-60 cultures were induced to form granulo-
cytoid cells by treatment with retinoic acid
(table 2). These "granulocytes" display some of
the functional characteristics of normal PMN,
e.g. the ability to reduce nitroblue tetrazolium
(NBT) after stimulation with phorbol ester
(table 2). We wanted to know if they also
released HP into their culture medium.

EFFECTS OF RA-HL-60 CONDITIONED MEDIUM ON IN VITRO HEMOPOIESIS

The used medium of RA-treated HL-60 cultures
exerts a strong inhibitory effect on granu-
locyte/macrophage colony formation (table 3).
The data also indicate that this inhibitory
action is confined to cells of the myeloid
lineage (CFU-GM and HL-60). Non-myeloid cells
(RAJI, Friend) showed strong stimulations under
identical conditions.

ISOLATION OF THE RA-PEPTIDE

The crude RA-HL-60 conditioned medium was
deproteinated by ultrafiltration (MW < 10 kDa)
and fractionated by gel chromatography on a
Sephadex G-10 column. The eluate between
$V_e/V_o=1.2 - 1.6$ was further investigated because
it should contain HP (if present at all). This
fraction G1.2, when tested on colony formation
by CFU-GM and HL-60 was inhibitory for normal
cells (27.5 +- 5.3 % of control) but had no
effect on the leukemic cells (102.3 +- 7.8 % of
control), while purified HP did produce a strong
inhibition of HL-60 growth, e.g. a reduction in
the plateau level of the growth curve from
2.8×10^6 to 0.95×10^6 cells/ml. The RA-induced
HL-60 peptide is thus different from
HP in its biological properties.

The CFU-GM inhibitor contained in fraction G1.2
was further characterized by chromatography on a
Mono-Q anion exchange column. The elution
profile, together with bioassay data from selected fractions is given in fig.3. It is clear
from these data that the RA induced HL-60 peptide is different from normal HP.
The inhibitory peak and/or activity "A" (fig.3)
was absent when identically prepared extracts of
untreated HL-60 media were chromatographed, or
when the active G-10 fraction was treated with
2,2'-dipyridyldisulfide (oxidation of
thiol groups) prior to Mono-Q separation.
The apparent thiol content of the RA-peptide was
utilized for further purification of the ^{3}H-
carboxymethylated peptide. After rechromatography on Mono-Q and separation on a Sepha-
sorb-HP column a pure peptide was obtained

(homogeneous in HPLC) which was sequenced by Chang's DABITC/PITC double coupling Edman-type method (31). After each degradation cycle the colored DABTH derivatives were separated and identified by HPLC as described previously (32), yielding the N-terminal sequence GlN-asp-pro-...
. The RA-peptide is thus also different from HP on the primary structural level.

POSSIBLE CONSEQUENCES FOR DIFFERENTIATION INDUCTION THERAPY

Several workers have recently discussed the idea to control certain kinds of myeloid leukemia by differentiation induction in vivo (see also other articles in this volume). This strategy is more or less based on induction experiments with the HL-60 cell line and on the assumption that the artificially matured progeny of the leukemic population will behave in a normal way. Our results indicate that this may not always be the case. Differentiation induction will generate a large population of

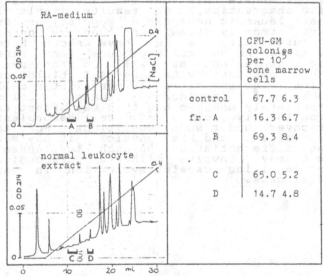

	CFU-GM colonies per 10^5 bone marrow cells
control	67.7 6.3
fr. A	16.3 6.7
B	69.3 8.4
C	65.0 5.2
D	14.7 4.8

Fig.3:High resolution anion exchange chromatography of prepurified (Sephadex G-10) RA-HL-60 conditioned medium or normal human leukocyte extract. Column: Pharmacia Mono-Q 5x50 mm, 20 mM Tris, pH 7.0, Gradient to 0.4 M NaCl. The table gives bioassay data for fractions A and B of each chromatogram. No CFU-GM growth modifying activity was found in any other fraction.

cells which produce regulatory peptide(s) which
are chemically and biologically different from
their normal counterparts. These still
"malignant" producer cells will, due to their
finite life span, remain in the body for some
time. Their aberrant regulatory behaviour may
lead to severe disturbances in the hemopoietic
control system.
Besides the widespread observation that differentiation induction never involves all cells,
thereby permitting the eventual regrowth of the
leukemic population, our results point to other
aspects which should be carefully evaluated
before and during such therapy forms. It is well
known that leukemic cells in vivo suppress
normal hemopoiesis, and that this is a major
problem for the host organism. It seems to be
quite important to clarify whether differentiation induction will allow the restoration of
normal hemopoiesis. Steinberg et al. (33) have
recently shown with induced HL-60 and K562 cells
that in vitro CFU-E and BFU-E are released from
a block that was exerted by the uninduced parent
HL-60 line. While this may be regarded as a
promising observation, our results (table 3)
show that leukemic nonmyeloid populations are
even more strongly stimulated than are normal
CFU-E. Furthermore, as we have shown here,
differentiated HL-60 cells produce (and other
leukemic populations may well do the same)
regulatory peptides with aberrant biological
properties, e.g. inhibition of normal stem cells
but not of (residual) leukemic cells.
It is completely unknown how this may affect the
situation in vivo, e.g., if normal hemopoiesis
could recover under such conditions. For the
leukemia patient and his physician it may mean
that the differentiation approach to leukemia
treatment may involve hitherto unrecognized
problems requiring careful evaluation in each
individual case.

REFERENCES

1. Pierce G.B.(1974) Am. J. Pathology 77: 103-117
2. Markert C.L.(1968) Cancer Res. 28: 1908-1914
3. Scott R.E., Florine D.L.(1982)
   Am. J. Pathology 107: 342-348
4. Reiss M., Gamba-Vitalo Ch., Sartorelli A.C.(1986)
   Cancer Treatment Rep. 70: 201-218
5. Strickland S., Sawey M.J.(1980)
   Developmental Biol. 78: 76-85
6. Chang J.H.T., Prasad K.N.(1976)
   J.Pediatr.Surg. 11: 847-858
7. Helson L., Helson C., Peterson R.F., et al.(1976)
   J.Natl.Cancer Inst. 57: 727-729
8. Lotem J., Sachs L.(1984) Int.J.Cancer 33:147-154
9. Honma Y., Kasukabe T., Okabe J., et al. (1979)
   Cancer Res. 39: 3167-3171
10.Rytömaa T.(1976) In: Chalones (J.C.Houck, ed.)
   pp 289-309, North Holland - Elsevier
11.Moore M.A.S., this volume
12.Metcalf D.(1984) The hemopoietic colony stimulating
   factors,Elsevier - North Holland
13.Walker F., Nicola N., Metcalf D., Burgess A.W.(1985)
   Cell 43: 269-276
14.Broxmeyer H.(1984) Blood Cells 10: 397-426
15.Paukovits W.R., Laerum O.D., Guigon M. (1986)
   In: Biological Regulation of Cell Proliferation,
   Baserga R., Foa P., Metcalf D., Polli E., (eds),
   pp. 111-119, Raven Press, New York
16.Collins S.J., Gallo R., Gallagher R.F.(1977)
   Nature (London) 270: 347-349
17.Harris P., Ralph P.(1985)
   J.Leukocyte Biol. 37: 407-422
18.Perkins S.L., Andreotti P.E., Sinha S.K., Wu M.C.,
   Yunis A.A.(1984) Cancer Res. 44: 5169-5175
19.Ascensao J.L., Mickman J.K.(1984)
   Exp.Hematol.12:177-182
20.Burgess A., Nicola N.(1984) Growth Factors and
   Stem Cells. Academic Press, New York
21.Paukovits W.R.(1971) Cell Tissue Kinet. 4: 539-547
22.Paukovits W.R., Laerum O.D. (1982)
   Z. Naturforschung Sect.C Biosci 37: 1297-1300
23.Paukovits W.R., Laerum O.D. (1984)
   Hoppe Seyler's Z.Physiol.Chem. 365: 303-311
24.Paukovits W.R., Laerum O.D., Paukovits J.B.,
   Hinterberger W., Rogan A. (1983) Hoppe Seyler's
   Z.Physiol.Chem.364: 383-396
25.Laerum O.D., Paukovits W.R.(1984) Exp.Hematol.12:7-17
26.Laerum O.D., Paukovits W.R.(1984)
   Differentiation 27:106-112
27.Laerum O.D., Paukovits W.R., Sletvold O.(1986)
   In: Biological Regulation of Cell Proliferation
   (Baserga R., Foa P., Metcalf D., Polli E., eds.)
   pp.121-129, Raven Press, New York
28.Paukovits W.R.(1983) J.Nat.Ca.Inst.Monogr.38:147-155
29.Rytömaa T., Kiviniemi K.(1968)
   Cell Tissue Kinet. 1: 341-350
30.Herman S.P., Golde D.W., Cline M.J.(1978)
   Blood 51: 207-219
31.Chang J.Y.(1983) Methods Enzymology 91: 455-466
32.Paukovits J.B., Paukovits W.R., Laerum O.D. (1986)
   Cancer Res. 46: 4444-4448
33.Steinberg H.N., Tsiftsoglu A.S., Robinson S.H. (1985)
   Blood 65: 100-106

BETA-ADRENERGIC RECEPTORS OF NORMAL, TRANSFORMED

AND IMMATURE HUMAN LEUCOCYTES

Georg Sager, Berit E. Bang,
Mona Pedersen and Jarle Aarbakke.

Department of Pharmacology,
Institute of Medical Biology,
University of Tromsø, Tromsø, Norway.

The physiological effects of beta-adrenergic stimulation are mediated through the activation of adenylate cyclase. The subsequent increase of intracellular cyclic AMP may play a regulatory role in hematopoiesis in normal bone marrow tissue culture (1-3) and has also been related to differentiation of leucemic cells (4-7). In polymorphonuclear leucocytes, these receptors are involved in the regulation of lysosomal enzyme release (8). The mononuclear leucocyte beta-adrenergic receptors participate in the modulation of immune and inflammatory responses (9).

The catecholamine sensitive adenylate cyclase complex consists of three different moieties: 1) The guanine nucleotide regulatory protein which functionally links 2) the beta-adrenergic receptor to 3) the catalytic unit. The stimulated enzyme activity is modulated by a change in receptor coupling to the catalytic unit and/or by a change in the number of beta-adrenergic receptors present at the plasma membrane. Mononuclear as well as polymorphonuclear leucocytes have beta-adrenergic receptors functionally linked to adenylate cyclase (10,11). The receptor number of polymorphonuclear leucocytes ranges from approximately 300 to 1,800 per cell (12-17). Normal mononuclear leucocytes consist of different subpopulations and most studies have shown a lower number of <u>beta</u>-adrenergic receptor on T-cells than on B-cells (17-19). The number of receptors on T-cells ranged from approximately 200 to 1,500 per cell and on B-cells from approximately 600 to 3,800 per cell. The large variations in binding capacity reflect the biological variability in addition to the differences in experimental procedures.

Lymphocytes in chronic lymphocytic leucemia have markedly lower number of <u>beta</u>-adrenergic receptors than normal B-cells (17,20). The high binding capacity reported by Sheppard and co-workers (20) is probably due to the experimental conditions which include non-specific binding. Paietta and Schwarzmeier (17) found values of 470 and 2,000 sites/cell for chronic lymphocytic leucemic lymphocytes and normal B-lymphocytes, respectively. In functional studies, the chronic lymphocytic leucemia lymphocyte adenylate cyclase responsiveness to <u>beta</u>-adrenergic stimulation was lowered (17,20,21), probably explained by down-regulation and not by uncoupling of the <u>beta</u>-adrenergic receptors (17). In acute lymphocytic leucemia and acute myelogenic leucemia the receptor number showed great variation, but did not differ from normal cells. The acute myelogenic monocytic leucemia/acute monocytic leucemia cells possessed 3,170 receptors compared to monocytes with 1,300 receptors (17). The degree of <u>beta</u>-adrenergic stimulation in acute leucemic cells appeared to reflect the number of <u>beta</u>-adrenergic receptors (17). These observations show that the malignant transformation of human leucocytes, in vivo, may affect the catecholamine sensitive adenylate cyclase complex. It is not known whether this modulation occurs before, during or after the transformation. The <u>beta</u>-adrenergic receptors in leucemic cells have possibly a functional role, but this has to be determined.

Changes have been observed in the catecholamine sensitive adenylate cyclase complex after differentiation of the human promyelocytic cell line HL-60 (22), but whether these occur before during or after differentiation is unknown. As a first step in answering this question, we characterized the beta-adrenergic receptors of the HL-60 cell.

The number of HL-60 cell beta-adrenergic receptors was 1,970 sites/cell ($\overline{\text{Kd}}$: 0.24 nM, Fig. 1), determined at 37° by use of the radioligand ^{3}H-CGP 12177. We found that propranolol inhibited the radioligand binding stereospecifically with the levoform more potent (Kd: 0.51 nM) than the dextroform (Kd: 38 nM). The radioligand binding was inhibited by an order of agonist potency: (-)-Isoproterenol (Kd: 58 nM) > (-)-Epinephrine (Kd: 270 nM) > (-)-Norepinephrine (Kd: 8,600 nM).

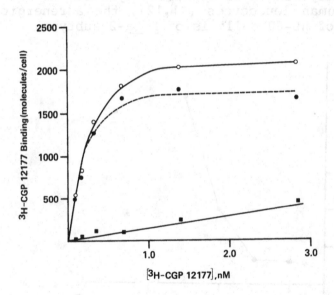

Fig.1: Binding of ^{3}H-CGP 12177 to HL-60 cells at 37° as a function of radioligand concentrations. Total binding (○) and non-specific binding (■) represent radioligand binding in absence or in presence of 100 nM (-)-alprenolol, respectively. Specific ^{3}H-CGP 12177 binding (●) is given as the difference between total and non-specific binding. The results from one representative experiment are shown.

Under the present experimental conditions the
basal cyclic AMP level was 5.5 pmol/10^6 cells.
(-)-Isoproterenol caused a concentration dependent increase of cyclic AMP accumulation with
maximum level 810 % of basal (Fig. 2). The EC50
values were 270 nM and 3,300 nM, respectively,
for the levoform and the dextroform of isoproterenol. The adrenergic agonists raised the cyclic
AMP levels by an order of potency: (-)-Isopro-
terenol (EC50: 270 nM) > (-)-Epinephrine (EC50:
990 nM) > (-)-Norepinephrine (EC50: 2,600 nM).
Propranolol inhibited the isoproterenol induced
cyclic AMP accumulation concentration dependently
and stereospecifically. These results show that
the HL-60 cells possess <u>beta</u>-adrenergic receptors
functionally linked to adenylate cyclase. As with
normal human leucocytes (11,12), the adrenergic
receptor of HL-60 cells is of <u>beta</u>-2 subtype.

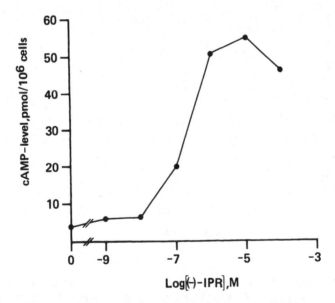

<u>Fig.2:</u> Cyclic AMP accumulation in intact HL-60
cells as a function of (-)-isoproterenol concentration. The cells were preincubated with 4 mM
theophylline for 30 min at 37° before 3 min
exposure to the indicated concentrations of (-)-
isoproterenol. The results from one representative experiment are shown.

In response to retinoic acid (23), the HL-60 cells mature into functional granulocytes with reduced isoproterenol stimulated cyclic AMP levels (22). However, the number of beta-adrenergic receptors did not decrease in response to retinoic acid (22) which indicates that the receptors become uncoupled from the catalytic unit. When treated with phorbol ester, the HL-60 cells differentiate into macrophage like cells (24) with a lowered isoproterenol responsiveness after differentiation (22). Receptor down-regulation, in addition to reduced cell surface area, can account for the 80 % decrease in the number of beta-adrenergic receptors after the exposure to phorbol ester (22).

In conclusion, human leucocytes, being normal, transformed or immature, have beta-adrenergic receptors functionally linked to adenylate cyclase. However, the following questions remain unanswered: 1) Do the change in catecholamine sensitive adenylate cyclase occur before, during or after cell transformation/maturation and 2) What is the functional role of beta-adrenergic receptors in transformed and in immature human leucocytes?

References.

1. Koeffler, H.P. and Golde,D.W. (1980) Cancer Res. **40**, 1858-1862.
2. Kurland, J.I., Broxmeyer, H.E., Pelus, L.M., Bockman, R.S. and Moore, M.A.S. (1978) Blood 52, 388-407.
3. Taetle, R. and Koessler, A. (1980) Cancer Res. **40**, 1223-1229.
4. Boynton, A.L. and Whitfield, J.F. (1983) Adv. Cycl. Nucleotide Res. 15, 193-294.
5. Friedman, D.L. (1976) Physiol. Rev. **56**, 652-708.
6. Rubin, C.S. (1978) J. Cell. Physiol. **94**, 57-68.

7. Chaplinski, T.J. and Niedel, J.E. (1982) J. Clin. Invest. 70, 953-964.

8. Zurier,R.B., Weissmann,G., Hoffstein,S., Kammerman, S. and Tai, H.H. (1974) J.Clin. Invest. 53, 297-309.

9. Parker, C.W. (1979) Ann. N.Y. Acad. Sci. 332, 255-261.

10. Bourne, H.R. and Melmon, K.L. (1971) J. Pharm. Exp. Ther. 178, 1-7.

11. Williams, L.T., Snyderman, R. and Lefkowitz, R.J. (1976) J. Clin. Invest. 51, 149-155.

12. Galant, S.P., Underwood, S., Duriseti, L. and Insel, P.A. (1978) J. Lab. Clin. Med. 92, 613-618.

13. Dulis, B.H. and Wilson, I.B. (1980) J. Biol. Chem. 255, 1043-1048.

14. Ruoho, A.E., DeClerque, J.L. and Busse, W.W. (1980) J. All. Clin. Immunol. 66, 46-51.

15. Davies, A.O. and Lefkowitz, R.J. (1980) J. Clin. Endocrin. Metab. 51, 599-605.

16. Lee, T-P., Szefler, S. and Ellis, E.F. (1981) Res. Commun. Chem. Pathol. Pharmacol. 31, 455-462.

17. Paietta, E. and Schwarzmeier, J.D. (1983) Europ. J. Clin. Invest. 13, 339-346.

18. Pochet, R., Delespesse, G., Gausset, P.W. and Collet, H. (1979) Clin. Exp. Immunol. 38, 578-584.

19. Landman, R.M.A., Burgisser, E., Wesp, M. and Buhler, F.R. (1984) J. Receptor Res. 4, 1-6.

20. Sheppard, J.R., Gomus, R. and Moldow, C.F. (1977) Nature 269, 693-695.

21. Carpentieri, U., Minguell, J.J. and Gardner, F.H. (1981) Blood 57, 975-978.

22. Paietta, E. (1983) Wiener Klinischer Wochenschrift 95, 336-344.

23. Breitman, R.T., Selonick, S.E. and Collins, S.E. (1980) Proc. Natl. Acad. Sci. USA 77, 2936-2940.

24. Rovera, G., O'Brien, T.G. and Diamond, L. (1979) Science 204, 868-870.

Vitamin Derivatives, Polyamines, and Differentiation

MOLECULAR AND CELLULAR ASPECTS OF
EMBRYONAL CARCINOMA CELL DIFFERENTIATION

JOEL SCHINDLER

DEPARTMENT OF ANATOMY AND CELL BIOLOGY
UNIVERSITY OF CINCINNATI COLLEGE OF MEDICINE
CINCINNATI, OHIO 45267

Embryonal carcinoma cells represent a subpopulation of undifferentiated stem cells contained within a mixture of differentiated cell phenotypes of teratocarcinoma tumors (1). Such tumors can develop spontaneously in gonadal tissue of certain mouse strains (2,3) and can be induced experimentally (4,5). The undifferentiated EC cells are the primary malignant cells of the tumor and are similar to early embryonic ectoderm morphologically (6), biochemically (7) and antigenically (8). Like early ectoderm cells, EC cells are pluripotent since injection of EC cells into host blastocysts leads to formation of chimeric mice (9-11).

Many EC cell lines have been isolated from in vivo tumors and successfully maintained in vitro. These various cell lines differ in their ability to differentiate in response to either physical or chemical stimuli (12). In vitro exponentially growing cells exhibit little tendency to differentiate, but as cultures reach high density, cells from some, but not all of the lines give rise to differentiated derivatives (13-16). Furthermore, cells from various EC cell lines can be induced to differentiate if they are allowed to form aggregates in vitro, rather than to attach to the substratum and grow as monolayer cultures (14,17,18). Several chemical inducers have been shown to be particularly effective in stimulating EC cell differentiation. These chemical compounds include retinoic acid (16,19), hexamethylene bisacetamide (20), and alpha difluoromethylornithine (21-23). A number of reports have indicated that if EC cells from certain cell lines are allowed to form aggregates in vitro and are treated with different chemical inducers of differentiation, combinations of inducers, or different concentrations of the same inducer, the expression of different cellular phenotypes can be stimulated (24-28).

Several recent studies have demonstrated that murine EC cells are particularly well-suited for studying molecular aspects of cell differentiation. A series of studies analyzing the expression of several cellular oncogenes has demonstrated that EC cells induced to differentiate in vitro exhibit a pattern of cellular oncogene expression that parallels expression of the same oncogenes in normal pre- and postnatal development (29,30). Transfection with the c-fos proto-oncogene led to the expression of several markers characteristic of differentiated cells, suggesting that c-fos may play a role in regulating cellular differentiation (31). In addition, it has been observed that RNA transcripts regulated during normal embryonic development and oncogenic transformation share a common repetitive sequence of DNA (32,33), the specific function of which is still unknown. This observation suggests that common developmentally regulated genes or genes induced coordinately may share common regulatory sequences. Such sequence homology has been identified in the co-inducible yeast enolase and glyceraldehyde phosphate dehydrogenase (34) genes and Drosophila heat shock genes (35).

Phenotype specific cDNAs have been isolated from cDNA libraries constructed from both undifferentiated EC cells and their differentiated derivatives. In particular, cDNAs isolated include a gene sequence expressed only in undifferentiated EC cells (36), a cDNA clone for an intermediate filament component specific to trophectoderm (37) and cDNAs for both type IV procollagen and laminin (38,39).

Transfection studies have shown that mouse EC cell lines can stably integrate exogenous genes and express them appropriately during differentiation into somatic tissue (40). A DNA sequence containing a homeo box sequence, a short DNA sequence conserved in most homeotic genes, the genes which specify segmentation in higher organisms, seems to respond to induction of differentiation (41). This provides further evidence that such DNA sequences are important in the development of multicellular organisms. Studies utilizing retroviral vectors have led to the expression of stably integrated recombinant genes flanked by retroviral long terminal repeats (42). Insertional mutagenesis studies (43) subsequently may be used for the genetic dissection of various cellular phenotypes.

Thus, embryonal carcinoma cells can serve as a useful model system for the study of the molecular basis of cellular differentiation. EC cells, which resemble stem cells of the early mouse embryo, can be induced to differentiate in vitro by known chemical and physical stimuli. The undifferentiated stem cells are malignant while their differentiated products are not. Differentiation involves changes in gene expression which can be monitored by molecular probes, including general markers of differentiation and probes specific to EC cells.

INDUCER-DEPENDENT PHENOTYPIC DIVERGENCE

Nulli-SCC1 EC cells fail to differentiate spontaneously in vivo or in vitro. When exposed to either retinoic acid (RA) or hexamethylene bisacetamide (HMBA) cells from this cell line differentiate extensively. Two distinct phenotypes can be identified depending on which inducer is utilized (44). These phenotypes are comparable to two of the earliest phenotypes expressed by cells that have themselves differentiated from blastocyst primitive ectoderm cells. These phenotypes are parietal endoderm-like and visceral endoderm-like. In addition to morphology, several different parameters demonstrate that the phenotypes of the treated cells are divergent. Table 1 shows the expression of several such characteristics. The data suggest that at least in the case of the specific parameters analyzed, RA- and HMBA-treated cells are divergent. Analysis of two dimensional gel electrophoresis profiles of untreated Nulli-SCC1 cells or cells treated with either RA or HMBA show a variety of differences. These differences include 1) new proteins expressed during differentiation in general, 2) new proteins that are RA-specific, 3) new proteins that are HMBA specific, 4) proteins which disappear as a result of differentiation, 5) proteins which disappear in response to RA alone and 6) proteins which disappear in response to HMBA alone. These six predicted classes of newly expressed proteins suggest that the phenotypic divergence of RA- or HMBA-treated cells is not unique to the specific characteristics identified in Table 1, but in fact influence broad changes in the expression of many different proteins.

TABLE 1

PHENOTYPIC DIVERGENCE IN AN EMBRYONAL CARCINOMA CELL LINE

Treatment	Expressed Characteristics			
	SSEA-1	Plasminogen Activator	Fibronectin	α-Fetoprotein
Untreated Controls	86%	8%	0%	0%
RA (1μm)	6%	79%	37%	0%
HMBA (5mM)	4%	8%	0%	96%
DFMO (2.1mM)	89%	10%	0%	0%

Nulli-SCC1 EC cells were treated for 48 hrs and the expression of the markers indicated was monitored. These results represent the percentage of positive cells recorded and are taken from previously published observations (23,44).

PHENOTYPE-SPECIFIC GENE EXPRESSION

A primary source of alphafetoprotein (AFP) during development is the visceral endoderm. Studies utilizing aggregates of F9 embryonal carcinoma cells have shown that the outer layer of cells differentiates into visceral endoderm and also expresses AFP (25). Our studies show that Nulli-SCC1 EC cells treated with HMBA in monolayer culture express a visceral endoderm-like phenotype. The different inductive and growth conditions of this alternative EC cell line suggested to us that it would be valuable to investigate the regulation of AFP gene expression. We have received an AFP cDNA probe (kindly provided by Dr. S. Tilghman, Institute for Cancer Research) to investigate AFP gene expression in HMBA-induced monolayer cultures of Nulli-SCC1 EC cells.

Kinetic analysis of AFP mRNA expression showed that within 1 hr of exposure to HMBA, AFP mRNA was detectable (45). After the initial appearance of AFP-specific mRNA, this mRNA disappears and reappears after 48 hrs of induction. No AFP-specific mRNA was detectable in either untreated Nulli-SCC1 EC cells or RA-treated cells. In vitro translation of the recovered mRNA and immunoprecipitation with AFP-specific antibody demonstrated that the identified AFP-specific mRNA encoded a protein that migrated with a molecular weight identical to AFP on SDS-PAGE. Some mRNA samples contained higher molecular weight species which did hybridize to the AFP cDNA. By in vitro translation analysis, this mRNA did not encode AFP protein. The specific nature and relationship between this high molecular weight mRNA and authentic AFP mRNA is currently under investigation.

Immunoprecipitation/SDS-PAGE was used to determine the appearance of AFP protein in HMBA-treated cells and media. AFP can be detected in cell extracts within 3-6 hrs after induction and remains at a constant level through 48 hrs of exposure to HMBA. In culture medium, no AFP was detectable until 48 hrs after treatment. These observations suggest a fairly long lag time between initial intracellular appearance of AFP and its secretion into the media. Pulse labeling of cells for 3 hr intervals followed by immunoprecipitation/SDS-PAGE analysis indicated that detectable AFP could only be synthesized at times corresponding to the presence of authentic 2.2 kb AFP mRNA (1,3,48 hrs).

While it is possible that the initial appearance of AFP-specific mRNA reflects a small subpopulation of cells that are differentially more mature or are at a sight in the cell cycle that facilitates the expression of a phenotype-specific marker, we feel that is unlikely since immunofluorescent detection of AFP indicates that at the time AFP protein can first be detected intracellularly,

low levels of protein are found in virtually all cells
rather than high levels of AFP in a small subpopulation of
HMBA-responsive cells.

POLYAMINES AND EC CELL DIFFERENTIATION

Extensive studies both _in vitro_ and _in vivo_ have
demonstrated that the role of polyamines during
differentiation is complex. Reduced levels of polyamines
clearly influence the normal development of many different
species (46-50). Bone, chondrocyte and adipocyte
differentiation all require increased levels of polyamines
while neuroblastoma cells and HL-60 cells require lower
levels of polyamines to induce differentiation (51-55).

With the use of α-difluoromethylornithine (DFMO), an
enzyme-activated irreversible inhibitor of the polyamine
biosynthetic enzyme ornithine decarboxylase (ODCase; see
Figure 1; 56), we have attempted to better understand the

FIGURE 1
POLYAMINE BIOSYNTHESIS

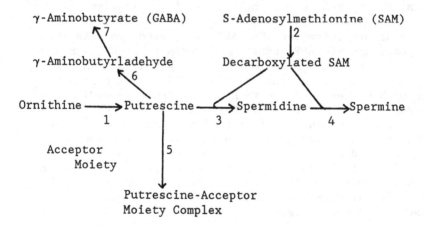

The enzymes involved in the biosynthesis of intracellular
polyamines are: 1) ornithine decarboxylase;
2) S-adenosylmethionine decarboxylase; 3) spermidine
synthase; 4) spermine synthase; 5) transglutaminase;
6) diamine oxidase; 7) aldehyde dehydrogenase. This
Figure is a modification of a previously published version
(58).

relationship between polyamine levels and EC cell differentiation. Several EC cell lines were exposed to DFMO and cell behavior was monitored. Studies analyzing morphological changes as well as changes in well-characterized antigenic and biochemical parameters, indicated that DFMO could influence EC cell behavior in a number of different ways (23). The EC cell lines which show large reductions in ODCase activity and polyamine levels show extensive morphological and biochemical differentiation. Cell lines which show limited reductions in both enzyme activity and polyamine levels show poor differentiation, while the cell lines that demonstrate little reduction in the levels of polyamines fail to respond to DFMO induction. These observations suggest that threshold levels of polyamines, that influence EC cells behavior, exist in all EC cell lines. In order to induce differentiation, polyamine levels must be reduced below these threshold levels to influence cell behavior. These studies suggest that reduced levels of intracellular polyamines do induce EC cell differentiation.

Retinoic acid (RA) is a potent inducer of EC cell differentiation (19). If reduced levels of polyamines are related to the induction of differentiation, we would predict that exposure to RA would lead to early decreases in intracellular levels of polyamines. Studies performed in our laboratory (57) indicate that while polyamine levels are important in determining the phenotypic state of EC cells, reduction in the intracellular levels of polyamines is alone insufficient to induce EC cell differentiation. Our data indicate that while RA does influence polyamine levels, this influence is not mediated through direct RA-ODCase interaction.

That RA and the polyamines do share common aspects of EC cell differentiation is demonstrated by studies using suboptimal levels of both inducers (58). These studies demonstrate that while suboptimal levels of either RA or DFMO have no effect on EC cell behavior, the two compounds together at similar suboptimal concentrations do synergize and induce EC cell differentiation.

A possible sight of RA-polyamine interaction could be the transglutaminase (TGase) enzyme (see Figure 1). Previous studies (59,60) have shown that RA can modulate TGase enzyme activity and changes in such enzyme activity

can cause changes in the levels of intracellular
polyamines. We therefore initiated studies to investigate
the possible effect of RA on TGase activity.

Our results show that RA modulates TGase activity
shortly after exposure of EC cells to the inducer. Levels
of enzyme activity change within 30 min after exposure to
retinoic acid (61). Additional observations using two
compounds which inhibit TGase activity are particularly
convincing with respect to a role for TGase enzyme
activity in mediating RA-induced EC cell differentiation.
The two compounds, cystamine and cadaverine, when added
simultaneously with concentrations of RA known to induce
EC cell differentiation, block that induction. This
observation provides strong evidence that TGase activity
may play a role in EC cell differentiation. The specific
site of RA-TGase interaction is not yet established, but
it is possible to suggest several alternatives. One could
consider 1) changes in the actual level of enzyme
activity; 2) changes in the level of the acceptor moiety
that participates in the TGase reaction; and 3) the
possibility that multiple forms of TGase exist, as has
been demonstrated in other experimental systems (62). RA
induction could cause a change in the nature of the TGase
enzyme. Studies are currently under way to distinguish
between these possible options.

DISSECTING THE MULTI-STEP NATURE OF EC CELL DIFFERENTIATION

Our earlier studies suggest that threshold levels of
polyamines dictate the state of EC cell phenotypic
expression. Table 2 clearly demonstrates that a high
degree of variability exists in the response of different
EC cell lines to different inducers, suggesting that each
cell line is "arrested" at a different developmental
stage. While all EC cells are considered to be
undifferentiated stem cells, it is clear that not all EC
cells are, in fact, alike, as reflected in the different
responsiveness of various EC cell lines to different
inducers. A series of studies using several inducers in
concert further confirms that the induction of EC cell
differentiation is a multi-step process. Either the
ability or inability of EC cells from different cell lines

TABLE 2

SPECTRA OF DIFFERENTIATIVE POTENTIAL

CONDITION

CELL LINE	TUMOR FORMATION	HIGH DENSITY GROWTH	AGGREGATE FORMATION	DFMO	HMBA	RA
OC-15	+	+	+	+	+	+
PCC3	+	+	+	+	+	+
PCC4aza1R	±	-	+	+	+	+
F9	±	-	±	±	+	+
NULLI-SCC1	-	-	-	-	+	+

Cells from the cell lines listed were induced to differentiate by the conditions indicated. (-) denotes no differentiation; (±) denotes 30-50% differentiation; (+) denotes >90% differentiation. This table is a composite of previously reported observations (12,23).

to respond to different inducers is a reflection of their developmental "arrest".

If one considers differentiation as a linear series of events (see Figure 2), it is possible to assign "transitional stages" to different EC cell lines. The relative location of these transitional stages is a reflection of the differing propensities of the various EC cell lines to differentiate. Figure 2 places several EC cell lines in such relative transitional positions.

The "dosage hypothesis" for differentiation suggests that cells progress through various stages of the differentiation process as a result of quantitative changes that concern the level of expression of certain intracellular modulator molecules. Our reported observations regarding threshold levels of polyamines, as well as the possible biosynthesis, through a TGase reaction of new regulator proteins, suggest that the

FIGURE 2

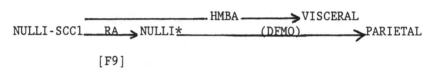

[F9]

                              HMBA
        PCCAaza1R____RA__→ PCC4aza1R*____DFMO__→ PARIETAL

                           [PCC3]

                           [OC-15]

UNDIFFERENTIATED————————(TRANSITIONAL) ———→ DIFFERENTIATED
(STEM CELL)

By considering differentiation as a multistep linear event, it is possible to "order" different EC cell lines along this linear path. The specific position along this path is a direct reflection of each cell line's "propensity to differentiate". The relative locations of RA, HMBA, and DFMO reflect their putative active sites in the multistep process.

"dosage hypothesis" may be valid for describing EC cell differentiation. By exploiting variable inducer responsiveness as a tool to dissect EC cell differentiation, it should be possible to identify the various steps involved in EC cell differentiation. While there are as yet no specific candidates for such intracellular regulatory moieties, it is possible to suggest the products of proto-oncogenes as possible candidates. Studies analyzing the relative quantitative levels of several different proto-oncogenes in different EC cells are currently under way.

OVERVIEW

The current report presents a variety of data at both the molecular and cellular levels that demonstrate the value of murine EC cells as a viable experimental system to investigate cytodifferentiation. Our studies focus on several interrelated issues central to stem cell differentiation. In particular, we are interested in 1) investigating the mechanism of action of specific chemical inducers, 2) defining the events which regulate phenotype-specific gene expression, and 3) identifying intracellular compounds whose level of expression is important in dictating phenotypic expression of EC cells. Our observations with various murine EC cell lines provide intriguing and useful information with respect to all of our expressed interests.

REFERENCES

1. Graham, C. (1977) In Concepts in Mammalian Embryogenesis. (ed., M.I. Sherman), M.I.T., Cambridge, Mass. pp. 315-394.
2. Stevens, L.C. (1959) J. Natl. Cancer Inst. 23:1249-1261.
3. Stevens, L.C., and Varnum, D.S. (1974) Develop. Biol. 37:369-380.
4. Stevens, L.C. (1968) J. Embryol. Exp. Morph. 20:329-341.
5. Solter, D., Skreb, N., and Damjanov, I. (1970) Nature 227:503-504.
6. Martin, G.R. (1977) In Cell Interactions in Differentiation. (eds., Kashinen-Jaaskelainen, M., Saxen, L., and Weiss, L.) Academic Press, New York. pp. 56-82.
7. Martin, G.R., Smith, S., and Epstein, C.J. (1978) Develop. Biol. 66:6-16.
8. Wiley, L. (1979) Curr. Topics Devel. Biol. 13:167-197.
9. Brinster, R.L. (1974) J. Exp. Med. 140:1049-1056.
10. Mintz, B., and Illmensee, K. (1975) Proc. Natl. Acad. Sci. USA 72:3585-3589.
11. Papaioannou, W.E., McBurney, M.W., Gardner, R.L., and Evans, M.J. (1975) Nature 258:70-73.
12. Sherman, M.I., Matthaei, K.I., and Schindler, J. (1981) Ann. N.Y. Acad. Sci. 359:192-199.
13. McBurney, M.W. (1976) J. Cell Physiol. 89:441-455.
14. Martin, G.R., and Evans, M.J. (1975) Proc. Natl. Acad. Sci. USA 72:1441-1445.
15. Sherman, M.I., and Miller, R.A. (1978) Develop. Biol. 63:27-34.
16. Jetten, A.M., Jetten, M.E.R., and Sherman, M.I. (1979) Exp. Cell Res. 124:281-291.

17. Sherman, M.I. (1975) In Teratomas and
     Differentiation. (eds., M.I. Sherman and D. Solter),
     Academic Press, N.Y. pp. 189-205.
18. Nicolas, J.F., Dubois, P., Jakob, H., Gaillard, J.,
     and Jacob, F. (1975) Ann. Microbiol. (Inst.
     Pasteur) 126A:3-22.
19. Strickland, S., and Mahdavi, V. (1978) Cell 15:393-
     403.
20. Jakob, H., Dubois, P., Eisen, H., and Jacob, F.
     (1978) C.R. Acad. Sci. Ser. D 286:109-111.
21. Schindler, J., Kelly, M., and McCann, P.P. (1983)
     Biochem. Biophys. Res. Commun. 114:410-417.
22. Heby, O., Oredsson, S.M., Olsson, I., and Marton,
     L.J. (1983) Adv. Polyamine Res. 4:727-742.
23. Schindler, J., Kelly, M., and McCann, P.P. (1985)
     J. Cell. Phys. 122:1-6.
24. Speers, W.C., Bridwell, C.R., Dixon, F.J. (1970)
     Am. J. Pathol. 97:563-577.
25. Hogan, B.L.M., Taylor, A., and Adamson, E. (1981)
     Nature 291:235-237.
26. McBurney, M.W., Jones-Villeneuve, E.M.V., Edwards,
     M.K.S., and Anderson, P.J. (1982) Nature 299:165-
     167.
27. Edwards, M.K.S., and McBurney, M.W. (1983) Dev.
     Biol. 98:187-191.
28. Rosenstrauss, M.J., Spadoro, J.P., and Nilsson, J.
     (1983) Dev. Biol. 98:110-116.
29. Muller, R., Verma, I.M., and Adamson, E.D. (1983)
     EMBO Journal 2:679-684.
30. Muller, R., Tremblay, J.M., Adamson, E.D., and Verma,
     I.M. (1983) Nature 304:454-456.
31. Muller, R., and Wagner, E.F. (1984) Nature 311:438-
     442.
32. Murphy, D., Brickell, P.M., Latchman, D.S., Willison,
     K., and Rigby, P.W.J. (1983) Cell 35:865-871.
33. Brickell, P.M., Latchman, D.S., Murphy, D., Willison,
     K., and Rigby, P.W.J. (1983) Nature 306:756-760.
34. Holland, M.J., Holland, J.P., Thrill, G.P., and
     Jackson, K.A. (1981) J. Biol. Chem. 256:1385-1395.
35. Ingolia, T.D., and Craig, E.A. (1981) Nucl. Acid
     Res. 9:1627-1642.
36. Stacey, A.J., and Evans, M.J. (1984) EMBO Journal
     3:2279-2285.
37. Vasseur, M., Duprey, P., Brulet, P., and Jacob, F.
     (1985) Proc. Natl. Acad. Sci. USA 82:1155-1159.

38. Wang, S-Y., LaRosa, G.J., and Gudas, L.J. (1985) Dev. Biol. 107:75-86.
39. Marotti, K.R., Brown, G.D., and Strickland, S. (1985) Dev. Biol. 108:26-31.
40. Scott, R.W., Vogt, T.F., Croke, M.E., and Tilghman, S.M. (1984) Nature 310:562-567.
41. Colberg-Poley, A.M., Voss, S.D., Chowdhury, K., and Gruss, P. (1985) Nature 314:713-718.
42. Taketo, M., Gilboa, E., and Sherman, M.I. (1985) Proc. Natl. Acad. Sci. USA 82:2422-2426.
43. King, W., Patel, M.D., Lobel, L.I., Goff, S.P., and Nguyen-Huu, M.C. (1985) Science 228:554-558.
44. Schindler, J., Hollingsworth, R., and Coughlin, P. (1984) Differentiation 27:236-242.
45. Coughlin, P., and Schindler, J. (1986) Submitted for publication.
46. Heby, O., and Emmanuelsson, H. (1981) Med. Biol. 59:417-423.
47. Brachet, J., Mamont, P., Boloukhere, M., Baltus, E., Hanocq-Quertier, J. (1978) C.R. Acad. Sci. [D] (Paris) 287:1289-1292.
48. Lowkvist, B., Heby, O., Emanuelsson, H. (1980) J. Embryol. Exp. Morphol. 60:83-89.
49. Fozard, J.R., Part, M.-L., Prakash, N.J., Grove, J., Schechter, P.J., Sjoerdsma, A., and Koch-Weser, J. (1980) Science 208:505-507.
50. Fozard, J.R., Part, M.-L., Prakash, N.J., and Grove, J. (1980) Eur. J. Pharmacol. 65:379-385.
51. Rath, N.C., and Reddi, A.H. (1981) Dev. Biol. 82:211-216.
52. Takano, T., Takigawa, M., and Suzuki, F. (1981) Med. Biol. 59:423-427.
53. Bethell, D.R., and Pegg, A.E. (1983) Biochem. Biophys. Res. Commun. 102:272-278.
54. Chen, K.Y., and Liu, A.Y.-C. (1981) FEBS Lett. 134:71-74.
55. Sugiura, M., Shafman, T., Mitchell, T., Griffin, J., and Kufe, D. (in press).
56. Mamont, P.S., Duchesne, M.-C., Grove, J., and Bey, P. (1978) Biochem. Biophys. Res. Commun. 81:58-66.
57. Kelly, M., McCann, P.P., and Schindler, J. (1985) Dev. Biol. 111:510-514.

58. Schindler, J., and Kelly, M. (1985) From: Vitamins and Cancer-Human Cancer Prevention by Vitamins and Micronutrients. Ed. by F.L. Meyskens and K.N. Prasad, The Humana Press, Inc., Clifton, NJ., pp.19-33.

59. Yuspa, S.H., Ben, T., and Steiner, P. (1982) J. Biol. Chem. $\underline{257}$:9906-9912.

60. Yuspa, S.H., Ben, T., and Lichti, U. (1983) Cancer Res. $\underline{43}$:5707-5712.

61. Uhl, L., and Schindler, J. (1986) Exp. Cell Biol. (in press).

62. Folk, J. (1986) Am. Rev. Biochem. $\underline{49}$:517-531.

The author wishes to acknowledge support for aspects of this work from a Biomedical Research Support Grant (NIH) and a grant from the National Science Foundation. The author also wishes to thank Dr. Peter P. McCann, Merrell Dow Research Institute, Cincinnati, Ohio for kindly providing α-difluoromethylornithine and performing polyamine analyses.

INTERACTION OF 1,25 DIHYDROXYVITAMIN D$_3$ WITH NORMAL AND ABNORMAL HEMATOPOIESIS

H. P. Koeffler, A. Tobler, H. Reichel*,
A. Norman*

University of California, LA; *University of
California, Riverside

Los Angeles, CA 90024; Riverside, CA 92502

EFFECT OF 1,25 DIHYDROXYVITAMIN D$_3$ ON NORMAL AND LEUKEMIC MYELOID CELLS IN VITRO

A diagram of the human hematopoietic system with their stem cells is shown on Figure 1. _In vitro_ clonogenic studies in the murine and human systems have shown that several lymphokines, known as colony stimulating factors (CSF), induce proliferation and differentiation of hematopoietic stem cells. The myeloid stem cell known as the granulocyte-monocyte colony forming cell (GM-CFC) can differentiate either to macrophage colonies when grown in the presence of macrophage or granulocyte-macrophage CSF or differentiate to granulocyte colonies in the presence of granulocyte or granulocyte-macrophage CSF. Few studies have examined the ability of other physiological substances to influence differentiation of myeloid stem cells. Recently 1,25 dihydroxyvitamin D$_3$ [1,25(OH)$_2$D$_3$] was found to induce cells from both a murine myeloid leukemia line known as M1 (1) and a human promyelocytic leukemia line (HL-60) (2-5) to differentiate to monocyte-macrophage like cells (Fig. 2, Table 1). The cells, when cultured in 1,25(OH)$_2$D$_3$ (10^{-7} - 10^{-10}M), become adherent to charged surfaces, develop long filamented pseudopodia, stained positively for nonspecific acid esterase (NAE), reduce nitro-blue tetrazolium (NBT), and acquire the ability to phagocytize yeast. The HL-60 cells cultured with 1,25(OH)$_2$D$_3$ also acquire the capacity to bind and degrade bone matrix _in vitro_ (3). The effective dose

137

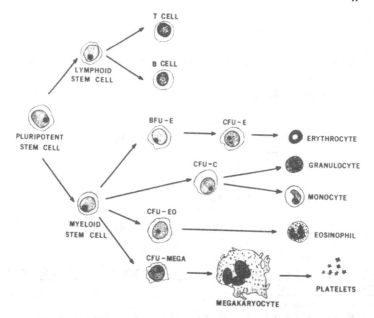

FIGURE 1: Hematopoietic system. Abbreviations: BFU-E, erythrocyte burst-forming unit; CFU-E, erythrocyte colony-forming unit; CFU-C, colony-forming unit in culture (synonymous with GM-CFC, granulocyte-monocyte colony forming cell); CFU-EO, eosinophil colony-forming unit; CFU-MEGA, (megakaryocyte colony-forming unit).

(ED_{50}) that induces approximately 50% of the cells to differentiate is about 6×10^{-9}M.

The mechanism by which HL-60 is induced to differentiate by $1,25(OH)_2D_3$ is not clear. These cells contain cellular receptors for the $1,25(OH)_2D_3$ as shown by sucrose density gradient analysis, DNA cellulose chromatography and by a specific monoclonal antibody which recognizes the $1,25(OH)_2D_3$ receptor (2, 5). Scatchard analysis shows that the HL-60 has about 4,000 $1,25(OH)_2D_3$ cellular receptors per cell with a Kd of ~ 5.4×10^{-9}M (Fig. 3).

Further indirect evidence that the vitamin D analogs mediate their induction of differentiation through $1,25(OH)_2D_3$ cellular receptors is shown in Fig. 4. We have found that $1,25(OH)_2D_3$ can inhibit clonal proliferation of HL-60 cells when plated in soft agar. We examined

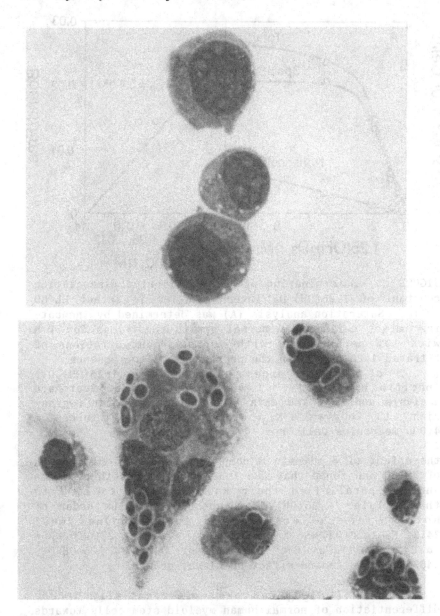

FIGURE 2: (A) HL-60 promyelocytes. (B) HL-60 cells
induced to macrophage-like cells after exposure to 10^{-7}
mol/L 1,25 dihydroxyvitamin D_3 for seven days. Cells are
adherent and have phagocytosed <u>Candida albicans</u>.

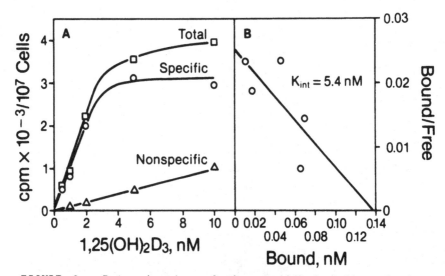

FIGURE 3.   Determination of the equilibrium dissociation
constant of $1,25(OH)_2D_3$ internalization in intact HL-60
cells.   Saturation analysis (A) was determined by incubating intact cells under normal growth conditions for 4 h
with 10% serum along with various concentrations of
titrated $1,25(OH)_2D_3$ in the presence (   ) or absence
(   ) of 100-fold excess nonradioactive $1,25(OH)_2D_3$.
Specific binding (   ) was transformed by Scatchard
analysis and then the data line-fitted by linear regression.   (B) to yield a K_{int} = 5.4 nM (abscissa intercept =
4,000 molecules/cell, r = -0.71).

the effect of 6 vitamin D compounds on the clonal growth
of HL-60 and found that the inhibition of growth by these
analogs parallelled their known ability to bind to
the cellular $1,25(OH)_2D_3$ receptor.   The rank order of
potency of the activity of the compounds was:
$24,24-F_2-1\alpha25(OH)_2D_3$ > $1\alpha,25(OH)_2D_3$ > $1\alpha,24R,25(OH)_3D_3$ =
$1\alpha,24S,25(OH)_3D_3$ (6).   In contrast $1\alpha-OH-D_3$, $25-OH-D_3$,
$24S25 (OH)_2D_3$ had no effect on clonal growth.

The $1,25(OH)_2D_3$ can also preferentially induce
differentiation of normal human myeloid stem cells towards
macrophages.   An initial study found that an increased
percent of monocytes and macrophages were present when
$1,25(OH)_2D_3$ was added to bone marrow cells in liquid
culture for 5 days as compared to control flasks
containing no $1,25(OH)_2D_3$ (4).   To further investigate

TABLE 1

Functional and Morphological Changes in HL-60 Cells
Induced by Various Concentrations of $1,25(OH)_2D_3$*

Added concentration of $1,25(OH)_2D_3$** (M)	NBT Reduction (%)	Phagocytic Cells (%)	Myeloblasts and Promyeloblasts (%)	Intermediate*** to mature cells (%)	Nonspecific acid esterase-positive (%)
0	2 ± 3	2 ± 2	99 ± 2	1 ± 2	2
10^{-11}	10 ± 2	2 ± 3	95 ± 3	5 ± 4	3
10^{-10}	18 ± 11	13 ± 7	82 ± 5	18 ± 7	10
10^{-9}	37 ± 19	20 ± 7	66 ± 9	23 ± 6	25
10^{-8}	64 ± 13	26 ± 4	45 ± 12	55 ± 9	54
10^{-7}	82 ± 8	44 ± 9	32 ± 5	67 ± 6	82
10^{-6}	86 ± 12	60 ± 3	27 ± 6	78 ± 14	98

* HL-60 and HL-60 blast cells were cultured in the presence or absence of various concentrations of $1,25(OH)_2D_3$; after 7 d, cells were assessed for the various differentiation parameters. All data are expressed as the percentage of total cells assayed and the data represent the mean ± standard deviation of triplicate assays.
** Basal $1,25(OH)_2D_3$ in 10% fetal bovine serum is 1.6×10^{-11} M.
*** Intermediate to mature cells include monocytes and macrophages.

this observation, $1,25(OH)_2D_3$ was added to soft agar cultures containing normal human bone marrow in the presence of GM-CSF (Table 2) (7). The GM-CFC stem cells proliferated and differentiated in soft agar and formed colonies. These colonies were plucked, cytochemically stained, examined by light microscopy and the absolute number and percent of monocyte, granulocyte and combined monocyte and granulocyte colonies was determined. The $1,25(OH)_2D_3$ induced human myeloid GM-CFC to differentiate to colonies containing macrophages. Nearly 95% of the colonies were composed of only macrophages in culture plates containing 10^{-8}M $1,25(OH)_2D_3$, and 55% of the colonies were composed of only macrophages in the plates containing 10^{-9}M $1,25(OH)_2D_3$. Control dishes of normal human bone marrow GM-CFC not containing $1,25(OH)_2D_3$ differentiated to approximately 55% neutrophil, 10% mixed neutrophil-macrophage and 25% macrophage colonies. The $1,25(OH)_2D_3$ increased the absolute number of macrophage colonies rather than merely increasing the relative proportion of macrophage colonies by selectively inhibiting granulocytic differentiation of GM-CFC (Table 2). Plates containing either 10^{-8} or 10^{-9}M $1,25(OH)_2D_3$

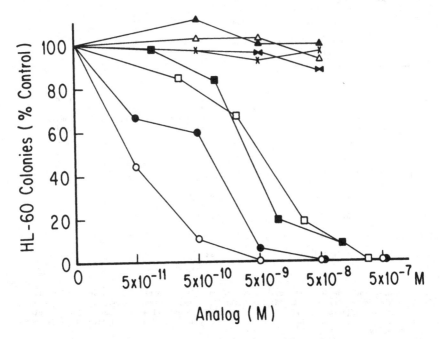

FIGURE 4: Effect of various concentrations of different
analogs of vitamin D on clonal growth of HL-60 promyelocytes. The analogs are: , $1\alpha,25(OH)_2D_3$;   ,
$1\alpha,24S25(OH)_3D_3$;   , $24S25(OH)_2D_3$;   , $1\alpha(OH)D_3$;   ,
$24,24-F_2-1\alpha,25(OH)_2D_3$;   x, $24R25(OH)_2D_3$;   , $25(OH)D_3$.
Cells were plated in soft agar with various vitamin D
analogs and the number of colonies enumerated after 10 d
of culture. Results are expressed as a percent of control
cells not exposed to the vitamin D analog. Each point
represents the mean of three experiments with triplicate
dishes per point.

developed approximately 90 and 65 macrophage colonies,
respectively, per 1 x 10^5 cultured marrow cells. In
contrast, 35 macrophage colonies per 1 x 10^5 cultured
marrow cells developed in control plates containing no
$1,25(OH)_2D_3$.

The paucity of GM-CFC in the bone marrow (approximately 1 per 2 x 10^3 marrow cells) prevents purification
of these cells in order to determine if they contain
$1,25(OH)_2D_3$ receptors. Nevertheless, extrapolation from
the data from the HL-60 promyelocytes suggest that

TABLE 2

Effects of 1,25(OH)$_2$D$_3$ on Differentiation and Proliferation
of Human Myeloid Colony Forming Cells

Cell Source [a]	(1,25(OH)$_2$D$_3$) (M)	No. of colonies (% of control)[a]	N	Colony morphology[b] (%) NM	M
Normal Volunteers (7)	0	100	56 ± 8	10 ± 1	34 ± 4
	10^{-10}	102 ± 6	58 ± 5	6 ± 1	36 ± 3
	10^{-9}	120 ± 5	29 ± 4	5 ± 1	56 ± 4
	10^{-8}	101 ± 5	2 ± 1	2 ± 1	96 ± 2
	10^{-7}	78 ± 6	0	0	100

[a] Marrow cells were obtained from 7 normal volunteers and the light density, nonadherent, mononuclear cells were cultivated in the presence of colony stimulating factor and various concentrations of the vitamin D metabolite 1,25(OH)$_2$D$_3$. Colonies were counted on day 10 of culture. Normal control cultures contained a mean of 94 ± 8 (± SE) myeloid colonies.

[b] Colony morphology was evaluated on day 10 of culture by dual esterase and luxol fast blue staining. N, neutrophilic colonies; NM, neutrophil-macrophage mixed colonies; M, monocyte-macrophage colonies; B, blast cells colonies.

1,25(OH)$_2$D$_3$ induces macrophage differentiation of hematopoietic progenitor cells by binding of the active vitamin D metabolite to 1,25(OH)$_2$D$_3$ receptors which presumably binds to DNA and alters transcriptional control. The differentiation may be regulated by 1,25(OH)$_2$D$_3$ itself, by local shifts in calcium transport mediated by 1,25(OH)$_2$D$_3$, or by induction of differentiation-inducing protein(s) by accessory cells in the culture plates.

The hypothesis that 1,25(OH)$_2$D$_3$ may be a possible differentiation inducer of GM-CFC to macrophages is appealing because of the known ability of 1,25(OH)$_2$D$_3$ to modulate bone resorption. Osteoclasts resorb bone. Evidence suggests that osteoclasts may develop from monocyte-macrophage cells (8) and one study suggested that 1,25(OH)$_2$D$_3$ may modulate the number of osteoclasts (9). Therefore, 1,25(OH)$_2$D$_3$ might modulate bone resorption by inducing GM-CFC to differentiate to monocytes and macrophages and eventually to osteoclasts. Likewise, in vitro the monocytes and macrophages can directly resorb bone (10).

The plasma concentration of 1,25(OH)$_2$D$_3$ in man is approximately 7.7 x 10^{-11}M (11). In vivo, concentrations of ≥ 10^{-9}M 1,25(OH)$_2$D$_3$ induce macrophage differ-

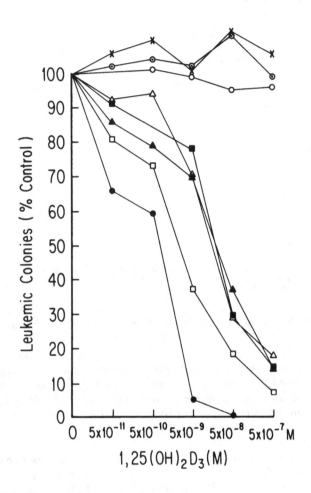

FIGURE 5: Effect of various concentrations of $1\alpha,25(OH)_2D_3$ on clonal growth of myeloid cell lines (, HL-60; , U937; , M1; , THP; , HEL; , HL-60 blast; , KG-1A; , K562). Cells were plated in soft agar containing different concentrations of $1\alpha,25(OH)_2D_3$ and the number of colonies were enumerated on day 12 of culture. Results are expressed as a percent of control cells not exposed to $1\alpha,25(OH)_2D_3$. Each point represents the mean of three experiments with triplicate dishes per point.

entiation of myeloid progenitor cells <u>in vitro</u>. Therefore, $1,25(OH)_2D_3$ may not have a physiological role in the induction of differentiation of human myeloid stem cells

TABLE 3

Effects of 1α,25(OH)$_2$D$_3$ on Clonal Growth of Cells Freshly from Myeloid
Leukemia Lines

Cell Line	Description	50% Inhibitory concentration M 1α,25(OH)$_2$D$_3$
HL-60	human promyelocytes	8 x 10^{-10}
U937	human monoblasts/histiocytes	4 x 10^{-9}
HEL	bipotent*	2 x 10^{-8}
THP-1	human monoblasts	3 x 10^{-8}
M1	mouse myeloid leukemia	1 x 10^{-8}
HL-60 blast	human early myeloblasts	no inhibition
KG-1A	human early myeloblasts	no inhibition
KG-1	human myeloblasts	no inhibition**
K562	bipotent*	no inhibition

*Monoblast and erythroblast characteristics.

**Stimulation at suboptimal concentrations of CSF.

to macrophages. Likewise, patients who received super-
physiological doses of 1,25(OH)$_2$D$_3$ have not been reported
to have an increased concentration of blood monocytes
(12). Also, patients with vitamin D resistant rickets
have not been reported to have low monocyte or macrophage
levels (13). The true hematopoietic role of vitamin D
metabolites _in vivo_ is unknown and will require careful
experimentation.

The effect of 1,25(OH)$_2$D$_3$ on both clonal proliferation and differentiation of cells from 8 myeloid leukemic
lines is shown on Fig. 5 and Tables 3, 4 (6). The 50%
inhibition of colony formation of the responsive lines
occurred in the concentration range of 3 x 10^{-8} - 4 x
10^{-10} M 1α,25(OH)$_2$D$_3$. These concentrations are comparable
to the concentrations required for induction of differentiation in liquid culture (1, 5, 14, 15). Cell lines
which were induced to differentiate by 1α,25(OH)$_2$D$_3$ were
always inhibited in their clonal growth by 1α,25(OH)$_2$D$_3$.
Differentiation was measured by their ability to reduce
nitroblue tetrazolium (NBT), which is a measure of
maturation. The responsive cells were relatively more

TABLE 4

Effect of 1α,25-Dihydroxyvitamin D₃ on the Ability of Cells from Leukemic Lines
to Reduce NBT

Percentage NBT-positive cells

Cell Line	HL-60	HL-60 blast	KG-1	KG-1a	U937	HEL	THP1
Control	2 ± 2	0 ± 1	0 ± 0	0 ± 0	1 ±	3 ± 2	35 ± 5
1,25(OH)₂D₃	60 ± 7	1 ± 1	0 ± 0	0 ± 0	49 ± 8	27 ± 9	48 ± 5

Results represent the mean of four separate experiments (±SD). Cells cultured in liquid
media containing 5 x 10⁻⁷M 1α,25(OH)₂D₃ for 5 d, washed, and tested for their ability to
reduce nitroblue tetrazolium (NBT).

mature (HL-60, U937, THP1, HEL, M1,) than the unresponsive
cells (KG1A, KG-1, HL-60 blast, K562). Our experiments
are supportive of the concept that myeloid blast cells
have limited capabilities for replication when induced to
differentiate. The vitamin D-responsive progenitor cells
differentiated in vitro and lost their potential for
clonal growth. The vitamin D-unresponsive leukemic cells
did not differentiate and remained in the proliferative
pool, giving rise to colonies of similar cells.

We also examined the effect of $1,25(OH)_2D_3$ on the
clonal growth of leukemic blast cells harvested from the
peripheral blood or bone marrow of 14 individuals with
myeloid leukemia (Fig. 6A, Table 5). Ten of the 14
leukemic patients had neoplastic cells that were at least
50% inhibited in their colony formation in the presence of
$5 \times 10^{-7}M$ $1,25(OH)_2D_3$ and 5 of the 14 leukemic patients
had a 50% inhibition of leukemic colony formation at $5 \times 10^{-9}M$ $1,25(OH)_2D_3$ (Table 5). Clonal growth of acute
myelogenous leukemia (AML) and chronic myelogenous
leukemia cells was inhibited approximately equally by
$1,25(OH)_2D_3$. However, $1,25(OH)_2D_3$ stimulated the clonal
proliferation of blast cells from an AML patient by
greater than 400%. This 33 year old patient had very
immature acute myeloblastic leukemia cells. The
$1,25(OH)_2D_3$ had little effect on clonal growth of normal
myeloid stem cells (GM-CFC) harvested from 12 myeloid
leukemia patients who were in remission (Fig. 6B). The
GM-CFC from leukemic patients in remission were not
inhibited more than 30% at any concentration of the
$1,25(OH)_2D_3$ (5×10^{-7} - $5 \times 10^{-11}M$).

Why $1,25(OH)_2D_3$ preferentially inhibits in vitro the

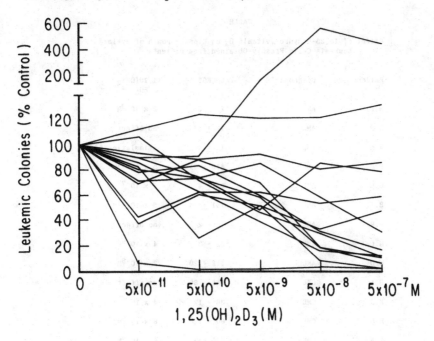

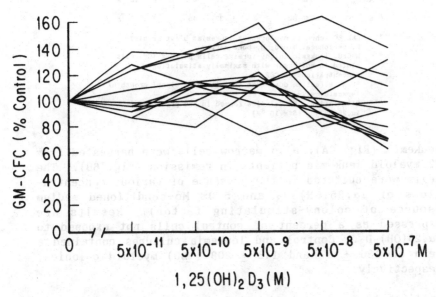

FIGURE 6. Effect of 1α,25(OH)₂D₃ on clonal growth of leukemic and normal myeloid colony-forming cells. Leukemic cells were obtained from 14 patient with myeloid

TABLE 5

Effect of 1α,25-Dihydroxyvitamin D_3 on Clonal Growth of Myeloid
Leukemia Cells Freshly Obtained from Patients

Patient	Diagnosis[+]	L-CFC[*]	1,25(OH)$_2$D$_3$ ED$_{50}$[**]
M.F.	AML	22 ± 5	2 x 10^{-9}M
W.P.	AML	72 ± 34	no effect
W.M.	AML	12 ± 4	stimulation[***]
P.O.	AML	810 ± 91	5 x 10^{-11}M
C.L.	AML	23 ± 4	5 x 10^{-7}
B.T.	AML	131 ± 34	5 x 10^{-11}M
K.R.	AML	16 ± 2	no effect
M.L.	AML	22 ± 3	4 x 10^{-9}M
W.D.	AML	112 ± 20	2 x 10^{-8}M
B.A.	CML	295 ± 89	no effect
H.J.	CML	36 ± 12	4 x 10^{-9}M
M.D.	CML	60 ± 11	8 x 10^{-9}M
C.A.	CML	129 ± 3	6 x 10^{-9}M
G.S.	CML-BC	337 ± 45	1 x 10^{-7}M

[+] CML-BC, chronic myelogenous leukemia, blast crisis;
B, peripheral blood; M, bone marrow
[*] L-CFC, leukemic colony-forming cells per 2 x 10^5 cells
plated in soft agar with maximally stimulating
concentrations of CSF
[**] ED$_{50}$, effective dose that inhibited 50% clonal growth of
leukemic cells.
[***] Stimulation: 62 colonies formed in the presence of
1α,25(OH)$_2$D$_3$ (5 x 10^{-8}M)

leukemia (Fig. 6A); also marrow cells were harvested from
12 myeloid leukemia patients in remission (Fig. 6B). The
cells were cultured in the presence of various concentrations of 1α,25(OH)$_2$D$_3$ and 5.0% Mo-conditioned medium
(source of colony-stimulating factor). Results are
expressed as a percent of control cells not exposed to
1α,25(OH)$_2$D$_3$. Control and leukemia cultures contained a
mean of 135 ± 67 and 148 ± 208 (±SD) myeloid colonies,
respectively.

proliferation of leukemic, but not normal human myeloid
stem cells is not clear. Differences in receptor number
or affinity, or the activation of different genes and
metabolic pathways may account for this differential

effect.

Further studies suggest that $1\alpha,25(OH)_2D_3$ can act as a hematopoietic cofactor that promotes clonal growth of certain myeloid stem cells (6). In the presence of submaximal concentrations of CSF, $1\alpha,25(OH)_2D_3$ stimulated the clonal growth of normal human bone marrow GM-CFC. A similar result was obtained with the human AML cell line known as KG-1 which is dependent on CSF for its clonal growth. The $1\alpha,25(OH)_2D_3$ did not stimulate the marrow or KG-1 cells to produce detectable CSF. The increased clonal growth in the presence of $1\alpha,25(OH)_2D_3$ and submaximal concentrations of CSF may reflect an increased responsiveness to CSF due to effects on the number and/or affinity of CSF receptors on the target cells.

A clinical study of 1,25-dihydroxyvitamin D₃ in patients with the myelodysplastic syndromes:

We initiated a trial of administering $1,25(OH)_2D_3$ to patients with myelodysplastic syndromes because of the ability of the vitamin D metabolite to induce differentiation and to inhibit the clonal proliferation of some human acute myelogenous leukemia cells. Studies also have shown that administration of $1\alpha,25(OH)_2D_3$ significantly prolonged the life of mice injected with the M1 trans-plantable murine leukemia cells (16). We chose to study myelodysplastic patients because the tempo of their disease allows scrutiny of therapeutic maneuvers. Patients with the myelodysplastic syndrome usually have their leukemic clone established; they have ineffective hematopoiesis, almost always with anemia and frequently thrombocytopenia, leukopenia, and often an increased number of marrow blast cells. We administered at least 2 μg of $1,25(OH)_2D_3$ to the patients orally, on a daily basis. Figure 7 summarizes the alteration of their granulocyte, red cell, platelet, blast cell and calcium concentrations during the study. All patients received weekly escalating (0.5 μg) doses of $1,25(OH)_2D_3$ until a daily dose of 2 μg was reached. The median duration of therapy with $1,25(OH)_2D_3$ was 12 weeks (range 4 to > 20). While on therapy, the granulocyte, monocyte, and platelet blood concentrations increased in most patients as compared to their starting values; and as a patient group, each of the peak blood values increased significantly as compared to beginning and ending blood values. In

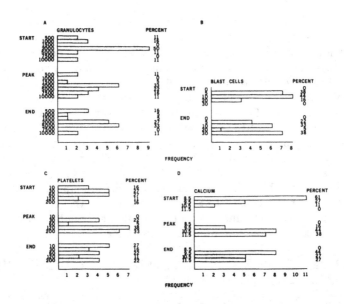

FIGURE 7. Effect of administration of 1,25 dihydroxy-vitamin D_3 on hematopoiesis in myelodysplastic (preleukemia) patients.

Panel A. Effect of $1,25(OH)_2D_3$ on peripheral blood granulocyte concentrations (per microliter of blood).

Panel B. Effect of $1,25(OH)_2D_3$ on percent of bone marrow myeloblasts.

Panel C. Effect of $1,25(OH)_2D_3$ on peripheral blood platelet concentrations (per microliter of blood).

Panel D. Effect of $1,25(OH)_2D_3$ on serum calcium concentrations (mg/dl); normal range of serum calcium is 8.2–10.5 mg/dl.

Start, baseline value; peak, highest value during study; end, value on last day of study.

contrast, the concentration of granulocytes, monocytes, and platelets in the blood was not significantly different between the beginning and the end of the study. The percent of myeloblasts in the marrow rose from a beginning median value of 10% (range, 3% - 20%) to a significantly (P<0.0136) elevated ending median value of 15% (range, 4% - 70%). Seven patients had an improvement of either their absolute granulocyte, monocyte, or platelet blood concentrations for > 4 sequential weeks of treatment. Wilcoxian statistics compared values for the patients at the end of the treatment period with the baseline values, and showed no significant improvement in any of the parameters. Of the 19 patients on the study, 6 of the 19 patients progressed to acute myelogenous leukemia by the end of the study.

The preleukemic patients received at least 2 μg/day of $1,25(OH)_2D_3$. This dose results in serum concentrations of $1,25(OH)_2D_3$ of about 2.0 x 10^{-10}M in normal individuals (17). A concentration of 2 x 10^{-10}M $1,25(OH)_2D_3$ induces maturation of <20% of HL-60 promyelocytes *in vitro* (5, 6, 18, 19). Theoretically, the obtainment of higher serum concentrations of $1,25(OH)_2D_3$ in our preleukemic patients would have been desired. During the study, however, nine of 18 patients became hypercalcemic. Three patients who independently increased their dose of $1,25(OH)_2D_3$ to 4-6 μg/day became symptomatically hypercalcemic. Somewhat higher concentrations of $1,25(OH)_2D_3$ could have been given if the patients had been placed on a low-calcium diet. In the future, vitamin D analogs that induce hematopoietic cell differentiation without inducing hypercalcemia might be medically useful compounds for selected patients with preleukemia and leukemia. Likewise, combinations of inducers of differentiation may be more effective than any one agent. The induction of differentiation of myeloid leukemic cells to functional end cells offers an appealing, but unproven, therapeutic prospect.

Macrophages and the Synthesis of 1,25-Dihydroxyvitamin D₃

Several lines of evidence suggest that cells, other than kidney cells, are capable of synthesis of $1,25(OH)_2D_3$. Normal circulating levels of $1,25(OH)_2D_3$ are in the 30-50 pg per ml range. The serum concentrations markedly decrease in nephrectomized patients; but have been reported to be detectable by several investigators, being in the 5-10 pg per ml concentrations (20). Twenty to 30 percent of patients with sacroidosis have hypercalcemia and elevated serum levels of $1,25(OH)_2D_3$. One study demonstrated increased serum $1,25(OH)_2D_3$ in a nephrectomized patient with sarcoidosis (21). These studies provide support that cells, other than cells from the kidney, can produce $1,25(OH)_2D_3$. Likewise, J. Adams et al reported that pulmonary alveolar macrophages harvested from patients with sarcoidosis are capable of constitutively converting the substrate $[3H]-25(OH)D_3$ to

[3H]-1,25(OH)$_2$D$_3$ (22).

Patients with sarcoidosis have activated T-lymphocytes which secrete large amounts of gamma interferon (Y-IFN). A reasonable hypothesis is that perhaps Y-IFN might stimulate normal human macrophages to produce 1,25(OH)$_2$D$_3$. We found that Y-IFN markedly enhanced the ability of normal human macrophages to synthesize a vitamin D metabolite that migrates on HPLC in exact identity with authentic, chemically synthesized 1,25(OH)$_2$D$_3$ (Figure 8) (23). We rechromatographed the putative 1,25(OH)$_2$D$_3$ using three other HPLC elution systems. In each system the [3H]-metabolite ran in exact identity with 1,25(OH)$_2$D$_3$ (Figure 8).

The 1,25(OH)$_2$D$_3$-like material produced by the macrophages was purified to homogeneity and was identified as 1,25(OH)$_2$D$_3$ by 1.) its characteristic affinity for the chicken intestinal 1,25(OH)$_2$D$_3$ receptor (25); 2.) comparison of its biological activity with that of chemically synthesized 1,25(OH)$_2$D$_3$ in vivo (intestinal calcium absorption and bone calcium mobilization in rachitic chickens) (24); 3.) mass spectroscopy which showed the typical spectral pattern of 1,25(OH)$_2$D$_3$ (25).

The examination of the ability of normal human pulmonary alveolar macrophages to synthesize putative 1,25(OH)$_2$D$_3$ has been examined from more than 20 normal volunteers. Although results varied quantitatively from patient to patient, we found that Y-IFN was able to enhance the synthesis of 1,25(OH)$_2$D$_3$ between 10 and 200 fold as compared to macrophages not exposed to the lymphokine. Dose-response studies showed that the ability of the macrophages to synthesize 1,25(OH)$_2$D$_3$ increased with exposure of the cells to increasing concentrations of Y-IFN with the earliest effects being noted at 200 units per ml Y-IFN (Figure 9). Maximally stimulated macrophages synthesized about 10-50 pmol 1,25(OH)$_2$D$_3$ per 10^6 cells. Time-response studies showed that maximal stimulation occured within 24 hours of exposure of the macrophages to Y-IFN (500 u/ml); stimulation of the macrophages was evident for at least six days (Figure 9). Inactivated Y-IFN did not stimulate macrophages to synthesize 1,25(OH)$_2$D$_3$. These studies suggest that Y-IFN can stimulate synthesis of 1,25(OH)$_2$D$_3$ by macrophages. Further studies by Drs. Reichel, Norman and myself (24)

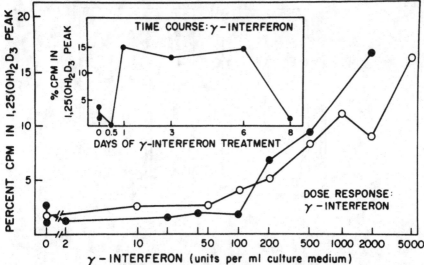

FIGURE 8. Rechromatography of [3H]-1,25(OH)$_2$D$_3$ produced by human pulmonary macrophages treated with recombinant human Y-interferon. Human pulmonary macrophages (1 x 10^6; 1 ml) were cultured with 500 units/ml of Y-interferon for 4 days. Ten hours before harvest, 1 x 10^{-7}M [3H]-25(-OH)D$_3$, 10 Ci/mmol was added to the cells in culture. Both the cells and conditioned media were removed and subjected to lipid extraction. The resulting chloroform layer was chromatographed successively on four HPLC systems with non-radioactive standards including 1,25(OH)$_2$D$_3$. Aliquots of each fraction were taken for liquid scintillation measurements to locate the peak regions of tritium; the peak of putative tritiated 1,25(OH)$_2$D$_3$ was then pooled for rechromatography. Panel A: Radial-Pak Porasil cartridge, eluted at 2 ml/min with a 4-to-60% isopropanol in hexane gradient. Panel B: Porasil column, eluted at 2 ml/min with 10% isopropanol in hexane. Panel C: Zorbax-Sil column, eluted at 1 ml/min with 10% isopropanol in dichloromethane. Panel D: Zorbax-ODS (reverse phase) column, eluted at 1 ml/min with 20% water in methanol.

showed that lipopolysaccharide was also a potent stimulator of the synthesis of 1,25(OH)$_2$D$_3$ by human macrophages.

1,25-Dihyroxyvitamin D₃ and the Immune System

Recent studies showed that low concentrations of

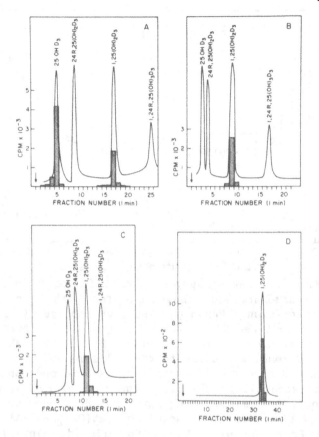

FIGURE 9. Treatment of human pulmonary macrophages with recombinant human Y-interferon: (Panel A): Y-IFN dose-dependent production of $1,25(OH)_2D_3$; (Panel B): Time course of appearance of $1,25(OH)_2D_3$ after treatment with Y-IFN. PAM in culture (1×10^6 cells; 1 ml) were treated with varying amounts of Y-IFN for 4 days (panel A) or with 500 units/ml of Y-IFN for the indicated time which varied between 0.5-8 days (panel B). Eight hours before harvest, $1 \times 10^{-7}M$ $[^3H]$-25(OH)D_3, 5 mCi/mmol, was added to the incubation. Cells and media were separated by centrifugation and either the media(0-0) or media + cells (0-0) were subjected to Bligh and Dyer lipid extraction and high pressure chromatography. Data are expressed as percent of the total recovered tritium comigrating with non-radioactive, chemically synthesized standard $1,25(OH)_2D_3$.

1,25(OH)$_2$D$_3$ can inhibit both the synthesis of interleukin-2 (IL-2) by activated T-lymphocytes (26). Concentrations as low as 10^{-11}M 1,25(OH)$_2$D$_3$ have been reported to have an inhibitory effect on IL-2 synthesis.

We showed that 1,25-dihydroxyvitamin D$_3$ [1,25(OH)$_2$D$_3$] modulated sensitively, rapidly and specifically both the mRNA and protein accumulation of the multilineage growth factor granulocyte-macrophage colony stimulating factor (GM-CSF) and gamma interferon (Y-IFN) in both normal human mitogen-activated T lymphocytes and T lymphocytes from a line (S-LB1) transformed with human T lymphocyte leukemia virus-1 (HTLV-1) (27, 28). Concentrations around 10^{-10}M 1,25(OH)$_2$D$_3$ decreased both mRNA and protein levels for both of these lymphokines about 50% as compared to control cultures not exposed to the sterol. In contrast, a HTLV-1 transformed T lymphocyte cell line (Ab-VDR) established from a patient with vitamin D resistant rickets type II contained undetectable 1,25(OH)$_2$D$_3$ cellular receptors and was resistant to the action of 1,25(OH)$_2$D$_3$. In these cells, concentrations as high as 10^{-8}M had no effect on levels of either GM-CSF or Y-IFN. Further studies showed that inhibition of GM-CSF and Y-IFN gene expression by 1,25(OH)$_2$D$_3$ occurred independently of interleukin-2 regulation and is probably mediated through cellular 1,25(OH)$_2$D$_3$ receptors (28, 29).

These studies provide support for our hypothesis that hypercalcemia present in patients with sarcoidosis may be secondary to stimulation by Y-IFN of 1,25(OH)$_2$D$_3$ synthesis by macrophages (and granulomatous tissue) in these patients. Likewise, our studies are consistent with the hypothesis that macrophages may be a normal physiologic source of 1,25(OH)$_2$D$_3$ causing local bone reabsorption through osteoclasts and enhancing proliferation and differentiation preferentially down the macrophage pathway. Likewise, synthesis of 1,25(OH)$_2$D$_3$ may play a significant role in communication between T-lymphocytes and macrophages.

A hypothesis of the interaction of 1,25(OH)$_2$D$_3$ with the hematopoietic system might be: Macrophages may be moderately activated to synthesize and release interleukin-I (IL-1) after exposure to an antigen. Both IL-1 and antigen-presentation by the macrophages stimulates the T-lymphocytes to produce IL-2 and other lymphokines including Y-IFN. Gamma interferon may enhance the macrophages to produce $1,25(OH)_2D_3$. Locally elevated levels of $1,25(OH)_2D_3$ might produce local bone resorption, preferentially induce differentiation of the myeloid stem cells to macrophages, and possibly augment the function of macrophages, including phagocytosis and killing of microbial organisms. As a negative feedback mechanism, high concentrations of $1,25(OH)_2D_3$ could diminish synthesis of lymphokines by activated T-lymphocytes. This would decrease Y-IFN synthesis which would diminish the activation of the macrophages causing a decrease in production of $1,25(OH)_2D_3$. Therefore, the macrophage and T-lymphocyte might interact through positive and negative feedback loops using $1,25(OH)_2D_3$ and Y-IFN.

REFERENCES

1. Abe, E., Miyaura, C., Sakagami, H., Takeda, M., Konno, K., Yamazaki, T., Yoshiki, S., and Suda, T. (1981) Proc. Natl. Acad. Sci. USA 78, 4990-4994.
2. Tanaka, H., Abe, E., Miyaura, C., Kuribayashi, T., Konno, K., Nishi, Y., and Suda, T.. (1982) Biochem. J. 204, 713-719.
3. Bar-Shavit, Z., Teitelbaum, S.L., Reitsma, P., Hall, A., Pegg, L.E., Trial J., and Kahn, A.J. (1983) Proc. Natl. Acad. Sci. USA 80, 5907-5911.
4. McCarthy, D.M., San Miguel, J.F., Freake, H.C., Green, P.M., Zola, H., Catovsky D., and Goldman, J.M. (1983) Leukemia Res. 7, 51-55.
5. Mangelsdorf, D.J., Koeffler, H.P., Donaldson, C.A., Pike, J.W., and Haussler, M.R. (1984) J. Cell Biology. 98, 391-398.
6. Munker, R., Norman, A., and Koeffler, H.P. (1986) J. Clin. Invest. 78, 1-8.
7. Koeffler, H.P., Amatruda, T., Ikekawa, N., Kobayashi, Y., DeLuca, H.F. (1984) Ca. Res. 44, 5624-5628.
8. Burger, E.H., van der Meer, J.W.M., van de Gevel, J.S., Gribnau, J.C., Thesingh C.W., and van Furth, R. (1982) J. Exp. Med. 156, 1604-1614.
9. Holtrop, M.E., Cox, K.A., Clark, M.B., Holick M.F., and Anast, C.S. (1981) Endocrinology 108, 2293-2301.
10. Mundy, G.R., A.J. Altman, A.J., M.D. Gondek, M.D., and J.G. Bandelin, J.G. (1977) Science 196, 1109-1111.

11. Haussler, M.R., D.J. Baylink, D.J., M.R. Hughes, M.R., P.F. Buembaugh, P.F., J.E. Wegedal, J.E., F.H. Shen, F.H., R.L. Willsen, R.L., S.J. Counts, S.J., K.M. Bursac, K.M., and T.A. McCain, T.A. (1979) Clinical Endocrinology 5, 157S-165S.

12. Norman, A.W. (1979) 402-450.

13. Liberman, U.A., Eil, C., and Marx, S.J. (1983) J. Clin. Invest. 71, 192-200.

14. Rigby, W.F.C., Shen, L., Ball, E.D., Juyre, P.M. and Fanger, M.W. (1984) Blood 64, 1110-1115.

15. Matsui, T., Nakao, Y., and Kobayashi, N. (1984) Int. J. Cancer 33, 193-202.

16. Honma, Y., Hozumi, M., Abe, E., Konno, K., Fukushima, M., Hata, S., Nishii, Y., De Luca, H.F., and Suda, T. (1983) Proc. Natl. Acad. Sci. USA 80, 201-204.

17. Adams, N., Gray, R., and Lemann, J. (1982) Kidney Int. 21, 90-97.

18. Koeffler, H.P. (1983) Blood 62, 709-721.

19. Miyayra C., Abe, E., and Kuribauashi, T. (1981) Biochem. Biophys. Res. Commun. 102, 937-943.

20. Lambert P.W., Stern, P.H., Avioli, R.C., Brackett, N.C., Turner, R.T., Greene, A., Irene, Y.F., and Bell, N.H.. (1982) J. Clin. Invest. 69, 722.

21. Barbour, G.L., Coburn, J.W., Slatopolsky, E., Norman, A.W., and Horst, R.L. (1981) N. Engl. J. Med. 305, 440.

22. Adams, J.S., Sharma, O.P., Gacad, M.A., and Singer, F.R. (1983) J. Clin. Invest. 72. 1856.

23. Koeffler, H.P., Reichel, H., Bishop, J., and Norman, A. (1985) Biochem. Biophys. Res. Comm. 127, 596.

24. Reichel, H., Koeffler, H.P., Bishop, J.E., and Norman, A.W. (1986) J. Clin. Endocrin. & Metab.

25. Reichel, H., Koeffler, H.P., and Norman, A.W. (1986 submitted).

26. Tsoukas, C., Provvedini, D., and Manologos, S. (1984) Science 224, 1438.

27. Tober, A., Norman, A., and Koeffler, H.P. (1986 submitted).

28. Reichel, H., Koeffler, H.P., Tobler, A., Norman, A.W. (1986) Proc. Natl. Acad. Sci. (In press).

RETINOIC ACID-INDUCED DIFFERENTIATION OF HL-60:

STUDIES IN VITRO AND IN VIVO

Theodore R. Breitman

Laboratory of Biological Chemistry

Developmental Therapeutics Program

Division of Cancer Treatment

National Cancer Institute

National Institutes of Health

Bethesda, MD 20892

Recent studies on transformation of cells has been elucidating the regulation and mechanism of cell proliferation and differentiation at the molecular level. Malignant transformation characterized by immortality and indefinite cell proliferation can be considered as a blockade in or a lack of ability to differentiate terminally. In bone marrow, for example, the maintenance of haematopoiesis is obviously based on a balance between self-renewal and differentiation of stem cells. Furthermore, the diversity of more mature haematopoietic cells has to be maintained and controlled properly. Whatever are the primary causes of leukemia (i.e., viruses, oncogenes, chemical carcinogens, etc.), the normal regulation for haematopoietic maintenance is apparently disrupted in leukemia. In this context, an understanding of regulation and mechanism of cell proliferation and differentiation is indispensable for the eluciation of transformation of cells. In recent years, the development of human leukemia cell lines has provided useful models for studying cell proliferation and differentiation and has contributed to our understanding of growth factors, differentiation-inducing agents, intracellular mediators and modulators, and gene regulation. These studies have revealed that some oncogene products are involved in the signal transduction of growth factors, and that intracellular mediators or modulators play very important roles in cell proliferation and differentiation. Therefore, it is likely that some leukemia cells do not differentiate because of alterations of specific genes or their products that are obligatory for differentiation, or because of a disturbed cellular mechanism that is required for a response to exogenous differentiative factors.

In this article, previous work is reviewed and new data is presented on retinoic acid(RA)-induced differentiation of HL-60 and fresh cells from patients with acute promyelocytic leukemia(APL). This induction is modulated by agents increasing the intracellular level of cyclic adenosine 3':5'-monophosphate (cAMP) and/or by T-lymphocyte derived lymphokines named DIA. Clinical trials of retinoids for treatment of malignant diseases including certain types of leukemia, is also reviewed.

An extension of these studies suggest a new approach to the treatment of leukemia based on the principle of promoting leukemic cells to differentiate to a more normal and functional nongrowing cell type.

THE HL-60 CELL LINE

HL-60 was isolated from the blood of a patient with APL. It was the first human cell line with distinct myeloid features to be developed (1). HL-60 cells grow continuously in suspension culture and consist of promyelocytes predominantly. HL-60 is induced to differentiate into cells with morphologic features of mature granulocytes by treatment with a variety of compounds including dimethyl sulfoxide (DMSO), dimethylformamide (DMF), hypoxanthine, actinomycin D, and RA (2,3). Moreover, these induced cells have many functional characteristics of normal human peripheral granulocytes including phagocytosis, lysozomal enzyme release, complement receptors, chemotaxis, hexose monophosphate shunt (HMPS) activity, superoxide anion (O_2^-) generation, and the ability to reduce nitroblue tetrazolium (NBT)(2,4,5). Other compounds, such as 1,25-

dihydroxyvitamin D_3, butyrate, and 12-0-tetradecanoyl-phorbol-13-acetate (TPA), induce HL-60 to differentiate to cells with the features of monocytes/ macrophages such as morphology, adherence, and increases in cellular activities of nonspecific esterase and 5'nucleotidase (9-12, Breitman and Keene,unpublished experiments). Because of these inducible characteristics HL-60 provides a unique and useful model system, for studying mechanism and regulation of growth and differentiation of human myeloid cells in vitro.

INDUCTION OF HL-60 DIFFERENTIATION BY RA

Recently, it was found that all-trans-RA induces granulocytic differentiation of HL-60 (3). These findings were important for subsequent investigations of HL-60 differentiation, because RA induces differentiation of HL-60 at concentrations that are close to the physiological concentration of 30 nM (17) and because, before these findings, terminal differentiation of HL-60 had been known to be induced only either by non-physiological compounds such as DMSO or by physiological compounds such as hypoxanthine at concentrations markedly higher than physiological.

RA induces differentiation of HL-60 in a concentration-dependent, time-dependent process in which there is a sequential appearance of mature granulocytes assessed morphologically and functionally (18,19). RA-induced HL-60 cells undergo morphological changes corresponding to normal granulocytic maturation as well as acquire the capacities of NBT reduction, O_2^- production measured by ferricytochrome c reduction, and an increased activity of HMPS. These induced cells also show positive reactivity for chloroacetate esterase staining.

In the presence of 1 μM RA, the growth rate of HL-60 decreases after two days, and growth ceases by the fourth day (18). These cells no longer proliferate even when resuspended in growth medium without RA, indicating that morphologically and functionally matured HL-60 induced by RA has lost the capacity for further proliferation.

RA-induced morphological differentiation of HL-60 occurs at a much faster rate than does DMSO-induced differentiation even though relatively immature HL-60 cells induced by DMSO show increases in biochemical parameters related to the respiratory burst of mature granulocytes, such as O_2^- production and HMPS activity (19). An analysis of the appearance of biochemical parameters as a function of morphological differentiation indicates that the acquisition of biochemical functions of HL-60 induced by DMSO is associated with less mature cells than those induced by RA. In the development of normal granulocytes, the ability to reduce NBT is at a low level in metamyelocytes and increases in banded and segmented granulocytes (20). Thus, RA-induced differentiation of HL-60 is more similar to the normal pattern than that of DMSO-induced differentiation.

CHEMOTACTIC PEPTIDE RECEPTORS

In normal granulocytes and other phagocytic cells, chemotactic peptides such as N-formyl-methionine-leucine-phenyl-alanine (FMLP) bind to specific receptors on these cells and stimulate the respiratory burst (21-23). In RA-induced HL-60 cells there is no increase of FMLP receptors (24) and various concentrations of FMLP do not stimulate NBT reduction (25). However, in HL-60 induced by DMSO or DMF there is an increased concentration of FMLP receptors and dexamethasone synergistically increases the number of these receptors (24-26).

PRODUCTION OF METABOLITES OF ARACHIDONIC ACID

Metabolites of arachidonic acid, such as prostaglandins (PG), thromboxanes (Tx), and leukotrienes(LT), play important roles as chemical mediators or modulators in a variety of intra- and intercellular biological reactions and responses. We therefore examined, in collaboration with Dr. L. Levine, the capacity of HL-60 induced with RA or DMSO to produce arachidonic acid metabolites when stimulated with the calcium ionophore A23187. Noninduced cells are essentially inactive while RA- and DMSO-induced cells produce each of the metabolites although there is a marked difference in synthesis as a function of A23187 concentration. Maximum production by DMSO-induced cells occurs at 0.3 μM A23187 while maximum production by RA-induced cells does not occur until 10 μM A23187, the highest concentration studied. Calcium uptake studies with uninduced HL-60 cells cells indicate that after 1 hr incubation with concentrations of 0.1 μM, 1 μM, and

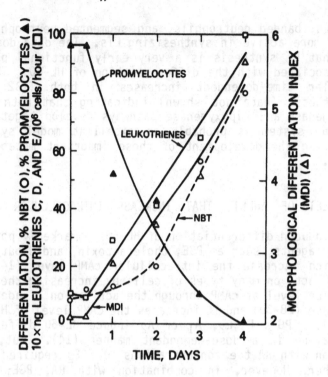

Fig. 1. The capacity of HL-60 to synthesize LT's C_4, D_4, and E_4 as a function of the extent of differentiation induced by 180 mM DMSO. The morphological differentiation index (MDI) was calculated as described in reference 33.

10 μM A23187 there are net increases in intracellular calcium (nmol/10^6 cells) of 0.31, 0.42, and 1.52, respectively (Breitman and Keene, unpublished results). It is possible that RA- and DMSO-induced cells are different from each other and/or from noninduced cells in regards to calcium uptake promoted by A23187.

The very low capacity of noninduced HL-60 to produce arachidonic acid metabolites prompted a study to determine at what stage during differentiation HL-60 cells gain this ability. The results shown in Fig. 1 indicate that this function is gained as the cells mature from promyelocytes to myelocytes and before the more mature function of NBT reduction is expressed. The data do not allow a determination if cells that are more mature than myelocytes (metamyelocytes, banded neutrophils, and segmented neutrophils) are even more active in synthesizing LTs. The data do indicate that LT synthesis is a very early functional parameter associated with the differentiation of HL-60. There are similar time-dependent increases in both TxB2 and PGE$_2$ synthesis (data not shown) indicating that both the cyclooxygenase and lipoxygenase pathways develop together. This HL-60 system is probably an excellent model system for studying the development of these important metabolic pathways.

EFFECTS OF AGENTS THAT INCREASE INTRACELLULAR cAMP

RA-induced differentiation of HL-60 is markedly potentiated by agents, such as PGE, cholera toxin, and dibutyryl cAMP, which increase the intracellular cAMP level (14,18, 27). PGE acts on many types of cells by increasing the intracellular level of cAMP through the activation of adenylate cyclase (28-30) and it increases the cAMP level of HL-60 cells (14). PG's E$_1$,E$_2$, A$_1$ or A$_2$ induce HL-60 differentiation alone in a dose-dependent manner (14). But, in comparison with RA the concentrations of PGE$_2$ required are much higher. However, in combination with RA, PGE$_1$ and PGE$_2$ induce differentiation of HL-60 very effectively in a synergistic, and not in an additive, manner (Fig. 2).

PGE$_2$ is routinely found in human peripheral blood at 1 nM (31) and can increase to 400 nM in localized areas of trauma, inflamation, or infection (32). Therefore, the conditions of the experiments in vitro, i.e., the combination of 10 nM RA and concentrations of 0.1 nM to 100 nM PGE$_2$, are likely to exist in the microenvironment in vivo.

PGF$_1$ and F$_2$, either alone or in combination with RA, are much less active than PGE in inducing HL-60 differentiation (33). These PG's are also much less potent than PGE in increasing the intracellular cAMP level of HL-60 (Breitman and Keene, unpublished experiments). These findings indicate that, for PG's, there is a positive correlation between the extent of the increase in intracellular cAMP and the potentiation of RA-induced differentiation.

Besides PG's, cholera toxin, which also increases intracellular cAMP levels of HL-60 (Breitman and Keene, unpublished experiments), synergistically potentiates RA-

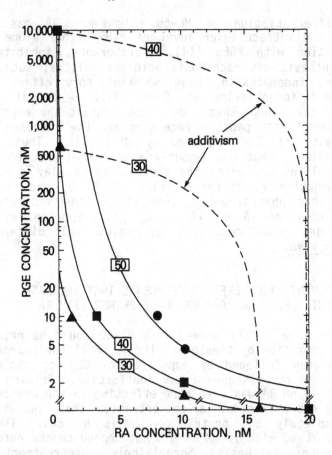

Fig. 2. Isobolograms showing synergy for induction of differentiation of HL-60 by combinations of PGE and RA. The
experimental points are the concentrations of PGE and RA in
combination inducing 30%, 40%, and 50% differentiation as
indicated by the boxed values on each curve. The dashed
lines connecting the values of PGE and RA alone would have
been obtained if the two compounds in combination were additive.

induced differentiation of HL-60 (27). Dibutyryl cAMP,
known to pass through the cell membrane and act like cAMP,
enhances HL-60 differentiation in combination with RA.
These findings suggest that there may be some protein(s)
in HL-60, which are phosphorylated by a cAMP-dependent
protein kinase and which mediate the potentiation of RA-

induced differentiation of HL-60. However, RA has no
effect on the intracellular level of cAMP either alone or
in combination with PGE_2 (14). Furthermore, inhibitors
of the synthesis of arachidonic acid metabolites, such as
aspirin and indomethacin, have no inhibitory effect on
RA-induced differentiation of HL-60 (33). Also, it has
been shown that indomethacin does not inhibit the expression of chemotactic peptide receptors and the increase of
HMPS activity of HL-60 induced by DMSO (34). Thus, it
appears unlikely that endogenously synthesized arachidonic
acid metabolites including the prostaglandins play a role
in the induction of differentiation of HL-60, and it is
suggested that physiological compounds in the microenvironment, including RA and PG's, may play important roles
in the mechanism and regulation of myeloid cell differentiation in vivo.

DIFFERENTIATION EFFECTS OF AGENTS THAT INCREASE
INTRACELLULAR cAMP ON HL-60 PRIMED WITH RA

Olsson et al. (27) showed that HL-60 could be primed
for differentiation by treatment with 10 nM RA for approximately one day followed by exposure to PGE_2 or cholera
toxin. The reverse sequence was ineffective. Priming of
HL-60 with 10 nM RA was even more effective in the presence
of 1 μg/ml cycloheximide, a concentration that inhibited
growth completely and protein synthesis by 86%. Thus,
priming of HL-60 with 10 nM RA did not depend on the normal
rate of protein synthesis. Surprisingly, pretreatment of
HL-60 with cycloheximide alone at 1 μg/ml primed for the
effect of PGE_2 and cholera toxin (27). However, the continuous presence of cycloheximide inhibited RA-induced differentiation of HL-60.

These findings suggest that a decrease in synthesis of
some protein(s) favors RA-induced differentiation. One possibility is that differentiation of HL-60 is inhibited by a
polypeptide, and the inhibition of protein synthesis by cycloheximide could diminish the production of this inhibitor
and facilitate the modulating activities on differentiation
by cAMP-inducing agents. Another possibility is that RA
induces the production of a mRNA whose translation initiates phenotypic changes characteristic of differentiated
cells, and that cycloheximide increases the production

and/or the half-life of this mRNA, as has been reported for human fibroblast interferon mRNA (35).

MONOCYTIC DIFFERENTIATION BY T-LYMPHOCYTE DERIVED LYMPHOKINES (DIA)

It has been reported that the conditioned media of activated peripheral mononuclear cells induce HL-60 to differentiate into cells with morphological and functional characteristics of mature monocytes/macrophages (36-40). Olsson et al. (40) showed that differentiation inducing factor(s) (DIF) released by mitogen-stimulated human blood mononuclear cells are distinct from colony-stimulating-activity (CSA) and that the human T-lymphocyte leukemia cell line HUT 102 is a constitutive producer of this factor(s)(27). This polypeptide has a molecular weight of 46,000 as determined by SDS-PAGE, an isoelectric point of approximately 5.2, and does not adhere to lectin-sepharose (41). We have named the differentiation inducing activity of these conditioned media "DIA" as a general term to refer to an activity that more than one protein may have. DIA purified partially from serum-free conditioned media of HUT 102 was used for the experiments described below.

MONOCYTIC DIFFERENTIATION BY A COMBINATION OF RA AND DIA

DIA alone induces HL-60 differentiation in a dose-dependent manner to a relatively small extent. However, in combination with 10 nM RA, DIA induces HL-60 differentiation to a remarkable extent (41). This combination of RA and DIA is synergistic in a manner similar to the synergy observed with combinations of RA and cAMP-inducing agents. However, DIA has no effect on the intracellular cAMP level (Breitman and Keene, unpublished experiments).

Three biochemical and functional parameters of differentiation; Fc receptors, immunophagocytosis, and NBT reduction, were studied in HL-60 induced by DIA alone and in combination with 10 nM RA (33). DIA alone increases the percentage of Fc receptor-positive cells beyond 80% at day 4, but the extent of the increase of immunophagocytosis and NBT reduction is much less than that of Fc receptors. RA alone (10 nM) has a very small inductive effect on

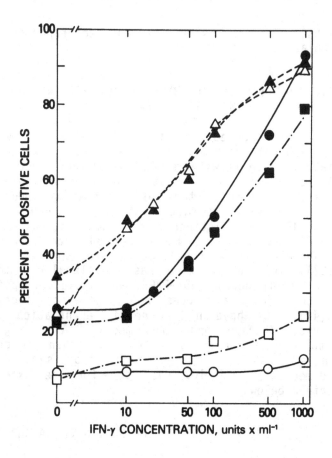

Fig. 3. Increases in biochemical and functional parameters of HL-60 treated with rIFN-γ and RA alone and in combination for 4 days. (△ , ▲), Fc receptors; (▢ , ■), immunophagocytosis; (○ , ●), NBT reduction. Open symbols , with no RA; closed symbols, with 10 nM RA.

these three parameters, whereas 1 μM RA induces approximately 90% cells positive for Fc receptor, immunophagocytosis, and NBT reduction at day 4. However, the combination of DIA and 10 nM RA increases phagocytosis and NBT reduction to a greater extent and at a greater rate than each agent alone. Also, two monocyte/macrophage specific enzymes, 5'-nucleotidase and nonspecific esterase, are increased in a manner similar to the increases in immunophagocytosis and NBT reduction.

Results qualitatively similiar to those described above have been found for combinations of 10 nM RA and recombinant human interferons gamma (rIFN- γ) or alpha (Fig. 3 and 42). Based on several criteria, including experiments with neutralizing antibody, the major DIA of HUT-102 conditioned medium is not IFN.

Recently, we studied the expression of receptors specific for the chemotactic peptide, FMLP, on HL-60 treated with the combination of DIA and 10 nM RA (25). As mentioned in a previous section, HL-60 treated with RA alone does not express FMLP receptors, and NBT reduction of the cells is not stimulated by FMLP. However, HL-60 treated with the combination of DIA and 10 nM RA reduces NBT in response to FMLP in a dose-dependent manner. Also FMLP receptors are detected on these cells and dexamethasone increases both the number of FMLP receptors and the responsiveness to FMLP in cells induced with DIA plus 10 nM RA. Dexamethasone alone has no effect on HL-60 differentiation (10,43). In addition, HL-60 cells induced with DIA plus 10 nM RA also have chemotactic activity in response to FMLP, and dexamethasone increases the chemotactic activity of HL-60 induced with DIA plus 10 nM RA. These findings indicate that the combination of DIA and 10 nM RA can induce HL-60 to differentiate to cells that possess functions and characteristics similar to normal mature monocytes/macrophages, and suggest that steroid hormones may modulate the induction of chemotactic peptide receptors of normal granulocytes and monocytes/macrophages during differentiation in vivo.

ONCOGENE EXPRESSION OF HL-60 INDUCED BY RA

Recent studies have been elucidating the mechanism of cell proliferation promoted by oncogenes. Several oncogene products are related to growth factors or their receptors (44-46). How the expression of oncogenes change during the induction of differentiation by RA and how RA influences gene regulation that may induce differentiation are questions that remain to be fully elucidated. Many studies on nucleic acids synthesis in vitamin A-deficient animals have suggested that vitamin A may be involved in the regulation of RNA (47-49) and DNA synthesis (50). HL-60 cells carry an unrearranged, but highly amplified c-myc oncogene (51,52) and they express RNA trans-

cripts of the myc, abl, and Harvey-ras genes (53). Westin
et al.(53) have reported that the amplified c-myc gene in
HL-60 is expressed at approximately a 10-fold greater level
compared with some other cell lines and is reduced 80-90%
by RA or DMSO during induction of differentiation. It has
recently been reported that 1,25-dihydroxyvitamin D₃ also
suppresses the expression of the c-myc oncogene in HL-60,
and that a marked decrement of the expression of the c-myc
gene preceded the phenotypic changes of the induced cells
(54). The cellular myc oncogene is amplified not only in
many human tumor cell lines and fresh malignant tumors (55,
56) but also in lectin-stimulated normal human lymphocytes
(57), and it appears that an increased level of c-myc expression and transcription is a relevant factor in determining transformation. More recently, it was shown that
the human c-myc protein is predominantly found in the cell
nucleus, suggesting that a DNA binding capability of the
c-myc product may correlate with cell proliferation (58).
Furthermore, the study on the appearance of a new nucleo-
somal protein in HL-60 suggests a rearrangement of chromatin structure during RA-induced differentiation (59).
Even though retinoids modify gene expression critical for
the promotion of differentiation (60), more research is
needed to reveal which genes are controlled by retinoids
and the mechanism for this control.

MECHANISM OF RA-INDUCED DIFFERENTIATION OF HL-60

Cellular retinoic acid-binding protein (CRABP) and
cellular retinolbinding protein (CRBP) have been detected
in the cytosol of many normal tissues, and tumor cells or
cell lines (61). While direct evidence has not been presented, many studies suggest that retinoid-binding proteins
mediate the biological activities of retinoids on growth
and differentiation (62-64). There is a good correlation between the relative biological activity of retinoids
and their relative affinities for retinoid-binding proteins
(61). In HL-60, however, CRABP has not been detected
either by a sucrose density gradient sedimentation assay
(65,66) or by a polyacrylamide gel electrophoresis technique (Jetten and Breitman, unpublished data). These findings indicate that RA-induced differentiation of HL-60
is unlikely to be mediated by retinoid-binding proteins.
Studies of the effect of various retinoids on HL-60
differentiation indicate that the most effective inducers

possess a carboxylic acid function at the C-15 terminal carbon (RA and 13-<u>cis</u>-RA). Substitutions at the C-15 position result in essentially a complete loss of activity (retinal, retinol, retinyl acetate). Even with some alterrations in the ring as in 4-hydroxy- and 4-keto-RA or α-RA the activities of those retinoids having a free carboxyl acid at C-15 retained some activity (18,67). The apparent critical role of the free carboxyl led to an hypothesis that RA is metabolized in a series of reactions analogous to the activation and transport of fatty acids (33). Thus, an acyl-CoA synthetase would catalyze the formation of a thioester bond between the carboxyl group of RA and the thiol group of coenzyme A: RA + ATP + CoA-SH ⟷ retinoyl-CoA + AMP + PPi. In the next reaction an oxygen ester is formed between the high energy retinoyl-CoA and an hydroxyl group of an acceptor: Retinoyl-CoA + R-OH ⟶ Retinoyl-O-R + CoA-SH. It is possible that the acceptor is an hydroxyl group of a macromolecule, e.g., the threonine, serine, or tyrosine moieties of a protein. This ester would be of low energy resulting in essentially a one-way reaction for its formation and the formation of a stable covalent bond.

An extension of this hypothesis is that retinoylation and another modification (phosphorylation, methylation, acetylation, etc.) occurs at the same site. When this other modification dominates, the cell continues to proliferate and does not differentiate. In a transformed or neoplastic cell, the balance is shifted even further in the direction of the other modification. This could be because of an increase in the cell's capacity to carry out the other modification or because the information for this modification, carried by an oncogene or an infective virus, is activated or amplified. Under these conditions, a higher than normal dose of RA may shift the balance back towards an increase in retinoylation, effectively blocking the competing modification, and allowing the cell to differentiate. With some cells, the higher than normal dose of RA may result in a retinoylation that competes with an essential modification, thus leading to cell death. This model, or one similar to it, can explain why treatment of cells with RA has chemoprevention, differentiation-inducing, and cytotoxic activities. More recently, evidence has been presented for a CoA mediated activation of RA (68).

RA-INDUCED DIFFERENTIATION OF APL CELLS IN PRIMARY CULTURE

The experimental findings that RA is a potent inducer of terminal differentiation of HL-60 raised a question of whether RA also promotes differentiation of fresh leukemia cells. In an initial study with fresh cells of 21 patients with various myeloid leukemias only the cells of two APL patients were induced by RA to differentiate (65). Since this initial study, 10 samples of fresh leukemia cells from peripheral blood and/or bone marrow of 6 APL patients were studied (19). The effects of PGE_2, DIA and two other inducers of HL-60 differentiation, DMSO and a vitamin D_3 analog, were also investigated. The cells from all patients differentiated in vitro in response to RA. The cells of two patients showed a very high response even to 10 nM RA. While PGE_2 (10nM) alone had no effect on differentiation, there was a small effect in combination with RA.

In contrast to the results with PGE_2, the combination of RA and DIA was synergistic in inducing differentiation of fresh APL cells. DIA alone had no effect on differentiation. However, the rate and/or extent of differentiation induced with a combination of RA and DIA was markedly greater than that induced with RA alone. Two other inducers of HL-60 differentiation were tested with the cells of one patient. DMSO had no effect even at 180 mM, a concentration that induces 40 % NBT-positivity of HL-60. Ro 22-9343 (24,24-difluro-1,25-dihydroxyvitamin D_3), which is approximately 10-fold more active on a molar basis than 1,25-dihydroxyvitamin D_3 in inducing HL-60 differentiation (Breitman and Keene, unpublished results), had essentially no effect, either alone or in combination with DIA, in inducing differentiation of this patient's cells.

INDUCTION BY RA AND CHEMOTHERAPEUTIC AGENTS

When it seemed possible that RA might have clinical utility, it became of interest to examine in vitro the effects of cell growth-inhibiting chemotherapeutic agents on RA-induced differentiation of HL-60. It was also felt that such studies might yield further insight into the mechanism of RA-induction and, more generally, into myeloid terminal differentiation. RA was tested in combination with two chemotherapeutic agents, hydroxyurea and arabinosylcytosine (ara-C). Both of these agents are known to in-

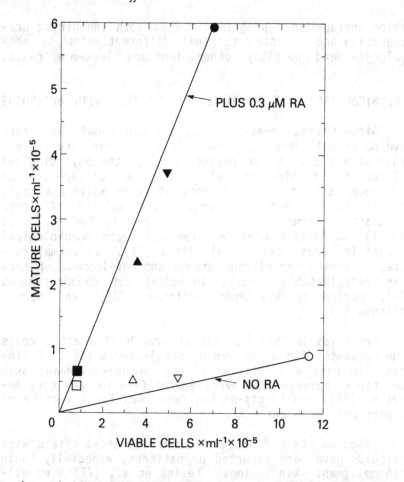

Fig. 4. RA-induced differentiation of HL-60 in the presence of ara-C. Cultures were incubated for 3 days with
(closed symbols) and without (open symbols) 0.3 μ M RA
and the following concentrations of ara-C: none (○ ,
●); 0.1 μ M (▽ , ▼); 0.3 μ M (△ , ▲); 1 μ M (□ ,
■). Mature cells were calculated by the formula: mature
cells/ml = (% NBT-positive cells x viable cells/ml) x
10^{-2}.

hibit cell growth by specifically inhibiting DNA synthesis.
It was found (18) that neither hydroxyurea nor ara-C interferes with the differentiative action of RA and that RA
does not interfere with their growth-inhibitory activity.
Thus, RA and other retinoids can be considered for combi-

nation therapy in a program aimed at both inhibiting proliferation and inducing terminal differentiation of promyelocytic and possibly other immature leukemia cells.

CLINICAL TREATMENT OF MALIGNANT DISEASES WITH RETINOIDS

Since the observations that vitamin A-deficient rats
develop premalignant epidermal lesions that are reversible with repletion of retinoids (69), the physiological
effects of retinoids on cell growth and differentiation
have been studied with a variety of fresh malignant cells
or cell lines. Retinoids reduce the ability of fresh
malignant melanoma cells and cell lines to form colonies
(70,71) and inhibit proliferation and cause morphological
changes in breast cancer cell lines (71). In animal cancers, retinoids inhibit the growth and development of certain transplantable tumors, including rat chondrosarcoma
(72), murine mammary adenocarcinoma (73), and murine
melanoma (74).

Retinoids inhibit the clonal growth of blastic cells
from patients with acute myelocytic leukemia (66). Retinoids also have a beneficial effect on non-malignant skin
conditions characterized by hyperproliferation and keratin-
ization (75), and 13-cis-RA has been used for a variety of
dermatologic problems (76).

Based on these findings, several clinical trials with
retinoids have been reported on patients, especially those
with malignant skin lesions. Levine et al. (77) used all-
trans-RA to treat multiple cutaneous metastasis in two
patients with malignant melanoma. There was a complete regression of the lesions in one case and a partial response
in the other. Kessler et al. (78) showed the clinical
effectiveness of 13-cis-RA in treatment of cutaneous T-cell
lymphoma (Mycosis fungoides). Claudy et al. (79) found
that treatment with an ethyl ester derivative of RA (Ro-
10-9359) improved the nodular lesions in a patient with
cutaneous T-cell lymphoma. Zachariae et al. (80) reported
complete remissions in eight of ten patients (Mycosis
fungoides) treated with the combination of retinoid and a
3-drug chemotherapy, while no response was seen in six
patients concurrently treated without additional retinoid.

In the field of clinical haematology, treatment of

leukemia and myelodysplastic syndrome with retinoids has been on trial. It has been reported that five of 15 evaluable patients with myelodysplastic syndrome showed improvement of pancytopenia and decrease in the marrow blasts after treatment with daily oral 13-cis-RA (81). Recently, a complete remission of a patient with this disease by therapy with RA has been reported (82). Flynn et al. (83) reported a therapeutic trial of 13-cis-RA in a patient with APL whose leukemic cells differentiated in vitro in the presence of 13-cis-RA, suggesting that RA-induced maturation of APL cells similar to that in vitro is also achievable in vivo. As we showed previously, there is a high specificity of a RA effect for APL cells when RA-induced differentiation of fresh leukemia cells is investigated. There are two other more persuasive cases of APL patients responding clinically to RA. In one case the patient responded to a combination of RA and anti-cancer drugs (84) and in the other case, the patient responded to RA alone (85). These reports and findings justify further clinical investigation of retinoids in the treatment of certain types of malignancy.

CONCLUSION

The development of human leukemia cell lines has made it possible to study the regulation and mechanism of cell proliferation and differentiation of specific haematopoietic cell types. RA is a potent inducer of terminal differentiation of the human promyelocytic leukemia cell line, HL-60, and the human monoblast-and monocyte-like cell lines, U-937 and THP-1. RA-induced differentiation of HL-60 is characterized with the morphological changes and functional acquisitions that occur during normal granulocytic maturation in vivo, and the combination of RA and agents that increase intracellular cAMP level (PGE_2 and cholera toxin) is synergistic in inducing granulocytic differentiation of HL-60. Furthermore, HL-60 cells are induced to differentiate to monocyte/macrophage-like cells by the combination of RA and T-lymphocyte derived lymphokines (DIA). While it is unclear what determines granulocytic or monocyte/macrophage differentiation of HL-60, some evidence suggests that different protein kinases are involved in the regulation of each course of differentiation of HL-60. The amplified expression of the c-myc oncogene in HL-60 is reduced by RA, DMSO, or 1,25-dihy-droxyvitamin D_3 during induction of differentiation.

From the evidence that HL-60 lacks cellular RA-binding protein and that the carboxyl group in the terminal carbon of retinoids is critical for biological activity in induc-ing differentiation of HL-60, it is speculated that RA may act after its activation in a reaction with CoA-SH to form retinoyl-CoA, and that an hydroxyl group of a macromolecule is an acceptor for the retinoyl moiety. This retinoylation may be the basis for the chemoprevention, differentiation-inducing, and cytotoxic activities of RA.

RA induces differentiation of fresh cells in primary culture of patients with APL. The combination of RA and DIA is synergistic also in inducing fresh leukemia cells of APL patients as it is in inducing differentiation of HL-60. RA has been on clinical trial in the treatment of certain types of malignancy including APL, suggesting the possibility of a new approach to the treatment of leukemia based on the promotion of differentiation to a more normal and functional nongrowing cell type.

Recent studies on cell transformation have emphasized that the mechanisms of transformation are closely related to that of cell proliferation and differentiation. Thus, we can anticipate that further studies on retinoids may lead to a better understanding of the relationship between cell differentiation and malignancy.

REFERENCES

1. Collins, S. J., Gallo, R. C., and Gallagher, R. E. (1977) Nature 270, 347-349
2. Collins, S. J., Ruscetti, F. W., Gallagher, R. E., and Gallo, R. C. (1978) Proc. Natl. Acad. Sci. U.S.A. 75, 2458-2462
3. Breitman, T. R., Selonick, S. E., and Collins, S. J. (1980) Proc. Natl. Acad. Sci. U.S.A. 77, 2936-2940
4. Collins, S. J., Ruscetti, F. W., Gallagher, R. E., and Gallo, R. C. (1979) J. Exp. Med. 149, 969-974
5. Newburger, P. E., Chovaniec, M. E., Greenberger, J. S., and Cohn, H. J. (1979) J. Cell Biol. 82, 315-322

6. Gallagher, R., Collins, S., Trujillo, J., McCredie, K., Ahearn, M., Tsai, S., Metzgar, R., Aulakh, G., Ting, R., Ruscetti, F., and Gallo, R. (1979) Blood 54, 713-733.

7. Fontana, J. A., Wright, D. G., Schiffman, E., Corcoran, B. A., and Deisseroth, A. B. (1980) Proc. Natl. Acad. Sci. U.S.A. 77, 3664-3688

8. Olsson, I., and Olofsson, T. (1981) Exp. Cell Res. 131, 225-230

9. Rovera, G., Santoli, D., and Damsky C. (1979) Proc. Natl. Acad. Sci. USA; 76, 2779-2783

10. Lotem, J., and Sachs, L. (1979) Proc. Natl. Acad. Sci. U.S.A. 76, 5158-5162

11. Newburger, P. E., Baker, R. D., Hansen, S. L., Duncan, R. A., and Greenberger, J. S. (1981) Cancer Res. 41, 1861-1865

12. McCarthy, D. M., San Miguel, J. F., Freake, H. C., Green, P. M., Zola, H., Catovsky, D., and Goldman, J. M. (1983) Exp. Cell Res. 7, 51-55

13. Breitman, T. R., Collins, S. J., and Keene B.R. (1980) Exp. Cell Res. 126, 494-498

14. Breitman, T. R., and Keene, B. R. (1982) in Growth of Cells in Hormonally Defined Media, (Cold Spring Harbor Conferences on Cell Proliferation, eds) pp. 691-702, Cold Spring Harbor Laboratory, New York

15. Ruscetti, F.W., Collins, S. J., Woods, A. M., and Gallo, R. C. (1981) Blood 58, 285-292

16. Taketazu, F., Kubota, S., Kagigaya, S., Motoyoshi, K., Saito, M., Takaku, F., and Miura Y. (1984) Cancer Res. 44, 531-535

17. Napoli, J. L., Pramanik, B. C., Williams, J. B., Dawson, M. I., and Hobbs, P. D. (1985) J. Lipid Res. 26, 387-392

18. Breitman, T. R. (1982) in Expression of Differentiated Functions in Cancer Cells (Revoltella, R. F., ed) pp. 257-273, Raven Press, New York

19. Hemmi, H., and Breitman, T. R. (1984) in Developments in Cancer Chemotherapy (Glazer, R. I. ed) pp. 247-280, CRC Press, Boca Raton, Florida

20. Zakhireh., B., and Root, R. K. (1979) Blood 54, 429-439

21. DeChatelet, L. R., Shirly, P. S., and Johnston, R. B. Jr. (1976) Blood 47, 545-554

22. Williams, L. T., Synderman, R., Pike, M. C., and Lefkowitz, R. J. (1977) Proc. Natl. Acad. Sci. U.S.A. 74, 1204-1208

23. Lehmeyer, J. E., Synderman, R., and Johnston, R. B. Jr. (1979) Blood 54, 35-45
24. Skubitz, K. M., Zhen, Y., and August, J. T. (1982) Blood 59, 586-593
25. Imaizumi, M., and Breitman, T. R. (1986) Blood 67, 1273-1280
26. Brandt, S. J., Barnes, K. C., Glass, D. B., and Kinkade, J. M. Jr. (1981) Cancer Res. 41, 4947-4951
27. Olsson, I. L., Breitman, T. R., and Gallo, R. C. (1982) Cancer Res. 42, 3928-3933
28. Gilman, A. G, and Nirenberg, M. (1971) Nature 234, 356-358
29. Kuehl, F. A. Jr, and Humes, J. L. (1972) Proc. Natl. Acad. Sci. U.S.A. 69, 480-484
30. Hittelman, K. J., and Butcher, R. W. (1973) in The Prostaglandins (Cuthbert, M. F., ed) pp. 151-165, J. B. Lippincott, Philadelphia
31. Jaffe, B. M., Behrman, H. R., and Parker, C. W. (1973) J. Clin. Invest. 52, 398-405
32. Berenbaum, M. C., Cope, W. A., and Bundick, R. V. (1976) Clin. Exp. Immunol. 26, 534-541.
33. Breitman, T. R., Keene, B. R., and Hemmi, H. (1983) Cancer Surveys 2, 263-291
34. Boser, R. W., Siegel, M. I., McConnell, R. T., and Cuatrecasas, P. (1981) Biochem. Biophys. Res. Comm. 98, 614-620
35. Cavalieri, R. L., Havell, E. A., Vilcek, J., and Pestka, S. (1977) Proc. Natl. Acad. Sci. U.S.A. 74, 4415-4419
36. Leung, K., and Chiao, J. W. (1985) Proc. Natl. Acad. Sci. U.S.A. 82, 1209-1213
37. Elias, L., Wogenrich, F. J., Wallace, J. M., and Longmire, J. (1980) Leukemia Res. 4, 301-307
38. Chiao, J. W., Freitag, W. F., Steinmetz, J. C., and Andreef, M. (1981) Leukemia Res. 5, 477-489
39. Todd, R. F. III, Griffin, J. D., Ritz, J., Nadler, L. M., Abrams. T., and Schlossman, S. F. (1981) Leukemia Res. 5, 491-495
40. Olsson, I., Olofsson, T., and Mauritzon, N. (1981) J. Natl. Cancer Inst. 67, 1225-1230
41. Olsson, I. L., Sarngadharan, M. G., Breitman, T. R., and Gallo, R. C. (1984) Blood 63, 510-517
42. Hemmi, H., and Breitman, T. R. (1987) Blood, in press
43. Collins, S. J., Bodner, A., Ting, R., and Gallo, R. C. (1980) Int. J. Cancer 25, 213-218

44. Waterfield, M. D., Scrace, G. T., Whittle, N., Stroobant, P., Johnsson, A., Wasteson, A., Westermark, B., Heldin, C., San Huang, J. S., and Deuel, T. F. (1983) Nature 304, 35-39
45. Downward, J., Yarden, Y., Mayes, E., Scrace, G., Totty, N., Stockwell, P, Ullrich A, Schlessinger J, and Waterfield, M. D. (1984) Nature 307, 521-527
46. Finkel, T., and Cooper, G. M. (1984) Cell 136, 1115-1121
47. Kaufman, D. G., Baker, M. S., Smith, J. M., Henderson, W. R., Harris, C. C., Sporn, M. B., and Saffiotti, U. (1972) Science 177, 1105-1108
48. Johnson, B. C., Kennedy, M., and Chiba, N. (1969) Am. J. Clin. Nutr. 22, 1048-1058
49. Zile, M., and DeLuca, H. F. (1970) Arch. Biochem. Biophys. 140, 210-214
50. Sherman, B. S. (1961) J. Invest. Dermatol. 37, 469-480
51. Collins, S., and Groudine, M. (1982) Nature 298, 679-681
52. Dalla-Favera RD, Wong-Staal F, and Gallo RC. (1982) Nature 299, 61-63
53. Westin, E. H., Wong-Staal, F., Gelmann, EP., Dalla-Favera, R. D., Papas, T. S., Lautenberger, J. A., Eva, A., Reddy, E. P., Tronick, S. R., Aaronson, S. A., and Gallo, R. C. (1982) Proc. Natl. Acad. Sci. U.S.A. 79, 2490-2494
54. Reitsma, P. H., Rothberg, P. G., Astrin, S. M., Trial, J., Bar-Shavit, Z., Hall, A., Teitelbaum, S. L., and Kahn, A. J. (1983) Nature 306, 492-494
55. Eva, A., Robbins, K. C., Anderson, P. R., Srinivasan, A., Tronick, S. R., Reddy, E. P., Ellmore, N. W., Galen, A. T., Lautenberger, J. A., Papas, T. S., Westin, E. H., Wong-Staal, F., Gallo, R. C., and Aaronson, S. A. (1982) Nature 295, 116-119
56. Slamon, D. J., deKernion, J. B., Verma, I. M., and Cline, M. J. (1984) Science 224, 256-262
57. Giallongo, A., Appella, E., Ricciardi, R., Rovera, G., and Croce, C. M. (1983) Science 222, 430-432
58. Persson, H., and Leder, P. (1984) Science 225, 718-721
59. Chou, R. H., Chervenick, P. A., and Barch, D. R. (1984) Science 223, 1420-1423
60. Sporn, M. B., and Roberts, A. B. (1983) Cancer Res. 43, 3034-3040
61. Lotan, R. (1980) Biochem. Biophys. Acta 605, 33-91

62. Jetten, A. M., and Jetten, M. E. R. (1979) Nature 278, 180-182
63. Sato, M., Hiragun, A., and Mitsui, H. (1980) Biochem. Biophys. Res. Comm. 95, 1839-1845
64. Takase, S., Ong, D. E., and Chytil, F. (1979) Proc. Natl. Acad. Sci. U.S.A. 76, 2204-2208
65. Breitman, T.R., Collins, S. J., and Keene, B. R. (1981) Blood 57, 1000-1004
66. Douer, D., and Koeffler, H. P. (1982) J. Clin. Invest. 69, 277-83
67. Hemmi, H., and Breitman, T. R. (1985) in Retinoids: New Trends in Research and Therapy (Saurat, J. H. ed) pp. 48-54, Karger, Basel
68. Miller, D. A., and DeLuca, H. F. (1985) Proc. Natl. Acad. Sci. U.S.A. 82, 6419-6422
69. Wolbach, S. B., and Howe, P. R. (1925) J. Exp. Med. 42, 753-777
70. Meyskens, F. L. Jr, and Salmon, S. E. (1979) Cancer Res. 39, 4055-4057
71. Lotan R. (1979) Cancer Res. 39, 1014-1019
72. Trown, P. B., Buck, M. J., and Hansen, R. (1976) Cancer Treat. Rep. 60, 1647-1653
73. Ruttura, G., Schittica, M., Hardy, M., Levenson, S.M., Demetriou, A., and Siefter, E. (1975) J. Natl. Cancer Inst. 54, 1489-1491
74. Flix, E. L., Lloyd, B., and Cohen, M.H. (1975) Science 189, 886-888
75. Lauharanta, J. (1980) Ann. Clin. Res. 12, 123-130
76. Peck, G. L., Olsen, T. G., Yorder, F. W., Strauss, J. S., Downing, D. T., Pandya, M., Butkus, D., and Arnaud-Battandier, J. (1979) N. Eng. J. Med. 300, 329-333
77. Levine, N., and Meyskens, F. L. (1980) Lancet, August 2, 224-226
78. Kessler, J. F., Metskens, F. L. Jr, Levine, N., and Lynch, P. J. (1983) Lancet, June 2, 1345-1347
79. Claudy, A., Delomier, Y., and Hermier, C. (1982) Arch. Dermatol. Res. 273, 37-42
80. Zachariae, H., Grunnet, E., Thestrup-Pedersen, K., Molin, L., Schmidt, H., Starfelt, F., and Thomsen, K. (1982) Acta Dermatovenereoloica 62, 162-164
81. Gold, E. J., Mertelsmann, R. H., Itri, L. M., Gee, T., Arlin, Z., Kempin, S., Clarkson, B., and Moore, M. A. S. (1983) Cancer Treat. Rep. 67, 981-986
82. Abrahm, J., Besa, E. C., Hyzinski, M., Finan, J., and Nowell, P. (1986) Blood 67, 1323-1327

83. Flynn, P. J., Miller, W. J., Weisdorf, D. J., Arthur,
    D. C., Brunning, R., and Brande, R. F. (1983) Blood
    62, 1211-1217
84. Nilsson, B. (1984) Br. J. Haematology 57, 365-371
85. Daenen, S., Vellenga. E., van Dobbenburgh, O. A., and
    Halie, M. R. (1986) Blood 67, 559-561

PLASMA MEMBRANE SIGNALS LINKED TO THE RETINOIC ACID-INDUCED DIFFERENTIATION OF HL-60 CELLS

J.P. ABITA, A. LADOUX, B. GENY, A. FAILLE, O. POIRIER, I. KRAWICE
U 204 INSERM Hôpital Saint Louis

75010 PARIS FRANCE

The HL-60 cell line of human acute promyelocytic leukemia origin, is composed of cells which express phenotypic characteristics of promyelocytes (1). It can be induced to differentiate into cells which have acquired many morphological, cytochemical and functional properties of mature granulocytes when cultured in the presence of retinoic acid (RA) (2).

The mechanisms by which RA induces these changes are not known. However, evidence exists which suggests that it might act through a signal (or signals) elicited at the level of the plasma membrane (3). We have already shown that RA increases the activity of the plasma membrane enzymes Na^+-K^+-ATPase (4) and adenylate cyclase (5) while decreasing the capacity of the latter enzyme to be stimulated by agents such as histamine (6).

In the present study we report that RA triggers an early increase in the intracellular concentrations of Na^+ and K^+ and in the intracellular pH (pHi). This latter event being due to the activation of a Na^+/H^+ exchange system. Moreover, RA changes the pattern of phosphoproteins in HL-60 cells.

MATERIAL AND METHODS

HL-60 cells were grown in RPMI 1640 medium supplemented with 15 % heat inactivated fetal bovine serum, glutamine and antibiotics. Differentiation was induced by addition of 1 µM all-trans-retinoic acid and was assessed by the changes

183

in morphology, estimated after May-Grunwald-Giemsa staining, and by the NBT reduction test. Cell viability, measured by trypan blue exclusion, was never less than 85 %.

The activity of the Na^+-K^+-ATPase was measured as the ouabain-inhibitable $^{86}RB^+$ (a K^+ tracer) uptake according to (4). For the determination of the intracellular Na^+ and K^+ content cells were incubated with either $^{22}Na^+$ or $^{86}Rb^+$ for 1 h at 37°. 0.2 ml aliquots were then taken, diluted in 1 ml ice-cold medium, and centrifuged through an oil phase composed of a mixture of 70 % dibutylphtalate and 30 % dinonylphtalate (density = 1.018) as described (4). For $^{22}Na^+$ counts, the cell lysate was homogenized in 10 ml of Instagel and for $^{86}Rb^+$ counts in 4 ml of distilled water.

pHi measurements, using the distribution of ^{14}C-benzoic acid or the fluorescent probe bis (carboxyéthyl)-5(6)carboxy-fluorescein (BCECF), and $^{22}Na^+$ uptake were performed as already described (7).

RESULTS

The activity of the Na^+-K^+-ATPase was measured by the difference between $^{86}Rb^+$ uptake with and without $10^{-3}M$ ouabain. Under physiological conditions, the activity of the sodium pump was found to be 1.05 fmoles K^+/cell/min in control HL-60 cells. As shown in Fig.1, RA induced a stimulation of the pump which reached a maximum (170 % of the initial value) after 7-8 hours. The pump activity returned to normal at about 12 hours. During this period the number of Na^+K^+-ATPase molecules, measured by the specific binding of ^3H-ouabaine, remained constant (4). Fig. 1 shows also that following RA addition to HL-60 cells, there was a transient increase in the intracellular concentrations of Na^+ and K^+. The maximum in $(K^+)i$ coincided with the maximum observed in the sodium pump activity whereas the maximum in $(Na^+)i$ preceded it.

Ouabain, the specific inhibitor of the Na^+-K^+-ATPase was found to be without effect on the differentiation of HL-60 cells at concentrations below $5. 10^{-8}M$ and cytotoxic at higher concentrations. When ouabain was added, at $2.5 .10^{-8}M$, 16 hours before addition of $10^{-7}M$ RA (a concentration which by itself induces the differentiation of 30-40 % of the cells in 4 days) there was an acceleration and a potentialyzation of the effect of RA (Fig.2). We have verified that not only the percentage but also the absolute number of NBT positive cells increased concomittently. On days 3 and

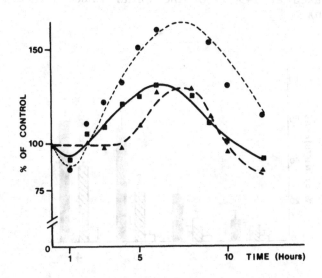

Figure 1

Intracellular Na^+K^+ contents in HL-60 cells during the first 12 hours after addition of 10^{-6}M retinoic acid. Measurements were made as described in Material and Methods using 20 μCi/ml of $^{22}Na^+$ and 3 μCi/ml of $^{86}Rb^+$ for $[Na^+]_i$ (▪) and $[K^+]_i$ (▲) determinations respectively. Results are expressed in percentages of each time value without drug and are the means of 3 different experiments made in triplicate.

The ouabain sensitive K^+ uptake (●) during the same period is also reported.

4 700,000 and 800,000 cells were NBT + in the presence of the combination of ouabain and RA, as compared to 250,000 and 500,000 with RA alone. Under these conditions, there was an early increase in the activity of the sodium pump which peaked at 145 % of the initial value after 3 hours (not shown).

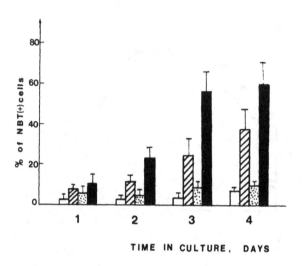

Figure 2

Percentage of NBT + cells for 4 days in the presence of drugs.

HL-60 cells were cultured as described in Material and Methods. Every day, aliquots were counted and examined for their ability to reduce NBT.

The percentage of cells reducing NBT were calculated for control cells (open columns) ; cells cultured with 10^{-7}M RA (cross-hetched columns) ; cells cultured with 2.5 X 10^{-8}M ouabain (dotted columns) ; and cells cultured with 2.5 X 10^{-8}M ouabain and 16 hours later 10^{-7} RA was added (dark columns).

Columns and bars represent the means $\pm$ S.D. of 4 different experiments made in triplicate.

The pHi value of undifferentiated HL-60 cells was 7.00 $\pm$ 0.03 as measured by the distribution of ^{14}C-benzoic acid and 7.04 $\pm$ 0.07 as measured by the fluorescence of BCECF. RA-differentiated HL-60 cells have a pHi of 7.37 $\pm$ 0.02 and 7.37 $\pm$ 0.1 when measured by both techniques. The time-course of the pHi change is presented in Fig. 3. No significant change could be observed during the first 3 hours of exposure to RA (inset). pHi values then rose to reach a maximum after 4 days of treatment with RA. Fig. 3 shows that the increase in pHi preceded the ability of the cells to reduce NBT. Fig. 4 shows that the dose-response curve for the effect of R A on pHi was similar to the dose-response curve for RA-induced differentiation of HL-60 cells.

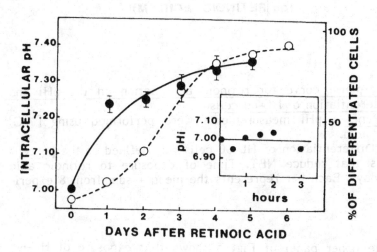

Figure 3
The time course of pHi changes during the differentiation of HL-60 cells
Main Panel : pHi measurements were performed using [^{14}C] benzoic acid (●). Differentiation of the cells into granulocytes was measured as the percent of cells reducing NBT (O). Retinoic acid was used at 1 µM. Each bar represents the mean $\pm$ sdm from 9-13 experiments.
Inset : pHi measurements of HL-60 cells during the first 3 hours following the addition of 1 µM retinoic acid.

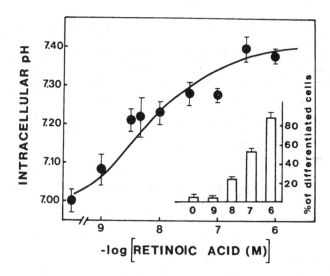

Figure 4
Dose response curve for retinoic acid action on the pHi and the differentiation of HL-60 cells
Main Panel : pHi measurements were performed using [^{14}C] benzoic acid.
Inset : Differentiation of HL-60 cells was defined as the percent of cells that reduce NBT. Time of exposure to retinoic acid was 5 days. Each bar represents the mean ± sdm from 8 experiments.

The upper panel of Fig. 5 shows that exposure of HL-60 cells to a Na^+ and bicarbonate-free, 5 mM K^+ medium, supplemented with 1 μM nigericin produced a rapid intracellular acidification from pHi = 6.95 to pHi = 6.3. After quenching of nigericin with BSA, the addition of 100 mM Na^+ to the external medium promoted the recovery of the pHi to its initial value. The lower panel shows that addition of ethylisopropoylamiloride (EIPA) to acidified cells prevented the pHi recovery induced by Na^+ readdition. EIPA is a potent and specific inhibitor of the Na^+/H^+ exchange system (9,10). Thus this simple experiment identified this exchange system as the major mechanism regulating pHi in HL-60 cells. When the same experiments were performed with fully differentiated

HL-60 cells (Fig. 6) it appeared that, in these cells, the Na^+/H^+ exchange system proceeded at a much faster rate than in control cells (Fig. 5).

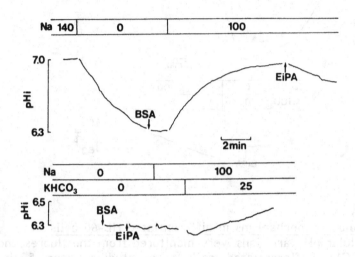

Figure 5
pHi regulating mechanisms in undifferentiated HL-60 cells
Intracellular pH variations were monitored from the fluorescence of BCECF.
Upper panel : Undifferentiated HL-60 cells were first incubated in a Na^+ free, 5 mM K^+ medium supplemented with 1 µM nigericin. After stabilization of the fluorescence, 5 mg.ml BSA was added to quench nigericin. The external solution was then made 100 mM Na^+ by the addition of a small volume of 4 M NaCl. After recovery of the pHi, 100 µM EIPA was added to the cells.
Lower panel : HL-60 cells, equilibrated in a Na^+ and bicarbonate free, 5 mM K^+ medium supplemented with nigericin, were added to the spectrometer's cuvette. BSA (5 mg/ml), EIPA (100 µM), NaCl (100 mM) and $KHCO_3$ (25 mM) were then added sequentially.

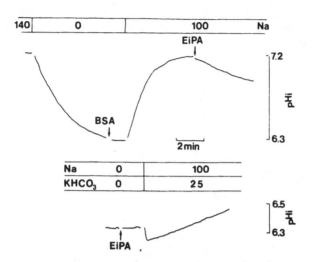

Figure 6

pHi regulating mechanisms in differentiated HL-60 cells

Intracellular pH variations were monitored from the fluorescence of BCECF. Differentiated cells were studied after 5 days of treatment with 1 µM retinoic acid.

Upper panel : Same experiment as in upper panel of Figure 5 using differentiated HL-60 cells.

Lower panel : Differentiated cells were acidified to pHi = 6.35 as described above and then sequentially treated with BSA (5 mg/ml) and EIPA (100 µM). The external solution was then made 100 mM NaCl and 25 mM $KHCO_3$.

Two-dimensional gel pattern of phosphoproteins revealed about 50 spots in undifferentiated HL-60 cells, from which 18 were highly reproducible on 4 successive experiments. RA-differentiated HL-60 cells possessed a different pattern of phosphoproteins characterized by a decrease of the overall phosphorylation, the decreased labeling or even extinction of the spots corresponding to pp2, pp3, pp8 (42 kDa), pp9 and 11 (33 to 25 kDa), pp12 (25 kDa), pp13 (21 kDa), pp14 and pp 18 (100 kDa), the appearance of a new heavily labeled protein pp22 (48 to 50 kDa) in the acid region of the gel. A clone of HL-60 cells resistant to RA-induced differentiation (11) presented a pattern of phosphoproteins very similar to that found in undifferentiated HL-60 cells, in particular pp8 and pp14 were still present whereas pp22 was absent. Though this resistant clone had been cultured continuously in the presence of 1 μM RA, indicating that the changes were a reflection of the differentiation process and not a side effect of RA.

DISCUSSION

All-trans-retinoic acid is one of the most powerful inducer of the granulocytic differentiation of HL-60 cells. However, the mode of action for eliciting the expression of the genes which control the differentiation process is still not known. Especially because in HL-60 cells a cellular binding protein (CRABP), which has been shown to carry RA to the cell nucleus in some systems (12), is apparently absent (13,14). Some results have suggested that the cellular signal initiating RA-induced HL-60 differentiation might originate at the plasma membrane (3). On the other hand, specific receptors for RA have been detected in brain membranes (15). Consistent with this hypothesis, the results presented in this study indicate that RA activates sequentially three systems located in the plasma membrane of HL-60 cells. The stimulation of a Na^+ transport system leads to an increase in the intracellular concentration of Na^+ and to the activation of the Na^+-K^+-ATPase which, in turn, increases the intracellular concentration of K^+. Concomitantly, RA stimulates the activity of the Na^+/H^+ exchange system leading to an alkalinization of the intracellular pH. On the other hand, we have previously, shown that RA-differentiated HL-60 cells, synthesized and accumulated less cyclic AMP than undifferentiated cells (6). Accordingly we show here that RA-induced differentiation of HL-60 cells is accompanied by a decrease of the overall protein phosphorylation.

Our experiments have shown that the major mechanism by which HL-60 cells are able to recover from a cellular acidosis is the Na^+/H^+ exchanger. This system is present in most, if not all, animal cells including rat and human lympho-cytes (16) and neutrophils (17,18). Its activity, measured both by the rate of $^{22}Na^+$ uptake and H^+ efflux, was increased two fold in RA-differentiated HL-60 cells. Considering that a steady state value of the pHi is attained when the rate of acide loading of the cells (via metabolic activity and the influx of protons) is balanced by the rate of acid extrusion (19), it was not surprising that increasing the activity of the Na^+/H^+ exchange system two fold produced an increase in pHi of the differentiated cells. We have recently determined the kinetics and pharmacological properties of the Na^+/H^+ exchange system of HL-60 cells (7) and found that it differs from that of other cell types in its weak affinities for Na^+ and Li^+. Previous studies have shown that this system is very sensitive to a variety of stimuly. Mitogens or phorbol esters elicit activations that are observed within seconds to minutes (20,21), whereas others such as metabolic acidosis (22), glucocorticoids (23) or thyroxine (24) induce responses that take hours or days to develop. Our results indicate that RA-induced activation of the Na^+/H^+ exchanger in HL-60 cells belongs to the category of slow responses. One question is whether the early events that we have described in this report are causally linked to the differentiation of HL-60 cells. The following arguments favor this hypothesis : 1) the stimulation of the Na^+-K^+-ATPase and of the Na^+/H^+ exchanger are also detected when HL-60 cells are treated with DMSO (4,7), whereas Etretinate, a synthetic retinoid with no differentiating activity (25), has no effect ; 2) an earlier stimulation of the sodium pump, by ouabain pretreatment of HL-60 cells, accelerates and potentiates RA -induced differentiation ; 3) the dose-response curves for RA-induced differentiation and pHi increase are observed in the same concentration range ; 4) these events precede the appearance of the differentiated phenotype.

The RA-induced differentiation of HL-60 cells is also accompanied by specific changes in the pattern of phosphoproteins characterized by : a) a decrease of the overall phosphorylation ; b) the disappearance of pp14 (17 kDa) ; c) the appearance of a new spot, pp22 of 48-50 kDa. It is highly probable that the decrease in overall phosphorylation is the result of the decreased intracellular concentration of cAMP (6) since treatment of RA-differentiated cells with histamine restores the phosphorylation of most of these proteins (31). pp14 is of particular interest in many respects : a) it disappears in HL-60 cells differentiated into granulocytes but remains present in cells differentiated to monocytes (26) ; b) its phosphorylation is enhanced when undifferentiated HL-60 cells are treated by either a short pulse of phorbol myristate acetate (PMA), which stimulates c-kinase (27,28), or by histamine, which increases the intracellular level of cAMP (29) ; c) it is present in a number of other cellular systems where its phosphorylation seems to be associated with growth arrest (30). However our data indicate that, in HL-60 cells, its phosphorylation state is rather linked to the differentiation pathway (26). The appearance of pp22 seems to be specific to the granulocytic phenotype since it was also detected in DMSO-differentiated HL-60 cells, but not in monocytic-differentiated cells (26) or in RA-resistant cells.

Taken together, the data presented in this and other studies (4,6,7,29) indicate that RA initiates, in HL-60 cells, a series of signals at the plasma membrane which seem to be causally related to the differentiation process. It remains to be seen how these signals are translated into the control of gene expression.

REFERENCES

1. Gallagher, R.E., Collins, S.J., Trujillo, J., Mc Credie, K., Tsai, M.S., Metzgar, R., Aulakh, G., Ting, R., Ruschetti, P. and Gallo, R.C. (1979) Blood **54**, 713-733.
2. Breitman, T.R., Selonick, S.E. and Collins, S.J. (1980) Proc. Natl. Acad. Sci. USA **77**, 2936-2940.
3. Yen, A., Reece, S.L. and Albricht, K.L. (1984) Exp. Cell Res. **152**, 493-499.
4. Ladoux, A., Geny, B., Marrec, N. and Abita, J.P. (1984) FEBS Letters **176**, 467-472.
5. Thomas, G., Chomienne, C., Balitrand, N., Schaison, G., Abita, J.P. and Baulieu, E.E. (1986) Anticancer Res. **6**, 857-860.
6. Abita, J.P., Gespach, C., Cost, H., Poirier, O. and Saal, F. (1982) IRCS Medical Science **10**, 882-883.
7. Ladoux, A., Cragoe Jr, E.J., Geny, B., Abita, J.P. and Frelin, C. (1987) J. Biol. Chem. in press.
8. Charron, D.J. and Mc Devitt, H.O. (1980) J. Exp. Med. **152**, 18s-36s.
9. Vigne, P., Frelin, C., Cragoe Jr, E.J. and Lazdunski, M. (1983) Biochem. Biophys. Res. Commun. **116**, 86-90.
10. Vigne, P., Frelin, C., Cragoe Jr, E.J. and Lazdunski, M. (1984) Mol. Pharmacol. **25**, 131-136.
11. Gallagher, R.E., Bilello, P.A., Ferrari, A.C., Chang, C.S., Chin-Yen, R.W., Nickols, W. and Muly, E.C. (1985) Leukemia Res. **9**, 967-986.
12. Chytil, F. and Ong, D.E. (1983) Adv. Nutr. Res. **5**, 13-29.
13. Breitman, T.R., Keene, B.R. and Hemmi, H. (1983) Cancer Surveys **2**, 263-291.
14. Douer, D. and Koeffler, H.P. (1982) J. Clin. Invest. **69**, 277-283.

15. Cope, F.O. and Boutwell, R.K. (1985) in "Retinoids" New trends in Research Therapy. (A. Saurat Ed.) pp 106-124, Karger, Basel.
16. Grinstein, S., Cohen, S., Lederman, H.M. and Gelfand, E.W. (1984) J. Cell Physiol. **121**, 87-95.
17. Grinstein, S., Furuya, W. and Biggar, W.D. (1986) J. Biol. Chem. **261**, 512-514.
18. Simchowitz, L. and Roos, A. (1985) J. Gen. Physiol. **85**, 443-470.
19. Roos, A. and Boron, W.F. (1981) Physiol. Rev. **61**, 296-434.
20. Frelin, C., Vigne, P. and Lazdunski, M. (1985) in Hormones and Cell Regulation (J.E. Dumont, B. Hamprecht and J. Nunez Ed.) Vol. **9**, 254-268.
21. Grinstein, S. and Rothstein, A. (1986) J. Memb. Biol. **90**, 1-12.
22. Kinsella, J.R., Cujdik, T. and Sacktor, B. (1984) J. Biol. Chem. **259**, 13224-13227.
23. Kinsella, J.R., Freiberg, J.M. and Sacktor, B. (1985) Am. J. Physiol. **248**, F233-F239.
24. Kinsella, J.R. and Sacktor, B. (1985) Proc. Natl. Acad. Sci. USA **82**, 3606-3610.
25. Chomienne, C., Balitrand, N. and Abita, J.P. (1986) Leukemia Res. **10**, 1079-1081.
26. Faille, A., Poirier, O., Turmel, P., Charron D., and Abita J.P. (1986) Anticancer Res. in press.
27. Castagna, M., Takai, Y., Kaibuchi, K., Sano, K., Kikhawa, U. and Nishizuka, Y. (1982) J. Biol. Chem. **257**, 7847-7851.
28. Niedel, J.E., Kuhn, L. and Vanderbark, G.R. (1983) Proc. Natl. Acad. Sci. USA **80**, 36-40.
29. Gespach, C., Saal, F., Cost, H. and Abita J.P. (1982) Mol. Pharmacol. **22**, 547-563.
30. Feuerstein, N., Sahai, A., Anderson, W.B., Salomon, D.S. and Cooper, H.L. (1984) Cancer Res. **44**, 5227-5233.

DOES INDUCTION OF DIFFERENTIATION HAVE A ROLE IN THE MAINTENANCE OF REMISSION IN ACUTE MYELOGENOUS LEUKEMIA IN CHILDREN?

Sverre O. Lie

Pediatric Research Institute

Rikshospitalet, 0027 Oslo 1, Norway

Acute myelogenous leukemia (AML) in children is considerably more resistant to chemotherapy than acute lymphoblastic leukemia where the progress is well known and well documented (1,2). In recent years, however, more aggressive chemotherapy has resulted in an increasing proportion of children who obtain a complete remission. With intensive consolidation therapy, the proportion of children remaining in complete remission is also increasing, but long-term survival figures of more than 40% has not been reported (3-5).

In a single institution study, we have obtained a high proportion of long-term relapse-free survivors in children using conventional induction therapy, but with high-dose cytosine arabinoside (Ara-C) as consolidation (6,7). In addition, we have used high-dose retinoids as maintenance. This paper describes our observations both on the effect and toxicity of the chemotherapeutic program and on the possible effects and toxicities of high-dose retinyl palmitate given to children with AML in first remission.

195

Patient material and methods

Nineteen consecutive children with AML below 15 years of age were enrolled in the study. Patient details and characteristics are depicted in table 1. Age at diagnoses varied from 3 months to 13 years and the patients were classified according to conventional FAB-morphology, histochemistry and monoclonal anti-bodies.

Therapy was initiated with Ara-C i.v. and 6-thioguanine (6TG) p.o. in a dose of 100 mg pr square meter q 12 hours days 1,2,3 and 4 followed by adriamycin, 75 mg per square meter given as the DNA complex (8,9), on day 5. This induction course was repeated 3 times. Consolidation was given as high dose Ara-C 2 g per square meter q 12 hours for 3 days repeated 4 times at approximately monthly intervals.

Retinyl palmitate in arachidonic oil was given in a dose of 50.000 IU per square meter p.o. daily once remission was achieved. The children were followed closely with regard to clinical signs of retinoid toxicity in addition to monthly determinations of total serum retinol, retinyl ester, retinol binding protein (RBP) vit. D metabolites, lipids and liver enzymes. Skeletal surveys were performed in 5 patients after 2 years of retinol therapy.

Results

Complete remission was obtained in 17 of the 19 patients. One boy died two days after admission with a severe cerebral hemorrhage. Another boy died after the second induction course of an overwhelming fungal infection.

The rest of the patients (88%) achieved a complete remission and could go through consolidation and maintenance therapy. The number of months in relapse-free survival are depicted in the table. We have seen three relapses at 7, 19 and 37 months from diagnoses.

Details of Children with AML Treated with High-dose Ara-C as consolidation Therapy and retinyl palmitate as maintenance therapy (as of September 1, 1986)

Patient	Age at Diagnosis (years)	WBC at diagnosis (x10^9 ul)	FAB morphology	Months of A-vit. Medication[1]	Months of Relapse-Free Survival
1	13	200.0	M1-M2	34	37 +
2	9	29.4	M4	43	58 +
3	1.5	13.0	M1	44	56 +
4	2	13.0	M1	41	45 +
5	3/12	88.0	M1 (M6 ?)	39	40 +
6	3/12	158.0	M6	38	39 +
7	2	18.0	M2	38	39 +
8	12	98.0	M4	36	37 +
9	10/12	203.0	M4	32	33 +
10	23/12	55.4	MS	Died the second day	
11	1	10.4	M1	20	24 +
12	10	10.0	M6	20	19 +
13	1.5	6.6	M6	20	24 +
14	4/12	95.0	M4	Died after 2. induction course	
15	1.5	7.2	M1	12	13 +
16	4	172.0	M5	6	7
17	12	47.3	M1	3	4+
18	6	1.9	M4	6	7+
19	9	21.1	M1	6	7+

1) : Retinyl palmitate - 50.000 IU/m^2 daily

Fourteen children (73%) remain in complete
remission with a median follow-up of 30 months
(range 4-58).

Toxicity has been acceptable. One
therapy-related death was observed during
induction (see above). No significant problems
were encountered after 68 courses of high-dose
Ara-C given as consolidation. Details of this
therapy are outlined elsewhere (7).

Particular attention was given to the
possible toxic effects of high-dose retinoids
which have been given for more than three years
to 8 children. No clinical signs of toxicities
were seen. No signs of accumulation of retinyl
ester in the blood were observed, neither any
change over time in serum lipids, liver enzymes
or D-vitamin metabolites. Bone surveys were
done on 5 patients who had been on vitamin A
supplementation for more than 3 years. No
signs of hyperostosis were observed (10,11).

Discussion

Leukemia originates in the transformation and subsequent clonal expansion of a
hemopoietic precursor somewhere early in the
hemopoietic hierarchy. Most evidence support
the notion that the disease is monoclonal, i.e.
originating from one transformed cell that has
an abnormal proliferative capacity coupled with
a maturation arrest (12,13).

Common sense dictates that successful
chemotherapy of the disease should eliminate
all the malignant cells, allowing the proliferation of normal cells to a stage of complete
remission. However, even in complete remission
we do know that malignant clones persist in the
patients. These clones, in spite of various
efforts to maintain the remission, will expand
and lead to a relapse of the disease in the
majority of patients.

The finding that the block in maturation in leukemic cells is not complete (13a)
has led to the speculation that inducers of

differentiation may play some role in hematological malignancies (14,15). In 1982, we
decided to test the effects of retinoids on the
maintenace of remission in children with AML.
We chose to use retinol and not the synthetic
analogs, in order to take advantage of the
homeostatic mechanism in the body that governs
the metabolism of this vitamin (11). The
dosage used was close to the toxic dose.

Of 19 consecutive children treated,
17 went into a complete remission. Of these,
only three have relapsed, with a median observation time of more than 30 months. This com-
pares very favourably with the best results
published so far, and three possible explanations should be considered:

First, it should be emphasized that
our results should not be overinterpreted. The
terror of small number - reflecting the small
population of our country - may still be with
us. We know that AML is many diseases and we
should expect a heterogeneity in response. In
a way we may have been very "lucky" with the
types of patients we have treated.

Secondly, the cytostatic agents used,
and the doses used (in particular the high-dose
Ara-C) may account for most of our results.
However, high-dose Ara-C has been with us for a
long time, and even though relatively few studies have used high-dose Ara-C as consolidation
therapy in first remission, the results have
not approached 50 per cent long term survival.

Thirdly- high-dose daily retinol may
have something to do with what we have
observed. We know today that retinol exerts
profound effects on the growth and differentiation of a wide variety of cells and tissues
(16). Myeloid cells in particular seem to be
targets of retinoid action. Retinol stimulates
the growth of normal myeloid progenitors cells
while inducing differentiation in a substantial
number of leukemic cells (17-20). Malignant
clones freshly isolated from patients can be
induced to differentiate using a variety of

compounds such as retinoids, vitamin D metabolites, phorbol esters and interferons (21). For
example, in a recent study by Findley et al
from the Pediatric Oncology Group in USA, 16 of
24 children with AML had leukemic cells that
were shown to mature in vitro upon exposure to
retinoids (22). In pilot studies retinoids
have been active in myelodysplastic syndromes
and induced remission in promyelocytic leukemias that have been resistant to cytostatic
agents (23-26). However, in full blown
malignancies they are unlikely to be effective.

I would also like to return to my
initial statement that agressive cytostatic
therapy is unlikely to erradicate the last
malignant cell. Recently, Dharmasena and
Galton (27) have shown that with proper techniques and patience, circulating blasts can
certainly be detected in patients with acute
myeloid leukemia in socalled remission. Consolini et al from Mathes group in Villejuif
have demonstrated the presence of abnormal and
probable leukemic clonogenic cells in ALL in
remission (28). Very recently, exciting
results have been published from Johns Hopkins
Hospital where Fearon et al (29) have convin-
cingly demonstrated that mature functioning
granulocytes originate from the leukemic clone
in some patients, and that the leukemic DNA
polymorphic pattern may persist years after
remission was obtained. In an accompanying
editorial (30) it was indeed speculated that
both cytocidal chemotherapy and cytodifferentiation agents should be explored further on
the basis of these findings.

The fact that malignant clones persist in patients in remission demonstrate that
there are factors in the body that prevent
these cells from entering the leukemic pathway.
Retinoids may be one of many such factors. We
have shown that retinyl palmitate in a dose 100
times the recommended daily allowances can
safely be given to children in remission for
periods up to 3 years. This may be of impor-

tance, especially since aggressive cytostatic therapy invariably results in a fat malabsorption state. A tissue deficiency may therefore well exist even when serum levels are normal (11).

Finally: The optimal therapy of cancer today may well be the best of modern, aggressive chemotherapy, followed by an inducer of differentiation as a continuous, long-term chemoprophylaxis.

REFERENCES

1. Riehm, H., Feickert, H.-J. and Lampert, F. (1986). Acute lymphoblastic leukaemia. In cancer in children. Clinical management (P.A. Voute, A. Barrett, H.J.G. Bloom, J. Lemerle M.K., Neiderhardt eds.). Heidelberg: Springer-Verlag, 101-18

2. Lampkin, B.C., Woods, W., Strauss, R. et al (1983) Blood 61,215-28

3. Weinstein, H.J., Mayer, R.H., Rosenthal, D.S. et al (1980) N Eng J Med 303, 473-484

4. Preisler, H.D., Brecher, M., Browman, G. et al (1982) Am J Haematol 13, 189-198

5. Creutzig, U., Ritter, J., Riehm, H. et al (1985) Blood 65,298-304

6. Lie, S.O. and Slørdahl, S.H (1984) Scand J Haematol 33,256-259

7. Lie, S.O. and Slørdahl, S.H. (1985) Seminars in Oncology 12, suppl. 3, 160-165

8. Trouet, A., Deprez-de Campeneere, D. and Duve, C. de. (1972) Nature 239,110-111

9. Lie, S.O., Lie, K.K. and Glomstein, A. (1979) Cancer Chemother Pharmacol 2, 61-66

10. Olson, J.A. (1983) Seminars in Oncology 9, 290-293

11. Goodman, S.D. (1984) New Engl J Med 310, 1023-1031

12. McCulloch, E.A. (1983) Blood 62, 1-13
13. Greaves, M.F., Chan, L.C., Furley, A.J.W.,
     Watt, S.M. and Molgaard, H.V. (1986)
     Blood 67, 1-11
13a. Breitman, T.R., Selonic, S.E. and Collins,
     S.J. (1980) Proc Natl Acad Sci USA 77,
     2936-2939
14. Sachs, L. (1985) Haematol Blood Transf
     29, 353-362
15. Koeffler, H.P. (1983) Blood 62, 709-21
16. Sporn, M.B., Roberts, A.B. and Goodman,
     D.S. (1984) The Retinoids, Vol 1 & 2,
     Academic Press Inc.
17. Douer, D. and Koeffler, H.P. (1982) Exp
     Cell Res 138, 193-198
18. Findley, H.W. jr., Steuber, C.P., Ruymann,
     F.B., Culbert, S. and Ragab, A.H.
     (1984) Exp Hematol 12, 768-773
19. Lotan, R. (1980) Biomed Biophys Acta 605,
     33-91
20. Lotem, J., Berrebi, A. and Sachs, L (1985)
     Leukemia Res 9, 249-258
21. Reiss, M., Gamba-Vitalo, C. and
     Sartorelli, A.C. (1986) Cancer
     Treat Rep 70, 201-218
22. Findley, H.W. jr., Steuber, C.P., Buymann
     F.B., McKolanis, J.R., Williams, D.L.
     and Ragab, A.H. (1986) Leukemia Res
     10, 43-50
23. Flynn, P.J., Miller, W.J., Weisdorf, D.J.,
     Arthur, C.C., Brunning, R. and Branda,
     R.F. (1983) Blood 62, 1211-1217
24. Fontana, J.A., Rogers, J.S. and Durham,
     J.P. (1986) Cancer 57, 209-217
25. Gold, E.J., Mertelsmann, R.H., Itri, L.M.,
     Gee, T., Arlin, Z., Kempin, S.,
     Clarkson, B. and Moore, M.A.S (1983)
     Cancer Treat Rep 67, 981-986
26. Daenen, S., Vellenga, E., Dobbenburg,
     O.A. van and Haile, M.R. (1986) Blood
     67, 559-561
27. Dharmasena, F. and Galton, D.A.G (1986)
     Brit J Haematol 63, 211-213
28. Consolini, R., Breard, J., Bourinbaiar,

A., Goutner, A., Georgoulias, W., Canon,
C., Bruserie, E. and Mathé, G. (1986)
Blood 67, 796-801

29. Fearon, E.R., Burke, P.J., Schiffer, C.A.,
Zehnbauer, B.A. and Vogelstein, B.
(1986) N Engl J Med 315, 15-23

30. Rifkind, R.A. (1986) N Engl J Med 315,
56-57

THERAPEUTIC EFFECTS OF LOW-DOSE CYTOSINE ARABINO-SIDE, α -INTERFERON, 1,25-DIHYDROXYVITAMIN D₃ AND RETINOIC ACID IN MYELODYSPLASTIC SYNDROMES AND ACUTE LEUKEMIA.

Eva Hellström, Karl-Henrik Robèrt, Gösta Gahrton[1], Håkan Mellstedt, Christina Lindemalm, Stefan Einhorn[2], Magnus Björkholm, Gunnar Grimfors[3], Ann-Mari Udén, Jan Samuelsson, Åke Öst[4], Andreas Killander[5], Bo Nilsson[6], Ingemar Winqvist and Inge Olsson[7].
Departments of Medicine at Huddinge University Hospital[1], Karolinska Hospital[2], Danderyd Hospital[3], Southern Hospital[4], University Hospital, Uppsala[5], Helsingborg Hospital[6] and Lund Hospital[7].

ABSTRACT

Fifty-six patients with myelodysplastic syndrome or with acute leukemia were treated with low-dose Ara-C, a combination (IDR) of α-interferon, 1,25-dihydroxyvitamin D₃ and retinoic acid or a combination of all drugs. Complete remissions were obtained only when treatment included Ara-C, but long-lasting and clinically stable partial remissions and significant responses were achieved in 7 of 16 patients treated with IDR. Bone marrow hypoplasia was not necessary for remission in any of the treatment groups. Our data indicate that these substances exert their action via mechanisms different from those seen in conventional chemotherapy. Possible mechanisms involve tumor-cell differentiation, a slow-acting cytotoxicity or a combination of these two mechanisms.

INTRODUCTION

Advances in the development of drug regimens, bone marrow transplantation and a better supportive care have significantly improved the treatment of acute leukemia during the last years. However, there is still a group of hematological malignancies which respond poorly to conventional chemotherapy and in which the patients are not suitable for bone marrow transplantation. This group includes the myelodysplastic syndromes (MDS) (1) and some forms of acute myelogenous leukemia (AML).

Differentiation of leukemic cells and cell lines have been observed in vitro with retinoic acid (2,3,4), vitamin D_3, (4,5,6,7), interferons (8,9,10) and low concentrations of Ara-C (11,12). The optimal ligand for induction of differentiation in vitro varies between different cell clones and different ligands can sometimes drive the same cell line into different hematopoietic lines of differentiation (13). This strongly indicates that the inducers of differentiation can exert their effects via different metabolic pathways. This is further emphazised by reports of synergistic effects in vitro, when two or more agents are used simultaneously (14,15,16). The successful attempts to activate and differentiate leukemic cells from patients in vitro provide a possible basis for new modes of therapy.

The recently observed capacity of IFN to induce remissions in hairy-cell leukemia, is possibly due to induction of differentiation in the leukemic cells (17). A few clinical studies using retinoic acid (18,19), vitamin D_3 (20) and IFN (21,22) in the treatment of AML and MDS have been reported. Positive effects have been achieved, but the frequency and magnitude of those clearly indicate that these agents do not provide a powerful therapeutic alternative when given as monotherapy.

A considerable number of reports concerning treatment with low doses of cytosine arabinoside seem more promising (23,24,25,26). However, whether the remissions achieved with low-dose Ara-C are due to the induction of differentiation or to a direct cytotoxic activity is not clear.

On the basis of data from synergistic effects in vitro, we have investigated whether a combination of drugs having differentiating effects in vitro could have a therapeutic effect on MDS and AML.

In a pilot study eight patients with AML of unfavourable prognosis were treated with combinations of low doses of Ara-C, retinoic acid, 1,25-dihydroxyvitamin D_3 and α-interferon (27). Three complete remissions and two partial reponses were achieved. Marrow hypoplasia was only noted in two of the responders, indicating a mechanism of action different from that in conventional chemotherapy.

Based on these results, a multicenter study was designed where consecutive patients with MDS and AML were treated with different combinations of the substances used in the pilot study. The aim was to study systematically the tumor-cell response rather than comparing the efficacy between the different treatment protocols. However, in order to avoid problems with selection, the patients were randomised to the different therapeutic alternatives. In the present paper we report interim results from the first 61 patients.

PATIENTS AND METHODS

Consecutive patients with myelodysplastic syndrome (MDS), acute myelogenous leukemia (AML) following MDS, acute leukemia in patients with age >75 years or acute leukemia refractory to chemotherapy were included in the study. Depending on the severity of disease patients were divided into three groups (Table 1) and in each group patients were randomised to either of two treatments (Fig. 1). The first 20 patients entering the study were grouped in a different way. Due to this 4 patients in group 2 were treated with CIDR and two patients in group 3 were treated with IDR (Tables 3 and 4).

The following treatments were used: IDR: α -interferon, 3 million units s.c. per day (28), retinoic acid, 1 mg per kilogram body weight p.o. per day, 1,25-dihydroxyvitamin D_3 p.o. in increasing doses p.o. until mild hypercalcemia started to develop. C: AraC subcutaneously, starting at a dose of 15 mg per m^2 per day. CIDR: A combination of all four drugs, given stimultaneously.

Treatment with Ara-C and IFN was given continuously, but was stopped if the bone marrow started to become hypoplastic. If the cellularity increased again and the blasts were still in excess, the drugs were reinstated. Treatment with Ara-C and IFN was also withdrawn if the patient entered partial

Table 1. Patient groups

1.	MDS 1 and 2, transfusion dependant
2.	MDS 3 and 4
3.	MDS 5 and acute leukemia

Figure 1. Randomisation of patients

IDR	—— Patient group 1	——	No active therapy
IDR	—— Patient group 2	——	C
CIDR	—— Patient group 3	——	C

or complete remissions. In remission or partial remission, patients were examined regularly with bone marrow samples and with peripheral blood counts every second week. A new cycle of treatment was initiated if bone marrow blasts started to increase again or if a need for transfusion appeared. Treatment with retinoic acid and vitamin D_3 was continued also in remission. If the disease progressed, in spite of a higher dose of Ara-C, therapy was withdrawn.

Responses were divided in CR, PR and SR (Table 2).

RESULTS

So far 61 patients have been included in our study. Forty-five had a myelodysplastic syndrome (MDS) (RA 8, RAS 2, RAEB 25, CMML 3, RAEB-t 7), 7 had acute leukemia following MDS, 7 were elderly patients with acute leukemia and 2 had refractory leukemia. Secondary MDS was found in 25% of the patients.

Nine patients were withdrawn from the analysis of tumor response. Five of these died within ten days from randomisation, two were diagnostic errors, two had major protocol violations.

In the MDS 1 and 2 group, 1/5 patients showed a significant response (SR) to active therapy. Five patients were randomised to no treatment, three of these deteriorated and two have a steady course of their disease.

In the MDS 3 and 4 group 5/9 patients improved on treatment with IDR, 7/10 on treatment with Ara-C and 2/4 on treatment with CIDR (Table 3). CR was achieved only when the treatment included Ara-C.

Table 2. Criteria for response

	AML	MDS
CR	BM blasts <5% Hb >100, plt >100 WBC >1.5	Normal BM Hb >100, plt >100 WBC >1.5
PR	BM blasts <10% >50% improved peripheral blood counts	BM blasts <5% >50% improved peripheral blood counts
SR	>50% decreased BM blasts or >25% improved peripheral blood counts	>50% decreased BM blasts or >25% improved peripheral blood counts

Of all patients with MDS 5 and AML, 4/8 patients treated with CIDR responded favourably, 3/9 of those treated with Ara-C and 1/2 of patients only treated with IDR (Table 4).

Looking at the whole material, 49% of the patients responded to therapy. In 6 patients (13%) CR, in 9 patients (19%) PR and in 8 patients (17%) SR was obtained. Response rates in the different diagnostical groups were 20% for MDS 1 and 2, 61% for MDS 3 and 4 and 42% for MDS 5 and AML. When looking separately at patients with primary and secondary MDS, the former responded in 54% and the latter in 27% of the cases. Duration of responses is shown in Table 5.

DISCUSSION

Patients with myelodysplastic syndromes and certain acute leukemias respond favourably to treatment with different combinations of low doses of Ara-C, α-interferon, retinoic acid and 1,25-dihydroxyvitamin D_3. In our material, when looking at the subgroups, the best results were found in patients

Table 3. Results of treatment in patient group 2 (MDS 3 and 4)

	n	CR	PR	SR	NR	Tot pos R	%
C	10	2	3	2	3	7	70
IDR	9	0	3	2	4	5	56
CIDR	4	1	1	0	2	2	50

Table 4. Results of treatment in patient group 3 (MDS 5 and AML)

	n	CR	PR	SR	NR	Tot pos R	%
C	9	2	9	1	6	3	33
IDR	2	0	0	1	1	1	50
CIDR	8	1	2	1	4	4	50

Table 5. Duration of reponses in months.
+: still in response; -: relapse or dead

CR : 2-,4-,6-,6-,8-,15+
PR : 1-,1+,3-,4-,8+,12+,12+,19+,22+
SR : 2+,3-,3-,4-,10-,12+,16-

with MDS 3, 4, and 5, and AML following MDS. The response rate of 49% may have been lowered by the high proportion of secondary MDS.

The possibility of achieving positive results with low doses of Ara-C is well known and the response rate in our material of 53% (10/10 pts) corresponds well with other studies recently published (23,24). Bone marrow hypoplasia was observed in less than half of the patients responding to the drug and no deaths related to therapy were seen. Our results do not tell us whether an additive or a synergistic effect was obtained when Ara-C was combined with IDR, but the combination of IDR in itself had a therapeutic effect (7/16 responded favourably). The mechanism of action of this combination is unclear, although the choice of therapy was based on the ability of these drugs to induce differentiation in vitro. A generally moderate descrease in hemoglobin, WBC and platelets was sometimes seen when initiating therapy, but a mild marrow hypoplasia was only observed in one of the patients responding to IDR.

Patients were selected because of their low probability of responding to conventional chemotherapy. The high response rate in itself and the fact that bone marrow hypoplasia was not necessary for complete or partial remission indicate that the mode of action of both the combination of IDR and low-dose Ara-C is different from that in conventional chemotherapy. Alternative explanations to this mechanism are differentiation, a slowly acting cytostatic mechanism or a combination of these two mechanisms.

To address these questions further, laboratory techniques need to be developed. We are therefore currently comparing differentiation and colony growth in vitro with the clinical results of treatment. These in vitro studies may be helpful to elucidate the mechanisms of the clinical responses. If successful, they might also provide useful tools for the design of a clinical therapy in the individual case.

REFERENCES

1.   Benett, J.M., Catovsky, D., Daniel, M.T., Flandrin, G., Galton, D.A.G., Gralnick, H.R., and Sultan, C. (1982) Br. J. Haematol. **51**, 189–199
2.   Breitman, T.R., Selonick, S.E., and Collins, S.J. (1980) Proc. Natl. Acad. Sci. U.S.A. **5**, 2936–2940

3. Breitman, T.R., Collins, S.J., and Keene, B.R. (1981) Blood **57**, 1000-1004

4. Nagler, A., Ricklis, I., Gazit, E., Tatarsky, I., and Fabian, I. (1986) Eur. J. Clin. Invest. **16**, 297-301

5. Rigby, W., Shen, L., Ball, E., Guyre, P., and Fanger, M. (1984) Blood **64**, 1110-1115

6. Olsson, I., Gullberg, U., Ivhed, I., and Nilsson, K. (1983) Cancer Res. **43**, 5862-5867

7. Koeffler, H.P., Amatruda, T., Ikekawa, N., Kobayashi, Y., and DeLuca, H.F. (1984) Cancer Res. **44**, 5624-5628

8. Tomida, M., Yamamoto, Y., and Hozumi, M., (1982) Biochem. Biophys. Res. Commun. **104**, 30-37

9. Takei, M., Takeda, K., and Konno, K. (1984) Biochem. Biophys. Res. Commun. **124**, 100-105

10. Robèrt, K.H., Einhorn, S., Östlund, L., Juliusson, G., and Biberfeld, P. (1985) Clin. Exp. Immunol. **62**, 530-534

11. Griffin, J., Munroe, D., Major, P., and Kufe, D. (1982) Exp. Haematol. **10**, 774-781

12. Michalewicz, R., Lotem, J., and Sachs, L. (1984) Leukemia Res. **8**, 783-790

13. Graziano, R., Ball, E., and Fanger, M. (1983) Blood **61**, 1215-1221

14. Olsson, I., Breitman, T.R., and Gallo, R.C. (1982) Cancer Res. **42**, 3928-3933

15. Gullberg, U., Nilsson, E., Einhorn, S., and Olsson, I. (1985) Exp. Hematol. **13**, 675-679

16. Sachs, L. (1982) J. Cell. Physiology, **Suppl 1**, 151-164

17. Quesada, J.R., Rensen, J., Manning, J.T., Hersch, E.M., and Gutterman, J.V. (1984) N. Engl. J. Med. **310**, 15-18

18. Nilsson, B. (1984) Br. J. Haematol. **57**, 365-371

19. Gold, E., Mertelsmann, R., Irti, L., Gee, T., Arlin, Z., Kempin, S., Clarkson, B., and Moore, M. (1983) Cancer Treat. Rep. **67**, 981-986.

20. Koeffler, H.P., Reichei, H., Tobler, A., Munker, R., and Norman, A. (1986) The Biology and Pharmacology of Tumor Cell Differentiation, Tromso, Norway, June 29-July 1, meeting abstract.

21. Rohatiner, A.Z.S., Balkwill, F.R., Malpas, J.S., and Lister T.A. (1983) Cancer Chemother. Pharmacol. **11**, 56-58

22.   Hill, N.O., Loeb, E., Pardue, A.S., Dorn, G.L., Khan,
       A., and Hill, J.M. (1979) J. Clin. Hematol. Oncol. **9**,
       137
23.   Castaigne, S., Daniel, M.T., Tilly, H., Herait, P., and
       Degos, L. (1983) Blood **62**, 85-86
24.   Tricot, G., De Bock, R., Dekker, A.W., Boogaerts,
       M.A., Peetermans, M., Punt, K., and Verwilghen, R.L.
       (1984) Br. J. Haematol. **58**, 231-240
25.   Manoharan, A., Leyden, M.J., and Sullivan, J. (1984)
       The Medical Journal of Australia **10**, 643-646
26.   Leyden, M., Manoharan, A., Boyd, A., Ming Cheng,
       Z., and Sullivan, J. (1984) Br. J. Haematol, **57**, 301-
       307
27.   Robèrt, K.H., Hellström, E., Einhorn, S., and Gahrton,
       G. (1986) Scandj J. Haematol, **36** (Suppl 44), 61-74
28.   Cantell, K., and Hirvonen, S. (1978) J. Gen. Virol.
       39, 541-543

Nucleosides, Methylation, and Differentiation

SEQUENCE-SPECIFIC DNA METHYLATION: PROMOTER INACTIVATION AND RELEASE OF THE EXPRESSION BLOCK

Dagmar Knebel, Klaus-Dieter Langner, Arnd Hoeveler, Ursula Lichtenberg, Bernd Weisshaar, Doris Renz, and Walter Doerfler

Institute of Genetics, University of Cologne, Cologne, Germany

INTRODUCTION

In the chemical, though by no means genetic, monotony of nucleotide sequences in DNA, the function of the modified base 5-methylcytosine (5-mC) poses an exciting challenge to the investigator. This enigmatic signal may affect more than one elementary mechanism in the molecular biology of eukaryotic cells. In recent years, the influence of sequence-specific promoter methylations on the regulation of gene transcription has been studied in considerable detail. From many independent studies in a variety of eukaryotic systems a, sometimes tenuous, consensus has emerged

- that sequence-specific promoter methylations are associated with and can cause gene inactivation,

- that the mechanisms by which the modulating signal, 5-mC, exerts its functions are complex, and

215

- that the core of the regulatory problem is camouflaged in the establishment of specific patterns of promoter and/or gene methylation. In this respect, studies on the activity and sequence specificity of eukaryotic DNA methyltransferases and of the factors that regulate their function, will assume an important role.

The fascination with the subject of DNA methylation, its biochemistry, biology, and genetic significance has led to the publication of numerous reviews and book on these topics (1-6).

Since our laboratory has made contributions to many of these treatises, it would be superfluous to repeat here what has been described in previous reviews in books (see above) or in a series of review articles (7-14). Instead, we shall summarize in the present paper some of the results of work in progress or of some of the recently completed studies on the mechanisms by which promoter methylations might affect genetic activity.

CHOICE OF SYSTEM - VIRAL PROMOTERS

For a number of reasons, we have concentrated in our studies on the effect of DNA methylation on the activity of viral promoters. (i) Adenovirus and baculovirus systems have been investigated for many years in this laboratory. (ii) The activity of viral promoters can be studied in different biological systems. These promoters can be transferred into cells from different species either in the context of intact viral genomes or sometimes in promoter constructs which can be generated by the methods of gene technology, and in which the activity of a viral promoter can be assessed under various conditions through the function of a suitable reporter gene. (iii) In mammalian cells, the function of viral promoters can be determined in free viral genomes or after the integration of an entire viral genome or of fragments derived from it into the host genome. (iv) Inverse correlations between the extent of DNA methylation in viral promoters (genes) and the level of transcription of these genes have been among the first such correlations noted in eukaryotic systems and have already been studied in detail.

In a series of exemplary investigations, the late promoter of the E2A gene of human adenovirus type 2 (Ad2) DNA, the promoter of the E1A region of human adenovirus type 12 (Ad12) DNA, and of the p10 gene of the insect baculovirus Autographa californica nuclear polyhedrosis virus (AcNPV) were studied with respect to their sensitivities towards sequence-specific promoter methylations (15-19). The sites of in vitro promoter methylations have been selected according to the results of analyses on naturally occurring methylation patterns, notably on the E2A gene of Ad2 DNA in Ad2-transformed hamster cells. In one Ad2-transformed hamster cell line, HE1 (20), which contains parts of the Ad2 genome in the integrated state, the E2A gene is expressed. All fourteen 5'-CCGG-3' sequences in the E2A region in cell line HE1 are unmethylated (21). In two additional Ad2-transformed hamster cell lines, HE2 and HE3 (20), the E2A gene is not transcribed (22, 23), and all fourteen 5'-CCGG-3' sequences are methylated (21). It was, therefore, thought that the in vitro methylation of these sequences in the isolated E2A gene of Ad2 DNA would constitute a sensible attempt to mimick functionally relevant patterns of methylation in a viral promoter and to determine the consequences of this modification on gene activity (15, 17, 18). Similar studies have also been reported with the E1 promoters of Ad12 DNA (16, 24), with the human γ-globin promoter in mouse L cells (25, 26), with the genes for herpes thymidine kinase and adenosyl-phosphoribosyl-transferase (APRTase) in mouse cells (27), and with the p10 promoter of AcNPV DNA in insect cells (19).

SEQUENCE-SPECIFIC PROMOTER METHYLATIONS CAUSE
EUKARYOTIC GENE INACTIVATIONS

This notion has been amply documented in
the reports and reviews which have been cited
above. Inactivation of the late E2A promoter of
Ad2 DNA, e.g., by 5'-CCGG-3' methylation at the
three sequences at positions -215, +5, and +23,
relative to the downstream cap site, as the
site of transcription initiation, has been
demonstrated after microinjection into the
nuclei of Xenopus laevis oocytes, as well as
after transfection into mammalian cells (17,
18). In these experiments the authentic E2A
gene or the prokaryotic gene for chlorampheni-
col acetyl transferase (CAT) has been used as
reporter gene. In mammalian cells, the regulatory effect of sequence-specific methylations
on the activities of promoters of house-keeping
genes has been clearly documented (27). It has
been noted that in the gene for herpes
thymidine kinase, sequence-specific methylations even in the 3' flanking sequences of the
gene can cause gene inactivation (27). In the
E1A promoter of Ad12 DNA, several restriction
sites have been in vitro methylated, and the
effects of these modifications on gene activities have been measured. The CAT gene has been
used as reporter gene in these experiments in
which the unmethylated or methylated constructs
have been transfected into human HeLa cells
(24). It is apparent that there are several
sites located in different regions of the E1A
promoter that have proved quite sensitive
towards the introduction of 5-mC groups. Of
course, a promoter sequence as a linear representation of genetic information must also
be viewed as a three-dimensional structure.
Thus, nucleotide sequences at an apparent
distance from each other may, in actual fact,
be in closer proximity in a functional promoter
sequence that has been complexed with specific
host factors which are required for promoter
activity (for reviews, 28, 29). In that sense,
there may be critical sequences in a promoter
whose methylation is associated with the in-

activated state of this promoter. The distribution of these methylation-sensitive sites might reflect the three-dimensional arrangement of promoter sequences rather than a linear array of genetic signals in a eukaryotic promoter. Moreover, it will have to be considered that sequence-specific promoter methylations may affect the binding of specific host protein factors. Even if this binding would not be interfered with directly, the functionality of host factors bound to methylated sequences might be altered. Lastly, sequence-specific promoter methylations could change the structure of the promoter, either directly, by causing alterations in the fine structure of nucleotide sequences, or indirectly, by modifying complex formations with specific host factors. The preponderance of the conjunctive tense in this paragraph reflects limitations in our understanding of these mechanisms and signals the importance of future research.

PROMOTER METHYLATION - SIGNAL VALUE EVEN IN INSECT CELLS

As outlined above, viral systems offer the opportunity to test promoter activities under a wide gamut of experimental conditions. We have used the promoter of the late p10 gene of AcNPV in conjunction with the CAT gene as activity indicator. The p10 gene codes for a polypeptide of 10,000 kiloDaltons of unknown function. This polypeptide is abundantly synthesized in AcNPV-infected cells. The promoter construct was 5'-CCGG-3' methylated at one site upstream and at two sites downstream (3') from the cap site in the coding region. This methylated construct or its non-methylated equivalent was transfected into AcNPV-infected Spodoptera frugiperda cells, a lepidopteran insect cell line, and the activity of each of the constructs was measured. The methylated construct exhibited activity levels which were about 40 fold lower than those of the unmethylated DNA (19). This result was considered with particular interest,

because the DNA of Spodoptera frugiperda cells
was apparently devoid of 5-mC as a modified
nucleotide (Th. Müller and W. Doerfler, unpublished results). This latter finding was
in keeping with the absence of 5-mC from the
DNA of Drosophila melanogaster (30, 31). These
results taken together indicate that the genetic signal of a methylated 5'-CCGG-3' promoter sequence can be assigned the same regulatory
value in an insect cell system as in mammalian
cells, even though this genetic signal does not
seem to be ordinarily used in some insects, as
in Drosophila or in lepidopteran cells. It
would be interesting to investigate at what
stage in evolution 5-mC as a promoter-inacti-
vating modification occurs for the first time,
and at what stage in evolution this genetic
signal can first be recognized.

METHYLATION OF THE LATE PROMOTER OF AD2 DNA:
MINOR EFFECTS ON HOST FACTOR BINDING TO
SPECIFIC PROMOTER SEQUENCES

In many of the studies on the genetic
function of DNA methylation, that have been
performed in our laboratory, the late E2A
promoter of Ad2 DNA has been used as a model.
We have, therefore, determined host factors and
the specific promoter sequences at which these
factors bind. Considerable evidence has been
adduced that binding of host factors at specific promoter sites is one of the decisive pre-
conditions for the functional activation of
eukaryotic promoters (for reviews, see 28, 29).
It was therefore of interest to investigate
whether the binding of host protein factors to
the late E2A promoter was influenced by sequence-specific methylations at the three 5'-
CCGG-3' sequences.

Obviously, one would like to understand
the mechanisms by which 5-mC residues are
capable of interfering with regulatory functions in the late E2A promoter of Ad2 DNA. The
binding of these protein factors to unmethyl-

ated or 5'-CCGG-3' methylated late E2A promoter sequences (sites I to VI) has been compared by using the gel migration delay assay or DNase I protection (footprinting) analyses. At least six different promoter sequences have been identified by DNase I protection analyses, and these sites bind specifically to host proteins (32). Apparently, protein factor binding is only slightly affected by late E2A promoter methylations. In particular, the factor(s) interacting at or close to the non-canonical TATA sequence of the late E2A promoter, in protein binding site I and at or close to the 5'-CCGG-3' sequences are slightly influenced by promoter methylations. Even though major differences in host factor binding have not been detectable at late E2A promoter sites, it is conceivable that the functionality of promoter-bound host factors is altered when the three 5'-CCGG-3' sequences are methylated.

The effects of sequence-specific methylations in certain promoters on protein binding to specific sites in these promoters have been tested in a number of eukaryotic systems. In the ß-globin promoter of chicken, site-specific promoter methylations did not interfere with the binding of one of the specific, highly purified protein factors to this promoter (G. Felsenfeld, personal communication cited in 33). Protein factors specifically interacting with six different sites in the late E2A promoter of Ad2 DNA were only slightly affected in their capacity to interact with these sites when 5-mC was experimentally introduced in three 5'-CCGG-3' sequences of the late E2A promoter. The significance of these effects is not yet understood. Possibly, sequence-specific methylations in promoter sequences can or do not abolish the capacity of these promoter sequences to associate with specific proteins. The functional consequences of promoter methylations might depend on the specific promoter site, on the specific protein binding at a certain promoter site or on both factors.

FACTORS THAT CAN CANCEL THE INACTIVATING FUNCTION OF SITE-SPECIFIC PROMOTER METHYLATIONS

It appears that promoter methylations serve as a long-term inactivating function in eukaryotic systems. In what way can that transcription block be permanently or temporarily released? One way of changing patterns of DNA methylation would be to inhibit specifically, during or after DNA replication, the activity of DNA methyltransferases that are responsible for maintaining a certain pattern of methylation in dividing cells. Another possibility is offered by active demethylation mechanisms. Evidence for enzymatic demethylation (34) or for a repair-like mechanism by which a 5-mC residue is replaced by cytidine (35) has been published. Either of these mechanisms, if in fact operative, would lead to a permanent change in patterns of methylation.

However, there are alternative ways that can transiently override the inactivating capacity of 5-mC in a promoter sequence and may render permanent changes in methylation patterns less mandatory. In the present overview, three possible mechanisms will be discussed that have the capacity to release the stringency of a transcriptional block caused by promoter methylation: (i) Activation of alternate promoters. (ii) Reactivation of a methylation-inactivated promoter by E1 functions of adenovirus. (iii) A hemimethylated promoter is activated when the reading strand lacks 5-mC.

Activation of Alternate Promoters

Derivatives of the plasmid construct pSV0-CAT have been used to test adenovirus promoter activities in the unmethylated or methylated state. We have shown that the late E2A promoter of Ad2 DNA activates the CAT gene upon transfection of the pAd2E2A-CAT construct into mammalian cells, and this promoter is inactivated by specific methylations of three 5'-

CCGG-3' sites. Surprisingly, it has been found that the pSV0-CAT construct, which lacks eukaryotic promoter sequences, is able to express the CAT gene upon transfection into human or hamster cells that harbor and constitutively express the El region of Ad2 or Ad5 DNA. In these cells, the expression of the unmethylated pAd2E2A-CAT construct is enhanced in comparison to non-virus transformed cells, and this expression is only partly sensitive to DNA methylation, possibly because DNA methylation is counteracted directly or indirectly by El functions. The pSV0-CAT construct is also expressed in HeLa or BHK21 cells upon cotransfection with a plasmid carrying the HindIII-G fragment of Ad2 DNA that contains the ElA region and part of the ElB region. By mapping pSV0-CAT-specific RNAs, it has been demonstrated that pSV0-CAT activity in Ad2- or Ad5-transformed cells is mediated by prokaryotic promoter-like sequences in the pBR322 section of the construct. These sequences are presumably trans-activated by functions in the El region. This trans-activation of pSV0-CAT in adenovirus-transformed cells is partly insensitive to DNA methylation.

There is preliminary evidence for the notion that viral enhancers artificially introduced into the vicinity of the methylation-inactivated late E2A promoter of Ad2 DNA can lead to the reactivation of this promoter. Hence, it does not appear necessary to provide alternate promoters. An additional enhancer element by itself may suffice to overcome the methylation block in the late E2A promoter (K.-D. Langner, R. Rüger, B. Fleckenstein, and W. Doerfler, unpublished data).

Reactivation of the Methylation-Inactivated Late E2A Promoter by El Functions of Adenovirus

The late E2A promoter of Ad2 DNA is inactivated by the in vitro methylation of three 5'-CCGG-3' sequences both after microinjection

into Xenopus laevis oocytes (17) and after
transfection into mammalian cells (18). In
human 293 cells (36), in hamster BHK297-C131
cells (37), or in hamster HE7 cells (38), which
contain in an integrated form and constitutively express the E1A and part of the E1B regions
of Ad5 or of Ad2 DNA, the methylated late E2A
promoter is not completely shut down but re-
tains part of its activity. However, activity
levels are reduced in comparison to the unmethylated construct. In 293 cells, transcription from the methylated late E2A promoter is
initiated from the authentic cap site that is
used in a regular productive Ad2 infection of
human cells, and not from promoter-like sequences in the plasmid part of the construct
(39). It has been shown that the methylated E2A
promoter remains methylated after transfection
during the course of the experiment. Similarly,
when hamster BHK21 cells are cotransfected with
the cloned left terminal 7.9% fragment of Ad2
DNA (HindIII-G fragment) which carries the E1A
and part of the E1B regions, and the methylated
or the unmethylated late E2A promoter construct, both the methylated and the unmethylated promoters are active. The methylated
promoter exhibits lower levels of activity. The
prokaryotic CAT gene has served as a reporter
gene in all of these experiments. These data
demonstrate that E1 functions of adenoviruses
have the capacity to counteract the promoter
inactivating effect of site-specific methylations, at least to some extent. This trans-
activation could be effected directly or by the
mediation of cellular functions, but is not due
to demethylation of the inactivated promoter.
It is unknown whether this transactivation
involves changes in the interactions with proteins or structural alterations of methylated
promoters or a combination of both events.

In a similar system, it has been reported
that the E1A promoter of Ad12 DNA that has been
inactivated by 5'-CCGG-3' methylation at two
such sequences (16) can be reactivated by
transfection into BHK21 hamster cells that have

previously been infected with the frog virus FV3 (40). Here, it has also been demonstrated that transcription is reinitiated in the 5'-CCGG-3' methylated E1A promoter. Again, the mechanism of this reactivation remains obscure.

Hemimethylation of the Late E2A Promoter of Ad2 DNA

When DNA methylated in both strands is replicated, sequences will at least transiently be rendered hemimethylated, until DNA methyltransferases, which are responsible for the maintenance of a given methylation pattern remethylate the newly synthesized DNA strand. For a methylation-inactivated promoter, replication of DNA leads to the hemimethylated state. Is a promoter reactivated by this partial "demethylation" of the doubly methylated duplex?

We have started to investigate this problem and have again used the late E2A promoter of Ad2 DNA (K.-D. Langner, U. Lichtenberg, B. Weisshaar, D. Renz, and W. Doerfler, manuscript in preparation). The two hemimethylated constructs of the late E2A promoter, with the three 5'-CCGG-3' sequences in the methylated configuration in the reading strand or in the opposite strand, have been prepared and have been linked to the main part of the unmethylated E2A gene. These constructs carrying hemimethylated late E2A promoters have been microinjected into Xenopus laevis oocytes, and promoter activities have been tested by screening for Ad2-specific RNAs and by mapping their origins in the late E2A promoter by S1 protection analyses, as described earlier (17, 18). Preliminary results indicate that the promoter construct is inactive when the reading strand is methylated, and at least partly active when the opposite strand is methylated. Thus, depending on which of the two strands is methylated, a hemimethylated promoter may be active or inactive. Similar conclusions are corrobo-

rated by the results of studies on the induction of the estradiol-inducible avian vitello-
genin II gene, in which the reading strand has
been found demethylated upon induction (41).

In this chapter, several mechanisms have
been enumerated that might cause at least the
transient reactivation of promoters that have
been inactivated by sequence-specific methylations. Of course, it is unknown whether the
results elaborated in the adenovirus system
would be applicable to the situations in other
systems. The possibility of a (transient) release from inactivation by methylation would
also explain the apparent discrepancies which
have occasionally been reported on the presump-
tive activity of methylated promoters. Perhaps
the situation in these instances had not been
investigated in sufficient detail.

CONCLUSIONS

In a series of investigations, we have
used viral promoters, mainly the late E2A
promoter of Ad2 DNA or the E1A promoter of Ad12
DNA, to study factors that influence the
promoter inactivating function of sequence-
specific methylations. We have also initiated
work to evaluate conditions that afflict the
stability of in vitro preimposed patterns of
methylation in the late E2A promoter of Ad2 DNA
after this promoter has been fixed in the mammalian genome by integration. In another set of
experiments, we have tried to assess the influence, if any, that 5'-CCGG-3' methylations
in the late E2A promoter can exert on the sequence-specific binding of host protein factors. The answers emanating from these studies
to the questions posed are complex and often
open up new problems whose solution will require further efforts.

Among the most important questions with respect to promoter methylations and their role in gene inactivation are the following.

(i) What is the biochemical mechanism of gene inactivation by promoter methylation?

(ii) How is a given pattern of DNA methylation established, when and how is it altered?

(iii) What is the specificity of DNA methyltransferases and how is their activity controlled?

(iv) Which factors affect the patterns of methylation of foreign genes artificially integrated into the host genome?

There are more problems, but who would not consider themselves fortunate to be capabable of broaching those listed in this summary.

Acknowledgments

We are grateful to Petra Böhm for excellent editorial work.

Research performed in the authors' laboratory was supported by the Deutsche Forschungsgemeinschaft through SFB74-Cl, by the Ministry of Science and Research in the State of Nordrhein-Westfalen and by donations of the Hoechst Company and the Fonds der Chemischen Industrie.

REFERENCES

1. Razin, A., Cedar, H., Riggs, A.D. (eds) (1984) DNA Methylation. Biochemistry and Biological Significance, Springer Verlag, New York, Berlin, Heidelberg, Tokyo

2. Taylor, J.H. (1984) DNA Methylation and Cellular Differentiation, Springer Verlag, Wien, New York

3. Trautner, T.A. (ed) (1984) Methylation of DNA, Springer Verlag, Berlin, Heidelberg, New York, Tokyo

4. Adams, R.L.T., and Burton, R.H. (1985) Molecular Biology of DNA Methylation. Springer Series in Molecular Biology, Springer Verlag, Berlin, Heidelberg, New York

5. Cantoni, G.L., and Razin, A. (eds) (1985) Biochemistry and Biology of DNA Methylation, Alan R. Liss, Inc., New York

6. Borchardt, R.T., Creveling, C.R., and Ueland, P.M. (eds) (1986) Biological Methylation and Drug Design, Humana Press Clifton, N.J.

7. Doerfler, W. (1981) J. Gen. Virol. 57, 1-20

8. Doerfler, W. (1983) Ann. Rev. Biochem. 52, 93-124

9. Doerfler, W. (1984a), in Advances in Viral Oncology (Klein, G., ed) Vol. 4, pp. 217-247, Raven Press, New York

10. Doerfler, W. (1984b) in Methylation of DNA. Current Topics in Microbiology and Immunology (Trautner, T.A., ed) Vol. 108, pp. 79-98, Springer Verlag, Berlin, Heidelberg, New York, Tokyo

11. Doerfler, W. (1986) in Oncogenes and Growth Control (Kahn, P., and Graf, T., eds) pp. 235-240, Springer Verlag, Berlin, Heidelberg, New York, London, Paris, Tokyo

12. Doerfler, W., Langner, K.-D., Kruczek, I., Vardimon, L., and Renz, D. (1984) in DNA Methylation. Biochemistry and Biological Significance (Razin, A., Cedar, H., and Riggs, A.D., eds) pp. 221-247, Springer Verlag, Berlin, Heidelberg, New York, Tokyo

13. Doerfler, W., Langner, K.-D., Knebel, D., Weyer, U., Dobrzanski, P., and Knust-Kron, B. (1985) in Biochemistry and Biology of DNA Methylation (Cantoni, G.L., and Razin, A., eds) pp. 133-155, Alan R. Liss, Inc., New York

14. Doerfler, W., Langner, K.-D., Knebel, D., and Weyer, U. (1986) in Biological Methylation and Drug Design (Borchardt, R.T., Creveling, C.R., and Ueland, P.M., eds) pp. 139-150, Humana Press, Clifton, N.J.
15. Vardimon, L., Kressmann, A., Cedar, H., Maechler, M., and Doerfler, W. (1982) Proc. Natl. Acad. Sci. USA **79**, 1073-1077
16. Kruczek, I., and Doerfler, W. (1983) Proc. Natl. Acad. Sci. USA **80**, 7586-7590
17. Langner, K.-D., Vardimon, L., Renz, D., and Doerfler, W. (1984) Proc. Natl. Acad. Sci. USA **81**, 2950-2954
18. Langner, K.-D., Weyer, U., and Doerfler, W. (1986) Proc. Natl. Acad. Sci. USA **83**, 1498-1602
19. Knebel, D., Lübbert, H., and Doerfler, W. (1985) EMBO J. **4**, 1301-1306
20. Cook, J.L., and Lewis, A.M., Jr. (1979) Cancer Res. **39**, 1455-1461
21. Vardimon, L., Neumann, R., Kuhlmann, I., Sutter, D., and Doerfler, W. (1980) Nucleic Acids Res. **8**, 2461-2473
22. Johansson, K., Persson, H., Lewis, A.M., Pettersson, U., Tibbetts, C., and Philipson, L. (1978) J. Virol. **27**, 628-639
23. Esche, H. (1982) J. Virol. **41**, 1076-1082
24. Knebel, D., and Doerfler, W. (1986) J. Mol. Biol. **189**, 371-375
25. Busslinger, M., Hurst, J., and Flavell, R.A. (1983) Cell **34**, 197-206
26. Murray, E., and Grosveld, F. (1985) in Biochemistry and Biology of DNA Methylation (Cantoni, G.L., and Razin, A., eds) pp. 157-176, Alan R. Liss, Inc., New York
27. Keshet, I., Yisraeli, J., and Cedar, H. (1985) Proc. Natl. Acad. Sci. USA **82**, 2560-2564
28. Dynan, W.S., and Tjian, R. (1985) Nature **316**, 774-778
29. McKnight, S., and Tjian, R. (1986) Cell **46**, 795-805
30. Smith, S.S., and Thomas, C.A., Jr. (1981) Gene **13**, 395-408
31. Eick, D., Fritz, H.-J., and Doerfler, W. (1983) Anal. Biochem. **135**, 165-171

32. Hoeveler, A., and Doerfler, W. (1987) submitted
33. Keshet, I., Lieman-Hurwitz, J., and Cedar, H. (1986) Cell **44**, 535-543
34. Gjerset, R.A., and Martin, D.W., Jr. (1982) J. Biol. Chem. **257**, 8581-8583
35. Razin, A., Szyf, M., Kafri, T., Roll, M., Giloh, H., Scarpa, S., Carotti, D., and Cantoni, G.L. (1986) Proc. Natl. Acad. Sci. USA **83**, 2827-2831
36. Graham, F.L., Smiley, J., Russell, W.C., and Nairn, R. (1977) J. Gen. Virol. **36**, 59-72
37. Visser, L., Maarschalkerweerd, M.W., Rozjin, T.H., Wassenaar, A.D.C., Reemst, A.M.C.B., and Sussenbach, J.S. (1979) Cold Spring Harbor Symp. Quant. Biol. **44**, 541-550
38. Klimkait, T., and Doerfler, W. (1985) J. Virol. **55**, 466-474
39. Weisshaar, B., Knust, B., Langner, K.-D., Jüttermann, R., Zock, C., and Doerfler, W. (1987) submitted
40. Thompson, J.P., Granoff, A., and Willis, D.B. (1986) Proc. Natl. Acad. Sci. USA **83**, 7688-7692
41. Saluz, H.P., Jiricny, J., and Jost, J.P. (1986) Proc. Natl. Acad. Sci. USA **83**, 7167-7171

INDUCTION OF DIFFERENTIATION OF 3T3-L1 FIBROBLASTS TO ADIPOCYTES BY 3-DEAZAADENOSINE AND INSULIN

Peter K. Chiang, Nesbitt D. Brown, Felipe N.
Padilla and Richard K. Gordon
Department of Applied Biochemistry
Walter Reed Army Institute of Research
Washington, D.C. 20307-5100
U.S.A.

3-Deazaadenosine (dzAdo), an analog of adenosine, is a potent proximal inhibitor of S-adenosylmethionine-dependent transmethylation reactions (1-3). A variety of transmethylation reactions have been shown to be inhibited by dzAdo because of its ability to act as an alternative substrate and also as an inhibitor of S-adenosylhomocysteine hydrolase, which hydrolyzes S-adenosylhomocysteine to adenosine and L-homocysteine. A unique feature of S-adenosylhomocysteine hydrolase is that it can synthesize a novel S-nucleosidylhomocysteine analog by condensing a nucleoside with L-homocysteine because the equilibrium of the reaction favors the synthetic direction (1-5). When dzAdo is administered to cells or animals, the net result is the accumulation of S-adenosylhomocysteine and S-3-deazaadenosylhomocysteine, both of which are known potent inhibitors of transmethylation reactions (6-11).

Because of the current hypothesis that DNA hypomethylation may lead to gene expression and cellular differentiation (12-14), we examined the effect of 3-deazaadenosine on the differentiation of 3T3-L1 fibroblasts to adipocytes (fat cells). This subline of fibroblasts, 3T3-L1, can undergo spontaneous differentiation to become adipocytes upon confluency (15). In addition to insulin and many other inducing agents, dzAdo has been found to increase the frequency of conversion of the 3T3-L1 fibroblasts to adipocytes (16).

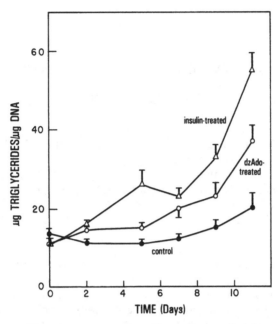

FIG. 1. Time course in the accumulation of total triglycerides in 3T3-L1 cells treated with 15 µM dzAdo or 10 µg/ml of insulin; culture media were changed every 2 days and supplemented with either inducer.

The culture of 3T3-L1 fibroblasts was as described previously (16); 2 to 3 days after the fresh seeding of cells, 15 µM dzAdo was added. It normally required a duration of about 7-9 days before the adipocytes were expressed morphologically and biochemically, with noticeable rise in cellular total triglycerides (Fig. 1). Similarly, the same time period was required for the appearance of adipocytes after treatment with 10 µg/ml of insulin (Fig. 1). Although the cells treated with dzAdo were lower in total triglycerides than those treated with insulin between 7-15 days, the total triglycerides in the dzAdo-treated cells were about equal to those of insulin-treated cells after 21 days. Comparable growth rates were observed among the control cells and the cells treated with dzAdo or insulin (Fig. 2). If dzAdo were withdrawn from the incubation medium after 10 days, the treated cells remained morphologically adipocytes and retained the same level of accumulated triglycerides (16). 3-Deaza-(±)aristeromycin, another inhibitor of S-

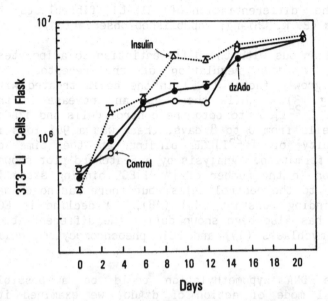

FIG. 2. Growth curves of 3T3-L1 cells treated with dzAdo or insulin.

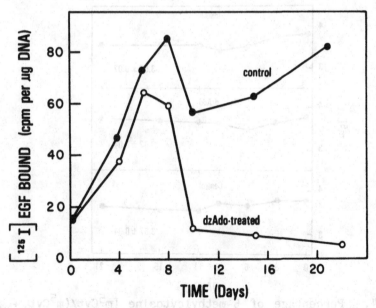

FIG. 3. Time course of the down regulation of epidermal growth factor (EGF) receptors (from ref. 18).

adenosylhomocysteine hydrolase (17), was also able to
induce the differentiation of 3T3-L1 fibroblasts to
adipocytes (P. K. Chiang, unpublished observation).

Simultaneous with the differentiation to adipocytes,
there was a down regulation of the receptors for
epidermal growth factor (EGF) in the cells treated with
dzAdo (Fig. 3). While there was an increase in the
binding of [^{125}I]EGF to both the control cells and dzAdo-
treated cells from 0 to 8 days, there was a 90% loss in
the capacity of [^{125}I]EGF binding at the time of
adipocyte formation. Analysis by a Scatchard plot showed
a reduction in the number of [^{125}I]EGF binding sites in
comparison to the control cells, but there was no change
in the binding constant (K_d) (18). A decline in EGF
receptors has also been shown during the differentiation
of mouse myoblasts (19) and PC12 pheochromocytoma cells
(20).

Since DNA hypomethylation could be a possible
biochemical mode of action of dzAdo, we examined its
effect on the status of DNA methylation in the cells
treated with dzAdo. As shown in Fig. 4, the percent of

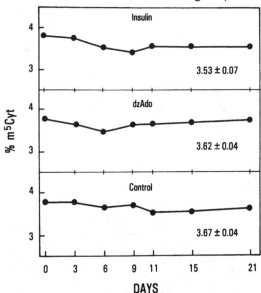

FIG. 4. Percentage of 5-methylcytosine [m^{5}Cyt/(m^{5}Cyt +
Cyt) x 100] in 3T3-L1 cells treated with dzAdo or
insulin.

5-methylcytosine (m⁵Cyt) in the cells treated with dzAdo
was the same as that of the control cells or insulin-
treated cells (3.53% as compared to 3.67 and 3.62,
respectively). Likewise, there was no discernible
difference in the ratio of [³H]m⁵Cyt/[¹⁴C]thymidine when
the cells, control vs those treated with dzAdo or
insulin, were labeled with [³H-methyl]methionine and [2-
¹⁴C]thymidine (Fig. 5). However, there appeared to be an
active methylation and demethylation process when the
cells were growing, regardless of treatments. The ratio
of [³H]methylcytosine/[¹⁴C]thymidine increased between 2-
14 days, during which there was active cell growth. The
ratio returned to about normal after 21 days when the
growth of cells reach a plateau phase.

Next, the levels of polyamines were measured in the
cells. Coincidental with the phenotypic expression of
adipocytes, putrescine increased tremendously on day 7 in

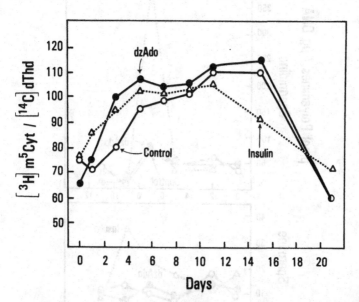

FIG. 5. Ratio of [³H]m⁵Cyt/[¹⁴C]thymidine (dThd) in 3T3-
L1 cells treated with dzAdo or insulin. At the indicated
time, the media were removed from triplicate flasks and
replaced with fresh media without methionine, containing
dzAdo or insulin, 25 μM [³H-methyl]methionine (200
mCi/mmol) and 3.4 μM [2-¹⁴C]thymidine (58 mCi/mmol) for 6
h.

both the cells treated with dzAdo and insulin (Fig. 6).
There was a 5-fold increase in putrescine in the cells
treated with dzAdo, and a 6-fold increase in the cells

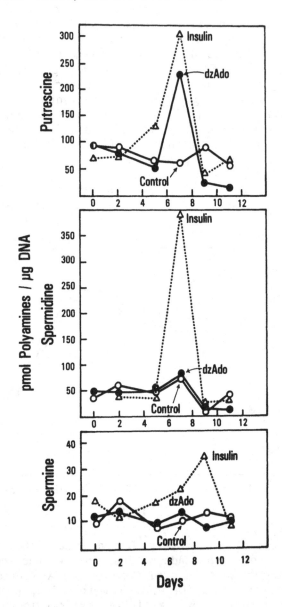

FIG. 6.   Levels of cellular polyamines in 3T3-L1 cells
treated with dzAdo or insulin.

treated with insulin. While there were also increases in spermidine (7-fold) and spermine (3-fold) in the cells treated with insulin, no changes in the levels of these two polyamines could be observed in the cells treated with dzAdo. Moreover, when the nondifferentiating 3T3-C2 cells were treated with dzAdo or insulin, the levels of polyamines remained unaltered (not shown), in contrast to the 3T3-L1 cells.

It is interesting that the levels of putrescine increased dramatically on day 7 in the cells treated with dzAdo or insulin. It has been reported that α-difluoromethylornithine, an irreversible inhibitor of ornithine decarboxylase, could block the differentiation of the 3T3-L1 cells (20). The inhibition of differentiation could be overcome completely by the provision of exogenous putrescine, spermidine or spermine, and it was concluded that polyamines were required for differentiation, although by themselves would not induce differentiation (20).

Coordinate expression of enzymes during the differentiation of 3T3-L1 cells has been reported (21-

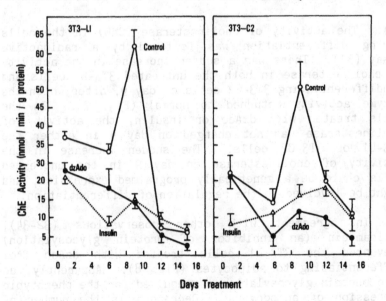

FIG. 7. Cholinesterase (ChE) activity in 3T3-L1 cells treated with dzAdo or insulin.

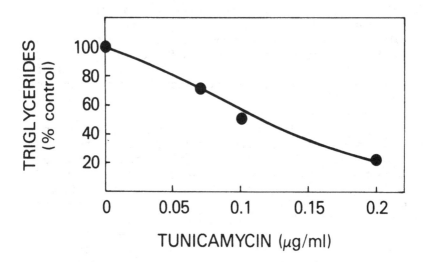

Fig. 8. Effect of tunicamycin on the accumulation of triglycerides in 3T3-L1 cells treated with dzAdo for 20 days. Each point is the mean of 5 flasks.

30). The activity of cholinesterase (ChE) in the cells during differentiation was followed by a radioactive assay (31). There was a sudden increase in the activity of cholinesterase in both the untreated 3T3-L1 cells and nondifferentiating 3T3-C2 cells on day 9, after which the enzyme activity returned to normal (Fig. 7). In the cells treated with dzAdo or insulin, the activity of cholinesterase was not changed on day 9 in either the 3T3-L1 or 3T3-C2 cells. The sudden increase in the activity of cholinesterase on day 9 in the untreated cells could be a genetically programmed expression, and might be involved in the regulation of differentiation.

In agreement with other observations (32-34), tunicamycin (an inhibitor of protein glycosylation) prevented the 3T3-L1 cells treated with dzAdo from differentiating to adipocytes (Fig. 8). Apparently, de novo protein glycosylation is required for the phenotypic expression of adipocytes. Decreases in the number of insulin receptors have been reported in 3T3-L1 cells treated with tunicamycin (32-34).

Our data showed that hypomethylation of DNA might not be involved in the differentiation of 3T3-L1 cells to adipocytes, whether dzAdo or insulin was used as an inducer. However, the hypomethylation of specific genes could not be ruled out at present; in this case, our assay methods were not sensitive enough to detect the differences. The induction of differentiation of 3T3-L1 cells by dzAdo, nonetheless, points to an effect on cellular transmethylation. The effect observed with tunicamycin suggests that receptor integrity is required, in addition to a hypomethylation step.

REFERENCES

1. Chiang, P. K. (1985) in Methods in Pharmacology, ed. Paton, D. M. (Plenum, New York), vol. 6, pp. 127-145.
2. Chiang, P. K. and Cantoni. G. L. (1979) Biochem. Pharmacol. 28, 1897-1902.
3. Guranowski, A., Montgomery, J. A., Cantoni, G. L. and Chiang, P. K. (1981) Biochemistry 20, 110-115.
4. Chiang, P. K., Richards, H. H. and Cantoni, G. L. (1977) Mol. Pharmacol. 13, 939-947.
5. Richards, H. H., Chiang, Pl K. and Cantoni, G. L. (1978) J. Biol. Chem. 253, 4476-4480.
6. Borchardt, R. T. and Pugh, S. G. (1979) in Transmethylation, ed. Usdin, E., Borchardt, R. T. and Creveling, C. R. (Elsevier, New York), pp.197-206.
7. Im, Y. S., Chiang, P. K. and Cantoni, G. L. (1979) J. Biol. Chem. 254, 11047-11050.
8. Pritchard, P. H., Chiang, P. K., Cantoni, G. L. and Vance, D. E. (1982) J. Biol. Chem. 257, 6362-6367.
9. Miura, G. A., Santangelo, J. R., Gordon, R. K. and Chiang, P. K. (1984) Anal. Biochem. 141, 161-167.
10. Ueland, P. M. (1983) Pharmacol. Rev. 34, 223-253.
11. Wiesmann, W. P., Johnson, J. P., Miura, G. A. and Chiang, P. K. (1985) Am. J. Physiol. 248, F43-F47.
12. Razin, A. and Riggs, A. D. (1980) Science 210, 604-610.
13. Doerfler, W. (1983) Ann. Rev. Biochem. 52, 93-124.
14. Jones, P. A. and Taylor, S. M. (1980) Cell 20, 85-93.
15. Green, H. and Kehinde, O. (1974) Cell 1, 113-116.
16. Chiang, P. K. (1981) Science 211, 1164-1166.

17. Chiang, P. K., Lucas, D. L. and Wright, D. G. (1984) N. Y. Acad. Sci. 435, 126-128.
18. Haigler, H. T., Gordon, R. K. and Chiang, P. K. (1985) N. Y. Acad. Sci. 463, 102-104.
19. Lim, R. W. and Hauschka, S. D. (1984) J. Cell Biol. 98, 739-747.
20. Erwin, B. G., Bethell, D. R. and Pegg, A. E. (1984). Am. J. Physiol 246, C293-C300.
21. Huff, K. and Guroff, G. (1981) J. Cell Biol. 88, 189-198.
22. Mackall, J. C., Student, A. K., Polakis. S. E. and Lane, M. D. (1976) J. Biol. Chem. 251, 6462-6464.
23. Kuri-Harcuch, W. and Green, H. (1977) J. Biol. Chem. 252, 2158-2160.
24. Wise, L. S. and Green, H. (1979) J. Biol. Chem. 254, 273-275.
25. Freytag, S. O. and Utter, M. F. (1980) Proc. Natl. Acad. Sci. USA 77, 1321-1325.
26. Pairault, J. and Green H. (1979) Proc. Natl. Acad. Sci. USA 76, 5138-5142.
27. Miller, R. and Carrrino, D. A. (1981) Archiv. Biochem. Biophys. 209, 486-503.
28. Lin, A. Y.-C. (1982) J. Biol. Chem. 257, 298-306.
29. Hu, C.-W. C., Utter, M. F. and Patel, M. S. (1983) J. Biol. Chem. 258, 2315-2320.
30. Zezulak, K. M. and Green, H. (1985) Mol. Cell. Biol. 5, 419-421.
31. Gordon, R. K., Doctor, B. P. and Chiang, P. K. (1982) Anal. Biol. Chem. 124, 333-337.
32. Rosen, O. M., Chia, G. H., Fung, C. and Rubin, C. S. (1979) J. Cell. Physiol. 99, 37-42.
33. Kohno, K., Hiragun, A., Takatsuki, A., Tamura, G. and Mitsui, H. (1980) Biochem. Biophys. Res. Commun. 93, 842-849.
34. Reed, B. C., Ronnett, G. V. and Lane, M. D. (1981) J. Biol. Chem. 78, 2908-2912.

DIFFERENTIATION OF HUMAN LEUKEMIA CELLS BY

NUCLEOSIDE ANALOGUES

Jarle Aarbakke, Per S. Prytz,
Peter K. Chiang* and
Atle Bessesen.

Institute of Medical Biology,
University of Tromsø, N-9001 Tromsø,
Norway and *Division of Biochemistry,
Walter Reed Army Institute of Research,
Washington D.C., 20307-5100, U.S.A.

Induction of differentiation in human leukemia
cells by nucleoside analogues was first reported
by Lotem and Sachs in the promyelocytic cell line
HL-60 (1). At concentrations causing a 50 %
inhibition of cell growth, bromodeoxyuridine
(BrdU) changed cell morphology, and cytosine
arabinoside (ara-C) and BrdU changed the number
of Fc and C3 rosettes. A wider range of nucleosides was tested in HL-60 cells, by means of
morphology and nitroblue tetrazolium test (NBT)
by Bodner, Ting and Gallo (2). 3-Deazauridine
(c^3urd), was the most potent while 5-azacytidine
(5-aza-Cyd) (for review see ref. 3) was only
moderately effective. Morphological criteria
indicated that the nucleosides had effects on
neutrophil maturation comparable to effects of
retinoic acid at concentrations of about 20 uM.

The nucleosides employed were selected because of
their general ability to interfere with purine
and pyrimidine metabolism and DNA synthesis.
Recently these and other variables have been
investigated in cells induced to differentiation
by nucleoside analogues. The majority of studies
have been conducted with HL-60 cells, comparing

241

untreated cells and cells induced to differentiation with respect to a number of biochemical
and biological variables.

Incorporation of analogues into DNA of differentiating HL-60 cells have been shown with BrdU
and fluoroadenine arabinoside (F-ara-A) (4,5).
Adenine arabinoside (ara-A), cyclopentenyl cytidine (cCyd) and cyclopentenyl adenosine (neplanocin A) inhibit DNA synthesis (6,7,8), while cCyd
and neplanocin A inhibit RNA synthesis (7,8).
Pertubation of nucleic acid methylation has been
demonstrated with a variety of compounds: reduced
DNA methylation by 5-aza-Cyd, 5-aza-2'-deoxycyti-
dine (5-aza-CdR) and neplanocin A (9,10,8), and
reduced RNA methylation by neplanocin A (8).

Expression of oncogenes changes during differentiation of HL-60 by nucleosides. cCyd,
neplanocin A and 5-aza-Cyd reduce the expression
of c-myc (7,8,11). On the other hand, 5-aza-Cyd
induces c-fos-expression and causes a transient
increase in c-ha-ras transcription (11).

The levels of guanosine nucleotides of HL-60
cells were decreased in maturing HL-60 cells by
a number of nucleoside analogues (12). Sialic
acid regeneration in membranes of HL-60 cells was
inhibited by ara-C (13), and glycoprotein synthesis of these cells was altered by tiazofurin
and selenazofurin (14). Finally pertubation of
cell cycle kinetics of HL-60 cells is observed
with ara-C and arabinofuranosyl-5-azacytosine
(ara-C) (15,16).

We have investigated differentiation inducing
effects of a number of nucleoside analogues which
perturb transmethylation reactions (17,18,19,20,
21,22,23). Morphology, NBT and in some studies a
newly developed quantitative assay for Fc receptors (18) were used to detect maturation of
cells.

The compounds neplanocin A,3-deazaneplanocin A
(c^3nep A), 3-deazaadenosine (c^3Ado) and 3-deaza-
aristeromycin (c^3Ari) inhibit AdoHcy hydrolase.
It has been stated that neplanocin A does not
inhibit the hydrolase of HL-60 cells (8). We have
shown (19) that neplanocin A inhibits the enzyme
of these cells with a K_i of 1nM (fig.1).

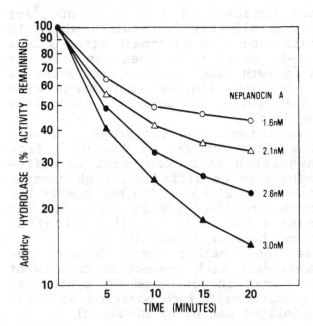

Fig.1: Time-dependent inactivation of HL-60
AdoHcy hydrolase by neplanocin A.

Inhibition of the enzyme causes a change in the
cellular levels of nucleosidyl methionine and
nucleosidylhomocysteine. Since homocysteine and
nucleosidylhomocysteine are potent inhibitors of
transmethylation reactions (for review, see 24),
the methylation of different cellular constituents are inhibited: DNA-methylation, RNA methylation, protein and phospholipid methylation.
These results make it tempting to put forward the
hypothesis that the induction of differentiation
by these compounds is causally related to pertubation of transmethylation reactions.

However, extensive work with c[3]Ado by Zimmerman
and coworkers have demonstrated biological
effects in additon to its effect on transmethylation reactions (25). We have therefore extended
our investigations of c[3]Ado and c[3]Ari in differentiating HL-60 cells.

The continuous presence of 1 to 5 uM of c³Ari
for four days was slightly cytostatic, while 10
uM was cytostatic and also cytotoxic after 3 days
exposure to HL-60 cells (21). When the drug was
removed normal growth rate was recovered after 24
and 48 hours exposure. Similar experiments with
c³Ado showed that growth was inhibited even after
removal of the drug.

The difference between the two drugs in growth
characteristics after removal of the drug from
the medium suggested that commitment to differentiation could also be different. High concentrations of c³Ari for 24 hours did not commit HL-
60 cells. Exposure to c³Ado for 24 and 6, but not
3 hours, committed the cells to differentiation
at concentrations between 10 and 100 uM.

We next questioned whether the difference between c³Ari and c³Ado with respect to commitment
mirrored a difference in action on DNA-synthesis.
Fig.2 shows results with incorporation of [³H]-
thymidine in isolated nuclei of HL-60 cells.

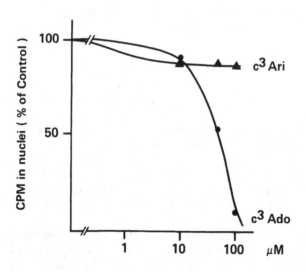

Fig. 2: Incorporation of [³H]-thymidine into
isolated nuclei of HL-60 cells.

Cells were exposed for 6 hours to the drugs and concomitantly exposed to [^{3}H]-thymidine. Only a slight decrease (about 10 %) in [^{3}H]-thymidine incorporation was noted with c^{3}Ari, and a very marked (90 %) reduction was found with c^{3}Ado. The steep shape of the dose response curve between 10 and 100 uM seen for most effects of c^{3}Ado was found also for this effect. The results may be indicative of a significant action of c^{3}Ado on DNA-synthesis while a slight effect was present for c^{3}Ari.

Similar experiments were performed with incorporation [^{14}C]-methyl from labelled [^{3}H]-methyl-methionine (fig.3). The shape of the dose respons curves were very similar to that of the curves for the thymidine incorporation. The extent of [^{14}C]-methylation of nuclear material with c^{3}Ado was dramatically decreased in comparison with controls and those treated with c^{3}Ari.

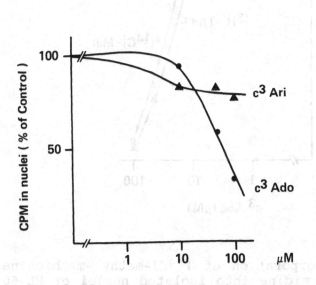

Fig.3: Incorporation of [^{14}C]-methyl-methionine into isolated nuclei of HL-60 cells.

Next we investigated whether the observed effects
were dependent upon the presence of c³Ado. After
6 hours incubation with c³Ado, and reincubation
in drug-free medium, followed by a six hour
period of incubation with [³H]-thymidine and
[¹⁴C]-methionine, a similar decrease in both
variables, compared to controls, was observed
(fig.4). Thus, 6 hours of incubation with c³Ado
causes a sustained decrease in [³H]-thymidine
incorpor-ation and methylation of nuclear
material.

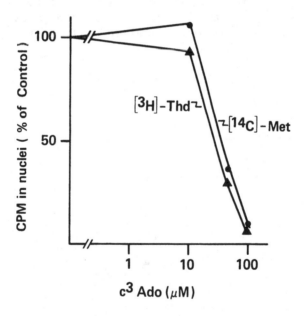

Fig. 4: Incorporation of [¹⁴C]-methyl-methionine
and [³H]-Thymidine into isolated nuclei of HL-60
cells. Cells were preincubated with c³Ado for 6
hours. Following washout and reincubation in drug
free medium cells were exposed to radiolabelled
compounds for 6 hours.

We have demonstrated additional important differences between the transmethylation inhibitors
c^3Ado and c^3Ari. Only c^3Ado commits HL-60 cells
to differentiation after short time exposure, and
c^3Ado has a much more pronounced effect on [^{3}H]-
Thymidine and [^{14}C]-methyl incorporation into
nuclei. Furthermore, the inhibition of incorporation by c^3Ado was not dependent on the
continuous presence of the drug. The results
obtained in differentiation of HL-60 cells fit
into a larger picture of the effects of c^3Ado and
c^3Ari. For instance, c^3Ado changes cyclic AMP-
levels in PGE_1 stimulated mouse lymphocytes (26)
and it interferes reversibly with microfilaments
in macrophages (27). The fact that the compound
is phosporylated, albeit to a very limited extent
(26), makes it a candidate for incorporation into
DNA. On the other hand, c^3Ari does not change
cyclic AMP-levels in PGE_1 stimulated platelets
(28), it is not phosphorylated by L1210 cells
(29) and it does not influence macrophage
microfilaments (27).

To summarize, c^3Ado and c^3Ari have been extensively characterized for the purpose of using
them as "non-pure" and "pure" transmethylation
inhibitors in the study of transmethylation
reactions in tumor cell differentiation.

REFERENCES

1. Lotem, J. and Sachs, L. (1980) Int. J. Cancer
    25, 561-564.
2. Bodner, A.J., Ting, R.C. and Gallo, R.C.
    (1981) J. Natn. Cancer Inst. 67,
    1025-1030.
3. Jones, P.A. (1985) Pharmac. Ther. 28, 17-27.
4. Koeffler, H.P., Yen, J. and Carlson, J.
    (1983) J. Cell. Physiol. 116, 111-117.
5. Spriggs, D., Robins, G., Mitchell, T. and
    Kufe, D. (1986) Biochem. Pharmacol. 35,
    247-252.

6. Munroe, D., Sugiura, M, Griffin, J. and Kufe, D. (1984) Leukemia Res. **8**, 355-361.
7. Glazer, R.I., Cohen, M.B., Hartman, K.D., Knode, M.C., Lim, M.-I. and Marquez, V.E. (1986) Biochem. Pharmac. **35**, 1841-1848.
8. Linevsky, J., Cohen, M, Hartman, K.D., Knode, M.C. and Glazer, R.I. (1985) Mol. Pharmacol., **28**, 45-50.
9. Christman, J.K., Mendelsohn, N., Herzog, D. and Schneiderman N. (1983) Cancer Res. **43**, 763-769.
10. Momparler, R.L., Bouchard, J. and Samson J. (1985) Leukemia Res. **9**, 1361-1366.
11. Brelvi, Z.S. and Studzinski, G.P. (1986) J. Cell. Biol. **102**, 2234-2243.
12. Lucas, D.L., Webster, H.K. and Wright D.G. (1984) J. Clin. Invest. **72**, 1889-1900.
13. Hindenburg, A.A., Taub, R.N., Grant, S., Chang, G. and Baker, M.A. (1985) Cancer Res. **45**, 3048-3052.
14. Sokoloski, J.A., Blair, O.C. and Sartorelli, A.C (1986) Cancer Res., **46**, 2314-2319.
15. Ross, D.W. (1985) Cancer Res. **45**, 1308-1313.
16. Dalal, M., Plowman, J., Breitman, T.R., Schuller, H.M., del Campo, A.A., Vistica, D.T., Driscoll, J.S., Cooney, D.A. and Johns, D.G. (1986) Cancer Res. **46**, 831-838.
17. Chiang, P.K., Lucas, D.L. and Wright, D.G. (1984) N.Y. Acad. Sci. **435**, 126-128
18. Aarbakke, J., Finbloom, D.S., Miura, G.A., Nacy, C.A. and Chiang, P.K. (1984). International Union of Pharmacology Ninth International Congress of Pharmacology, London. Abstr. 598.
19. Aarbakke, J., Gordon, R.K., Cross, A.S., Miura, G.A. and Chiang, P.K. (1985) Fed. Proc. **44**, 313.
20. Aarbakke, J., Miura, G.A., Prytz, P.S., Bessesen, A. and Chiang, P.K. (1985) Eur. Paediatr. Haematol Oncol. 2, 189-192.
21. Aarbakke, J., Miura, G.A., Prytz, P.S., Bessesen, A., Slørdal, L, Gordon R.K. and Chiang, P.K. (1986) Cancer Res. **46**, 5469-5472.

22. Glazer, R.I., Hartman, K.D., Knode, M.C.,
    Richard, M.M., Chiang, P.K., Tseng, C.K.H.
    and Marquez, V.E. (1986) Biochem. Biophy
    Res. Comm. **135**, 688-694.
23. Miura, G.A., Gordon, R.K., Montgomery, J.A.
    and Chiang, P.K. (1986) in Purine and
    Pyrimidine Metabolism in Man, Part B
    (Nyhan, W.L., Thompson, L.F. and Watts,
    R.W.E., eds.) pp 667-672, Plenum
    Publishing Corp.
24. Ueland, P.M. (1982). Pharmacol. Rev. **34**,
    223-253.
25. Zimmerman, T.P., Iannone, M. and Wolberg, G.
    (1984) J. Biol. Chem. **259**, 1122-1126.
26. Zimmerman, T.P., Wolberg, G., Stopford, C.R.,
    Prus, K.L. and Iannone, M.A. (1986) in
    Biological Methylation and Drug Design.
    Experimental and Clinical Roles of
    S-Adenosylmethionine (Borchardt, R.T.,
    Creveling, C.R. and Ueland, P.M. eds.) pp
    417-426, Humana Press, Clifton, NJ.
27. Stopford, C.R., Wolerg, G., Prus, K.L.,
    Reynolds-Vaughn, R. and Zimmerman, T.P.
    (1985) Proc. Natl. Acad. Sci. USA **82**,
    4060-4064.
28. Shattil,S.J., Montgomery, J.A. and Chiang,
    P.K. (1982) Blood 59, 906-912.
29. Montgomery, J.A., Clayton, S.J.,
    Thomas, H.J., Shannon, W.E., Arnett, G.,
    Bodner, A.I., Kion, I-K., Cantoni, G.L.
    and Chiang, P.K. (1982), J. Med. Chem. **25**,
    626-629.

EFFECTS OF PURINE NUCLEOSIDES ON DIFFERENTIATION IN LYMPHOHEMATOPOIETIC STEM CELL LEUKEMIA

Michael S. Hershfield, Joanne Kurtzberg,
Sara Chaffee, Michael L. Greenberg,
and Barton F. Haynes

Duke University Medical Center
Durham, North Carolina USA 27710

It is generally assumed that the antineoplastic effects of nucleoside analogues result from cytotoxicity that these agents or their metabolites exert through interference with various steps in nucleotide or nucleic acid metabolism. Nucleosides may also alter cellular differentiation, though the basis for this type of action remains to be established. Other papers will address the in vitro effects of purine nucleoside analogues on the maturation of myeloid leukemia cell lines and suggest some mechanisms that may be involved. I will review in vivo and in vitro evidence that abnormal concentrations of naturally occuring purine nucleosides, as well as their analogues, may affect the differentiation of leukemic stem cells.

Some indication that purine nucleosides might influence stem cell differentiation comes from the fact that certain inborn errors of purine nucleoside metabolism are associated with selective absence of lymphoid lineages. Inherited deficiency of adenosine deaminase (ADA) results in failure of both T and B cell development, causing severe combined immunodeficiency disease (SCID) (1), while absence of purine nucleoside phosphorylase (PNP) is associated with selective T lymphopenia and impaired cell mediated immunity (2). Selective toxicity of nucleosides to lymphocytes could account for lymphopenia in ADA and PNP deficiencies, but on a formal basis so could selective interference by nucleosides with a step specifically required for lymphoid differentiation.

    Impaired stem cell differentiation has always been
considered a potential cause of inherited immunodeficiency
diseases of unknown etiology, but in the case of ADA and PNP
deficiencies this possibility has received less attention
than nucleoside toxicity, largely for two reasons. First,
no compelling clinical observation has pointed directly
towards interference with stem cell differentiation, as
opposed to cytotoxicity, as the cause of lymphopenia.
Second, the ADA and PNP substrates adenosine (Ado),
2'-deoxyadensoine (dAdo), guanosine (Guo) and
2'-deoxyguanosine (dGuo) are toxic to mature and immature
cultured lymphoid cells and cell lines (3). While toxicity
is easily investigated in vitro, there has been no cell
model for systematically examining the effects of
nucleosides on lymphoid vs. nonlymphoid differentiation.
The near absence of lymphoid tissues in affected children is
a major obstacle to direct experimental studies of ADA or
PNP deficient lymphocytes or lymphocyte progenitors.

    Around 1980 clinical oncologists began to investigate
the use of a potent, tight binding inhibitor of ADA,
2'-deoxycoformycin (dCF) in the treatment of acute T
lymphoblastic leukemia. This provided a unique opportunity
to examine in vivo the biochemical consequences of
pharmacologically induced ADA deficiency in large numbers of
clonally related malignant lymphoid cells arrested at
several stages of differentiation. Since malignant
transformation may occur at the level of primitive stem
cells, these studies also offered the possibility of
acquiring specific insight into the effects of ADA
deficiency on stem cells as well as immature, but committed
lymphoid progenitors.

    The biochemical changes observed in circulating T
lymphoblasts associated with dCF treatment corresponded to
the effects of Ado and dAdo that had been observed in red
cells of ADA deficient patients or in vitro in studies with
cultured, ADA-inhibited T cell lines. These effects
included accumulation of dATP derived from dAdo (4-7) and
accumulation of S-adenosylhomocysteine (AdoHcy) (7-10), a
potent competitive inhibitor of S-adenosylmethionine
(AdoMet) dependent transmethylation, caused by inhibition by
Ado (8, 9) and inactivation by dAdo (10) of AdoHcy
hydrolase. In some patients these changes were small and no
clinical response resulted; in others systemic toxicity
occurred. In the majority, the metabolic effects of induced

ADA deficiency were significant and were accompanied by a selective, striking decline in circulating T lymphoblasts over a period of a few days. In contrast to this typical lymphocytotoxic response, in two patients a distinctly different phenomenon was observed, namely, an abrupt change in the leukemic phenotype from T lymphoblastoid to myeloid (11, 12). Each of these patients had originally been diagnosed as having acute T cell leukemia and the characteristics of their leukemic cells had been unaltered by prior cytotoxic therapy. However, the sudden change in lineage immediately following treatment with dCF led to the conclusion that malignant transformation had occurred in a pluripotent stem cell capable of both lymphoid and myeloid differentiation.

In one case, a decline in circulating T lymphoblasts several days prior to the appearance of myeloid leukemia suggested selective lymphocytotoxicity followed by outgrowth of a dCF-resistant myeloid clone (11). In the other patient, who was studied in considerably more detail, both before and on a daily basis during the 7 day period of dCF treatment and phenotypic conversion, evidence strongly indicated a direct effect of ADA inhibition on differentiation (12). Among other findings supporting this interpretation, the total number of circulating leukemic cells remained in the 60,000-80,000 range during the change in phenotype, suggesting a precursor-product relationship between the lymphoblastoid and myeloid cell populations. The same abnormal karyotype was present in T lymphoblasts obtained before treatment and in promyelocytic cells examined after conversion, proof that the two populations arose from the same malignant clone. Subsequent studies with a cell line derived from the patient's leukemic cells, called DU.528, supported the conclusion regarding the stem cell nature of the leukemia and have permitted direct studies of the effects of nucleosides on its differentiation (13).

We established DU.528 from leukemic cells that were cryopreserved at the time of diagnosis, prior to treatment. DU.528 and clones derived from it by limiting dilution had the same karyotype as the patient's circulating T lymphoblasts and promyelocytes. When first placed in culture, the cells had an undifferentiated lymphoblastoid morphology and expressed the 3A1 (now CD-7) surface antigen, a pan T cell marker that is expressed on prothymocytes in

the embryonic thymus (14, 15). Other T cell markers and
markers of nonlymphoid hematopoietic cells were initially
not expressed. Over the next two months, the cells
spontaneously underwent a gradual transformation to a
population of predominantly myeloid cells at various stages
of maturation. During this transformation cells were
observed to express simultaneously CD-7 (3A1) and
myeloid-specific markers, but eventually fully mature
neutrophils and monocytes appeared, which lacked lymphoid
markers. Following terminal myeloid differentiation,
undifferentiated T lymphoblasts expressing only CD-7 (3A1)
reemerged as the dominant cell population.

Over a 2 year period in continuous culture the DU.528
cell line (and clones derived from it) maintained the
undifferentiated T lymphoblastoid phenotype, but continued
to give rise spontaneously to mature cells of at least three
cell lineages, T lymphoid, granulocytic/monocytic, and
erythroid. Initially, 'waves' of differentiation affecting
most cells in a culture occurred, but this capacity for
multilineage differentiation gradually declined. By 24-30
months in culture, spontaneous differentiation ceased and
the line remained T lymphoblastoid. During the period when
spontaneous differentiation was occurring we also observed
that myeloid differentiation could be induced by treatment
with a number of agents, including dibutyryl cyclic AMP,
phorbol esters, 5-azacytidine, and of most interest to us,
by Ado and dAdo at concentrations that mimicked the effects
produced by dCF treatment. As the capacity for spontaneous
differentiation declined, so did sensitivity to induction of
differentiation by nucleosides and non-nucleosides (13).

EFFECTS OF NUCLEOSIDES ON DIFFERENTIATION OF DU.528

Inhibition of ADA alone did not alter growth or
phenotype of DU.528, but dCF potentiated the effects of Ado
and dAdo. The lowest concentrations of Ado and dAdo that
altered phenotype (2-20 uM) also inhibited growth of DU.528.
However, since the absolute numbers of cells expressing
myeloid surface antigens or other markers of mature myeloid
maturation increased by up to 5 fold over untreated control
cultures, the change in phenotype represented a real effect
on differentiation, and not simply selective killing of a
sensitive lymphoblastoid cell subpopulation (13). Uridine
and deoxycytidine, which diminish the formation or block the

cytotoxic effects of nucleotides derived from low concentrations of Ado and dAdo (reviewed in reference 3), also diminished effects of 2-20 uM Ado and dAdo on differentiation of DU.528. Thus, growth inhibition caused by Ado and dAdo nucleotide formation appeared to be necessary for induction of differentiation. However, since DU.528 remained sensititve to the cytotoxicity of Ado and dAdo after loss of its capacity to differentiate, cytotoxicity alone was not sufficient to induce differentiation.

During dCF treatment of the patient from whom the DU.528 cell line was derived, a marked accumulation of AdoHcy, as well as of dATP, occurred in malignant cells immediately prior to the onset of phenotypic conversion (12). The ratio of AdoMet to AdoHcy, an index of the ability to transmethylate, fell by 10 fold in leukemic cells. To selectively evaluate the in vitro effects of AdoHcy accumulation on differentiation of DU.528, we carried out some experiments using analogues of Ado that are neither phosphorylated nor deaminated, but which cause potent inhibition of AdoHcy hydrolase (16). 3-Deazaadenosine (c3Ado) is a substrate for the enzyme and causes accumulation in cells of 3-deazaadenosylhomocysteine as well as AdoHcy; the carbocyclic analogue of c3Ado, 3-deazaaristeromycin (c3Ari), inhibits but is not a substrate for AdoHcy hydrolase. During a 3 hour incubation, 5 uM c3Ari increased the concentration of AdoHcy in DU.528 cells by almost 10 fold, from 2.7 to 26 nmol/10^9 cells, decreasing the ratio of AdoMet to AdoHcy from 12 to 1.6. Incubation for 3 hours with 5 uM c3Ado increased AdoHcy by <2 fold, but 3-deazaadenosylhomocysteine accumulated to 12 nmol/10^9 cells.

The experiment summarized in Table 1 shows the effects of a 3 day exposure to 1 uM concentrations of these analogues (which caused <50% growth inhibition) on the differentiation of DU.528.37, a subline in culture for less than a year, which was still undergoing periodic spontaneous differentiation, and on DU.528.101, a subline in culture for over 3 years, which no longer showed spontaneous differentiation. The effects of c3Ari and c3Ado are compared with 2 kinds of positive controls, a) with cells treated with 50 uM dibutyryl cAMP, and b) with the combination of 5 uM dCF, 10 uM dAdo, 5 uM Ado and 20 uM uridine. The effects of this combination are primarily due

TABLE 1. INDUCTION OF DIFFERENTIATION BY PURINES

DU.528.37	Morphology		Function	Antigen	expression	
	Blasts	Myeloid	NBT	3A1	HL60-3	My10
Control	*83*	*16*	*1*	*85*	*10*	*2*
C3Ari 1 uM	33	57	23	42	81	72
C3Ado 1 uM	29	60	15	58	74	21
dCF,dAdo,Ado*	16	64	42	45	86	15
DBcAMP 50 uM	22	48	40	48	89	12
DU.528.101						
Control	*100*	*0*	*3*	*92*	*2*	*0*
C3Ari 1 uM	100	0	4	94	1	0
C3Ado 1 uM	100	0	3	94	0	0
dCF,dAdo,Ado*	100	0	11	94	1	0
DBcAMP 50 uM	100	0	3	92	2	0

Values are percentages of cells positive after 3 days
NBT=nitroblue tetrazolium reduction
*5 uM dCF, 10 uM dAdo, 5 uM Ado, 20 uM Uri

to accumulation of dATP, but we had found that the addition of Ado with uridine (without effect by themselves) potentiated the effects of dAdo on differentiation while diminsihing its cytotoxicity (13). With DU.528.37, all 4 inducers caused a decrease in the percentage of 3A1 (CD-7) positive, undifferentiated lymphoblastoid cells and an increase in the percentage of myeloid cells that reduced NBT and expressed the HL60-3 (17) myeloid surface antigen. c3Ari caused a strong induction of the My10 antigen, which is characteristic of myeloid progenitors (18). None of the 4 inducers altered the phenotype of the DU.528.101 subline. These results suggest that accumulation of AdoHcy (or an AdoHcy analogue) is able to induce differentiation of DU.528, and this effect may not necessarily involve inhibition of growth. As with nucleotide-dependent induction of differentiation, accumulation of AdoHcy alone is not sufficient to cause differentiation since the response is lost with loss of the capacity for spontaneous differentiation.

The fact that a differentiative response to dCF treatment has occurred in only two patients, as well as the fact that most leukemic T cell lines exhibit only a cytotoxic response to Ado and dAdo in vitro, suggest that the differentiative response that we have observed probably represents a unique property of a very primitive stem cell. This cell would appear to have some characteristics of an immature T lymphoblast (expression of CD-7), but unlike most leukemic T lymphoblasts, it has not become irreversibly committed to the T lineage. Ongoing efforts are aimed at identifying and characterizing other patients with CD-7 positive stem cell leukemia, and at isolating the normal counterpart of this cell. Ultimately, understanding the mechanisms that underly the effects of purine nucleosides and their analogues on differentiation of this stem cell may provide new approaches to the treatment of the earliest stage at which malignant transformation occurs in leukemia, and may provide a better understanding of the basis for selective lymphopenia in ADA and PNP deficiency.

REFERENCES

1. Giblett ER, Anderson PE, Cohen F, Pollara B, Meuwissen HJ (1972) Lancet ii, 1067-1069.
2. Giblett ER, Amman AJ, Wara DW, Sandman R, Diamond LK, (1975) Lancet i, 1010-1013.
3. Kredich NM, Hershfield MS (1983) in The Metabolic Basis of Inherited Disease, Stanbury JB, Wyngaarden JB, Fredrickson DS, Goldstein J, Brown M, eds. McGraw-Hill, 5th ed, pp 1157-1201.
4. Coleman MS, Donofrio J, Hutton JJ, Hahn L, Daoud A, Lampkin B, Dyminski J (1978) J Biol Chem 253, 1619-1626.
5. Cohen A, Hirschhorn R, Horowitz SD, Rubinstein A, Polmar SH, Hong R, Martin DW Jr (1978) Proc Natl Acad Sci 75, 472-476.
6. Mitchell BS, Koller CA, and Heyn R (1980) Blood 56, 556-559.
7. Hershfield MS, Kredich NM, Koller CA, Mitchell BS, Kurtzberg J, Kinney TR, Falletta JM (1983) Cancer Res 43, 3451-3458.
8. Kredich NM, Martin DW Jr (1977) Cell 12, 931-938.
9. Kredich NM, Hershfield MS (1979) Proc Natl Acad Sci 76, 2450-2454.
10. Hershfield MS (1979) J Biol Chem 254, 22-25.

11. Murphy SB, Stass S, Kalwinsky D, Rivera G (1983) Br J Haematol 55, 285-293.
12. Hershfield MS, Kurtzberg J, Harden E, Moore JO, Whang-Peng J, Haynes BF (1984) Proc Natl Acad Sci USA 81, 253-257.
13. Kurtzberg J, Bigner SH, Hershfield MS (1985) J Exp Med 162, 1561-1578.
14. Haynes BF, Eisenbarth GS, Fauci AS (1979) Proc Natl Acad Sci USA 76, 5829-5833.
15. Harden EA, Haynes BF (1985) Sem Hematol 22, 13-26.
16. Chiang PK, Miura GA in Biological Methylation and Drug Design Borchardt RT, Creveling CR, Ueland PM eds (1986) Humana Press, Clifton NJ, 239-251.
17. McKolanis JR, Borowitz MJ, Tuck FL, Metzgar RS (1984) in Leukocyte Typing Bernard A, Boumsell L, Dausset J, Milstein C, Schlossman SF eds. Springer-Verlag, Heidelberg, 387-394.
18. Civin CI, Strauss LC, Brovall C, Fackler MJ, Schwartz JF, Shaper JH (1984) J Immunol 133, 157-165.

EFFECT OF METHYLATION INHIBITORS ON

PHORBOL ESTER INDUCED DIFFERENTIATION OF

HL-60 PROMYELOCYTIC LEUKEMIA CELLS

John A. Duerre*, Lee D. Nelson†, William P.
Wiesmann† and Peter K. Chiang†
*Department of Microbiology and Immunology,
Ireland Research Laboratory, University of
North Dakota Medical School, Grand Forks, ND
58202
†Walter Reed Army Institute of Research,
Washington, DC 20307

INTRODUCTION

Cells of the promyelocytic leukemia line, HL-60,
differentiate into a macrophage-like cell in response to
phorbol-12-myristate-13-acetate (phorbol ester). The
discrete changes include adherence to surfaces, motility
and acquisition of macrophage-like characteristics,
including synthesis of discrete proteins (1-3). Of
particular interest has been the observation that the
methylation inhibitor, 3-deazaadenosine, blocked the
phorbol ester induction of the differentiation functions,
adherence and motility (3). Specifically,
3-deazaadenosine arrested the induction of a specific
differentiation protein but had no effect on the early or
late phosphorylation events initiated by phorbol esters
(3,4).

The role that methylation reactions play in
differentiation of cells remains unclear. Methylation of
phospholipids or carboxyl groups of proteins has been
implicated in the regulation of numerous cellular
processes including leukocyte chemotaxis (5), cellular
secretion (6,7), ion transport (8), signal transduction
(9) and cellular differentiation (10,11). Specific
relationships between phospholipid methylation and (or)
protein carboxyl methylation and cellular differentiation
also have been established through the use of the
methylation inhibitor, 3-deazaadenosine (12-14). Indeed,

one of the most sensitive targets for 3-deazaadenosine
appears to be the methylation of phospholipids (15,16).
This inhibition is brought about by increases in
intracellular S-adenosylhomocysteine, and the formation
of 3-deazaadenosylhomocysteine, both of which act as a
potent blocker of S-adenosylhomocysteine hydrolase (17).
Under conditions were the methylation of phospholipids is
markedly inhibited, the total amount of phospholipid
synthesized in 3-deazaadenosine treated cells remained
unchanged. Hence, blockage of phospholipid methylation
appears to be compensated for by increased synthesis of
phospholipids through the CDP-choline pathway (15,16).
Consequently, changes brought about by 3-deazaadenosine
need not be directed solely at phospholipids. Numerous
other methylation reactions could be perturbed by this
compound; i.e. methylation of nucleic acids or proteins.
Montgomery et al. (18), suggest that the antiviral
properties of 3-Deazaadenosine and its carboxcyclic
analogs may be due to inhibit methylation of 5' cap of
viral mRNA. Inhibition of the methylation of mRNA would
lead to a cascade of effects. Indeed, inhibition of the
synthesis of various proteins has been observed in the
presence of 3-deazaadenosine (3,14,17). Conversely, no
such effects were observed when the purine analog,
3-deaza-(±)aristeromycin, was used as a methylation
blocker (19). To gain further insight into the role that
methylation plays in differentiation, we examined the
effects that various purine analogs had on the growth,
protein synthesis, and the methylation of DNA, proteins
and phospholipids in HL-60 cells during phorbol ester
induced differentiation.

RESULTS

Effect of purine analogs on protein synthesis and
phospholipid methylation.

   The purine analogs, 3-deazaadenosine, 3-deaza-(±)-
aristeromycin and neplanocin A markedly inhibited the
transfer of methyl groups from L-[methyl-^{3}H]methionine to
phosphatidylethanolamine (Table 1). Of all the drugs
tested, 3-deaza-(±)aristeromycin appeared to be the most
specific. At a concentration of 20 µM, this drug
completely inhibited the methylation of phospholipids

TABLE 1

EFFECT OF PURINE ANALOGS AND PHORBOL ESTER ON SYNTHESIS OF PHOSPHATIDYCHOLINE

Drug	μM	Time Exposed to drug	Phosphatidycholine [³H] DPM/10⁷ cells^b	% Control	Phosphatidycholine [¹⁴C] DPM/10⁷ cells	% Control
None			4790		940	
dzAri	10	4 d	2090	44	1380	146
dzAri	20	4 d	0	0	485	52
dzAri	40	4 d	0	0	120	13
Nep A	0.5	4 d	195	4	1438	153
Nep A	2	4 d	80	2	1020	108
dzAdo	40	4 d	527	11	1993	212
dzAdo	100	3 h	170	4	1640	175
PMA	0.1	2 d	710	15	5500	585

aFrom 5-6 mg cells were suspended in 20 mL of RPMI 1640 medium containing 60 μCi of L-[methyl-³H]methionine, 20 μCi of [1,2-C¹⁴]choline and the same amount or purine analog as the growth medium. The reaction was terminated after 1 h with the addition of 10% Cl₃CCOOH. The cells were washed 5 times with 10% Cl₃CCOOH and suspended in 1 mL saline-0.1 M HCl. The lipids were extracted with methanol-chloroform (1:2 v/v) and fractionated on an Ultracil amine bonded column employing Gilson model 811 HPLC system (20).

b1 x 10⁷ cells contain approximately 1 mg protein.

with only marginal effects on the rate of growth and
protein synthesis (Table 2). Apparently the CDP-choline
pathway can supply sufficient phosphatidylcholine to
fulfill the requirements of the cell. When the
concentration of 3-deaza-(±)aristeromycin was held at 10
µM the incorporation of [1,2-^{14}C]choline into phospho-
tidylcholine was stimulated. The cells responded
similarly when 0.5 µM neplanocin A or 40 µM
3-deazaadenosine was added. However, when these two
drugs were added at concentrations sufficient to
completely inhibit phospholipid methylation, cytotoxic
effects were observed. This was most apparent when
3-deazaadenosine was used as a methylation blocker. To
completely block phospholipid methylation, this drug must
be added at concentration greater than 100 µM. However,
under such conditions growth is completely arrested, and
within 3 h protein synthesis was only 42% of the control
values (Table 2). After 6 h, the cells round up and cell
death became apparent as measured by trypan blue
exclusion test.

In both control and phorbol ester treated cells
[^{3}H]methyl groups from L-[methyl-^{3}H]methionine were
effectively transferred to phosphatidylethanolamine in a
linear manner with respect to time. However, 48 h after
adding phorbol ester the rate was only 15% of that of the
control cells (Table 1). Under similar conditions, the
rate of incorporation of L-[methyl-^{3}H]methionine into
proteins was essentially the same as the untreated cells
(Table 2). There was a 5-6-fold increase in the rate of
incorporation of [1,2-^{14}C]choline into phosphatidylcholine in the phorbol ester treated cells (Table 1).
Although the majority of the [^{14}C]choline was
incorporated into phosphatidylcholine, measurable amounts
also were incorporated into lysophosphatidylcholine in
the control cells (60 DPM/10^7 cells). No radioactive
lysophosphatidylcholine was observed in the phorbol ester
treated cells, nor were any [^{3}H]methyl groups detected in
phosphatidylmonoethanolamine or phosphatidyldimethyl-
ethanolamine in these cells. In the control cells,
detectable amounts of [^{3}H]methyl groups were incorporated
into phosphatidylmonoethanolamine and phosphatidyl-
dimethylethanolamine. Little or no [^{14}C]choline was
incorporated into sphingomyelin in the control or phorbol
ester treated cells.

TABLE 2

EFFECT OF PURINE ANALOGS AND PHORBOL ESTER ON GROWTH AND PROTEIN SYNTHESIS

Drug	μM	Time exposed to drug	Growth cells/mL x 10⁻³	Growth % Control	Protein synthesis DPM/mg x 10⁻³	Protein synthesis % Control
None			165		176	
dzAri	10	4 d	153	93	167	95
dzAri	20	4 d	122	74	125	71
dzAri	40	4 d	83	50	85	48
Nep A	0.5	4 d	86	52	153	87
Nep A	2	4 d	45	27	127	72
dzAdo	40	4 d	114	69	111	63
dzAdo	100	3 h	140	100	74	42
PMA	0.1	2 d	60	36	229	130

After lipids had been extracted with organic solvents as described under Table 1, the residual proteins were dissolved in 5 ml of 0.3% sodium dodecyl sulfate. Protein was estimated with Lowry reagent using bovine albumin as standard and radioactivity determined by scintillation spectrometry.

Effect of purine analogs on phorbol ester induced differentiation.

When the cells were cultured in the presence of the various purine analogs for 24 h prior to inducing differentiation, the results were quite surprising. 3-Deazaadenosine (40 μM), 3-deaza-(±)aristeromycin (20 μM) and neplanocin A (2 μM) completely blocked phospholipid methylation (Table 3). However, 90-95% of the cells adhered to surface and acquired the characteristics of macrophages. One of the most characteristic features of monocytes is the high level of nonspecific esterases (21). When α-naphthal acetate was used as a substrate, no significant difference was observed between the level of nonspecific esterase activity in cells pretreated with 3-deaza-(±)-aristeromycin and those without. The level of these enzymes appeared to be enhanced when the cells had been pretreated with neplanocin A or 3-deazaadenosine. However, more specific assays for the levels of the various lysosomal enzymes will have to be performed to confirm these results.

If the cells were pretreated with the purine analogs for 48 h prior to inducing differentiation with phorbol ester, the results were quite similar. However, increasing the time of exposure to these compounds for up to 3-4 days resulted in increased cytotoxicity and cell death as measured by the trypan blue exclusion test. Cell death and subsequent lysis resulted in release of autolytic enzymes which prevented attachment of the cell to the surface. However, many of the cells formed aggregates and acquired macrophage-like characteristics including a positive test for nonspecific esterases.

CONCLUSIONS

In conclusion, it is quite evident that the inhibition of phospholipid methylation has little or no effect on the growth and (or) phorbol ester induced differentiation of promyelocytic leukemia cells to macrophage-like cells. Of all the methylation blockers tested, 3-deaza-(±)aristeromycin appeared to be the most specific. This compound, at 20 μM, can be used to completely block phospholipid methylation without

TABLE 3

EFFECT OF PURINE ANALOGS ON PROTEIN SYNTHESIS AND PHOSPHOLIPID METHYLATION IN HL-60 CELLS INDUCED TO DIFFERENTIATE WITH PHORBOL ESTER[a]

Additions	Phosphatidylcholine		Protein synthesis	
	DPM/mg cells	% Control	DPM/mg x 10^{-3}	% Control
None	13700	0	595	0
PMA (0.1 μM)	2460	18	651	109
dzAri (20 μM) + PMA	0	0	380	65
dzAdo (40 μM) + PMA	550	4	380	65
Nep A (2.0 μM) + PMA	260	2	320	54

[a]Cells were cultured for 24 h in the presence or absence of purine analogs, after which time 0.1 μM phorbol ester was added to induce differentiation. After 48 h the cells were pulse labeled with 60 μCi of L-[methyl-^{3}H]methionine. The reaction was terminated after 1 h with the addition of 10% Cl_3CCOOH and the cells washed and fractionated as described under Table 1. Results are the average of two separate experiments.

effecting the rate of growth, as measured by cell count, protein or DNA synthesis. Contrarywise, 3-deazaadenosine, which has been extensively employed as a methylation blocker, markedly depressed the rate of growth of HL-60 cells. Unlike the mouse macrophage cell line, where only the synthesis of a few specific proteins are inhibited (19), total protein synthesis is markedly inhibited in HL-60. It may well be that methylation of mRNA is adversely effected by 3-deazaadenosine with the subsequent shut down of protein synthesis.

When the methylation inhibitors were added to HL-60 cells in culture there was a shift in synthesis of phosphatidylcholine from the methylation pathway to the CDP-choline pathway. Apparently the CDP-choline pathway can compensate for the lack of synthesis of phosphatidylcholine via the methylation pathway.

When promyelocytic cells were exposed to phorbol ester they adhere to the surface within 24 h and demonstrate characteristics of macrophages including elevated levels of nonspecific esterases. In agreement with the data of Cassileth et al. (22) the synthesis of phosphatidylcholine is shifted from the methylation pathway to the CDP-choline pathway. Furthermore, if the methylation pathway was completely blocked prior to addition of phorbol ester, the differentiation process was unaffected or even enhanced. Apparently the CDP-choline pathway can supply all the cellular requirements for phosphatidylcholine. Thus, lipid methylation appears to play no role in signal transduction in phorbol ester induced differentiation of HL-60 cells.

REFERENCES

1. Rovera, G., Santoli, D and Damsky, C. (1979) Proc. Natl. Acad. Sci. USA 76, 2779-2783.
2. Huberman, E. and Callahan, M.F. (1979) Proc. Natl. Acad. Sci. USA 76, 1293-1297.
3. Feuerstein, N. and Cooper, H.L. (1984) Biochim. Biophys. Acta 781, 247-256.
4. Feuerstein, N. and Cooper, H.L. (1983) J. Biol. Chem. 258, 10786-10793.

5. VenKatasubramanian, K., Hirata, F., Gagnon, C., Corcoran, B.A., O'Dea, R.F., Axelrod, J. and Schiffman, E. (1980) Mol. Immunol. 17, 201-207.
6. O'Dea, R.F., Viveros, O.H. and Diliberto, E.J., Jr. (1981) Biochem, Pharm. 30, 1163-1168.
7. Billingsley, M.L., Kim, S. and Kuhn, D.M. (1985) Neurosci. 15, 159-171.
8. Toyoshima, S., Saido, T., Makishima, F. and Osawa, (1983) T. Biochem. Biophys. Res. Commun. 114, 1126-1131.
9. Swanson, R.J. and Applebury, M.L. (1983) J. Biol. Chem. 258, 10599-10605.
10. Zuckerman, S.H., O'Dea, R.F., Olson, J.M. and Douglas, S.D. (1982) Mol. Immunol. 19, 281-286.
11. Fetters, H.A., Kelleher, J. and Duerre, J.A. (1985) Canad. J. Biochem. Cell Biol. 63, 1112-1119.
12. Zelenka, P.S., Beebe, D.C. and Fegans, D.E. (1982) Science 217, 1265-1267.
13. Aksamit, R.R., Falk, W. and Cantoni, G.L. (1982) J. Biol. Chem. 257, 621-625.
14. Pike, M.C., Kredich, N.M. and Synderman, R. (1978) Proc. Natl. Acad. Sci. USA 75, 3928-3932.
15. Chiang, P.K., Im, Y.S. and Cantoni, G.L. (1980) Biochem. Biophys. Res. Commun. 94, 174-181.
16. Pritchard, P.H., Chiang, P.K., Cantoni, G.L. and Vance, D.E. (1982) J. Biol. Chem. 257, 6362-6367.
17. Chiang, P.K. (1984) In "Purine metabolism in Man-IV," (DeBruyn, C.H.M., Simmonds, H.A. and Mueller, M., eds.) pp. 199-203, Plenum Publishing Corp.
18. Montgomery, J.A., Clayton, S.J., Thomas, H.J., Shannon, W.M., Arnett, G., Bodner, A.J., Kim, I.K., Cantoni, G.L. and Chiang, P.K. (1982) J. Med. Chem. 25, 626-629.
19. Aksamit, R.R., Backlund, P.S., Jr. and Cantoni, G.L. (1983) J. Biol. Chem. 258, 20-23.
20. Hanson, V.L., Park, J.Y., Osborn, T.W. and Kiral, R.M. (1981) J. Chromat. 205, 393-400.
21. Stuart, A.E., Habeshaw, J.A. and Davidson, A.E. (1978) In: D.M. Weir (ed.) Handbook of Experimental Immunology, Vol. 1, pp. 31.21-31.23, Oxford, Blackwell.
22. Cassileth, P.A., Suholet, D. and Cooper, R.A. (1981) Blood 58, 237-243.

PERTURBATION OF HOMOCYSTEINE METABOLISM BY PHARMACOLOGICAL AGENTS IN EXPERIMENTAL AND CLINICAL USE.

Per M. Ueland, Helga Refsum, Asbjørn M. Svardal, Rune Djurhuus and Svein Helland

Clinical Pharmacological Unit, Department of Pharmacology, University of Bergen, 5000 Bergen, Norway.

INTRODUCTION

Homocysteine, a sulfur amino acid, was discovered over 50 years ago by DuVigneaud as the product of demethylation of methionine This discovery was followed by reports that homocysteine could support growth of animals fed diets deficient in either cysteine, methionine or choline (1).

The possible involvement of homocysteine in human disease has stimulated the interest in this amino acid.

In 1962 homocystine was detected in urine from two mentally retarded children (2). Since then, homocystinuria has been defined as an inherited disorder of homocysteine metabolism. Children afflicted with this disease suffer from premature arteriosclerosis (for review, see ref. 3). This discovery was followed by research into the possible role of homocysteine in the development of arteriosclerotic lesions (4). Recent clinical studies in man strongly indicate a relation between elevated plasma homocysteine and arteriosclerotic disease (5).

During the last 10 years there have been numerous reports that malignant cells cannot use homocysteine instead of methionine to fully support growth. Non-transformed cells thrive under these conditions (6). The biochemical basis of the so-called methionine dependence of cancer cells is not understood, and this concept has been questioned by some workers (7). Nevertheless, the possible role of homocysteine in malignant growth is currently a subject of interest.

The possible centrality of homocysteine in pathological processes like arteriosclerosis and malignant growth, points to the possibility that pharmacological interference with homocysteine metabolism may have important implications. There are examples of pharmacological

269

agents that either block homocysteine production or perturb the metabolism of this amino acid. This article reviews some recent data on
this topic. Some central features of homocysteine metabolism and
recent advances in methods for quantitation of homocysteine in
biological material, are also reviewed.

METABOLISM AND DISPOSITION OF HOMOCYSTEINE

S-Adenosylmethionine functions as a methyldonor in numerous
transmethylation reactions. All these reactions produce stoichio-
metric amounts of S-adenosylhomocysteine (AdoHcy). This product
of transmethylation functions as a negative feed-back inhibitor of this
class of reactions. The inhibition is relieved upon metabolic
degradation of AdoHcy to homocysteine and adenosine. This reaction
is catalyzed by the ubiquitous enzyme, AdoHcy hydrolase (EC
3.3.1.1.) (8).

The structural formulae of homocysteine and related compounds
are shown in figure 1.

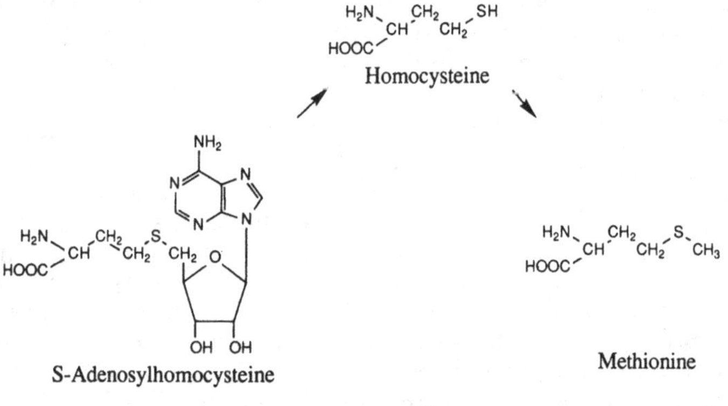

FIG. 1. **Structural formulae of homocysteine and related
compounds.**

The AdoHcy hydrolase reaction, the only known source of
homocysteine in vertebrates, is reversible and the equilibrium lies in
the direction of synthesis of AdoHcy. The metabolic flux *in vivo* is in
the hydrolytic direction because both adenosine and homocysteine are
continuously removed from the intracellular compartment (8).

Intracellular homocysteine is either methylated to methionine or
is condensed with serine to form the thioether, cystathionine. The
salvage to methionine is catalyzed by two separate enzymes. One,

betaine-homocysteine methyltransferase (EC 2.1.1.5.), requires betaine as methyl donor and this enzyme is confined to liver and kidney. The other enzyme, 5-methyltetrahydrofolate-homocysteine methyltransferase (EC 2.1.1.13., known as methionine synthase) uses 5-methyltetrahydrofolate, and is widely distributed in tissues of vertebrates. Notably, this enzyme is one of the two enzymes dependent on cobalamin, and homocysteine is thus linked both to the metabolism of reduced folates and vitamin B12 (3)

The methionine synthase reaction is the only known metabolic pathway common to folate, vitamin B12 and methionine. Based on both experimental and clinical evidence, Noronha and Silverman (9) and Herbert and Zalusky (10) advanced the so-called "methyl trap" hypothesis, which states that the consequences of vitamin B12 deficiency stem from reduced activity of the vitamin B12 dependent conversion of 5-methyltetrahydrofolate to tetrahydrofolate. Under these conditions, reduced folates are trapped as 5-methyltetra-hydrofolate, thereby causing slowdown in thymidylate and purine biosynthesis. Homocysteine is the methyl acceptor in this reaction, and this implies that the availability of intracellular homocysteine is critical for the quantitative relation between 5-methyltetrahydrofolate and other reduced folates.

Conversion of homocysteine to cystathionine represents the alternative pathway to methylation. This reaction, which is essentially irreversible, is catalyzed by cystathionine ß-synthase (EC 4.2.1.22). The bulk of this enzyme resides in the liver but human brain is also rich in cystathionine ß-synthase. The reaction is an important step in the conversion of methionine to cysteine, i.e. the so-called transsulfuration pathway (3)

The homocysteine content in tissues is low under physiological conditions (1-5 nmol/g,), and a significant amount is associated with proteins (11,12). Similarly, low concentrations can be detected in isolated or cultured cells (12-15). However, cells export large amounts into the extracellular medium (12-17) and the homocysteine egress seems related to the metabolic flux through homocysteine (12).

Homocysteine egress from cultured cells was proportional to the growth rate (16). This should be related to the finding that 5-methyltetrahydrofolate content in human breast cancer cells increased markedly during growth, whereas the levels of other reduced folates remained stable (18).

The efficient export of homocysteine is in accordance with the relatively high concentration of homocysteine in extracellular media like plasma and urine (19). Thus, urinary or plasma homocysteine may be a measure of altered homocysteine metabolism.

In conclusion, homocysteine can be metabolized by different routes (Fig. 2). The quantitative relations between these competing pathways have recently been evaluated by Finkelstein and Martin. (20). Homocysteine is a branch-point metabolite, with relations to the

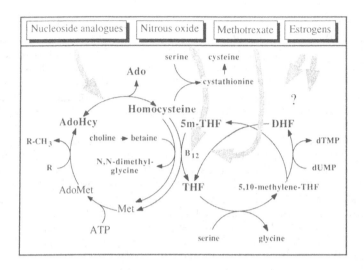

FIG. 2. **Metabolism of homocysteine and related compounds and the metabolic targets of various drugs.** Ado, adenosine; AdoHcy, S-adenosylhomocysteine; AdoMet, S-adenosylmethionine; Met, methionine; THF, tetrahydrofolate; DHF, dihydrofolate.

metabolic fates of several other compounds. This points to homocysteine metabolism as an important target for drug action

METHODS

Investigations into the biological roles of homocysteine have been hampered by lack of sensitive methods for the determination of the small amounts of this compound in biological material.

The homocysteine-cysteine mixed disulfide has been detected in plasma deproteinized by acid using modern amino acid analyzers (21). Homocysteine in plasma has also been determined with HPLC and electrochemical detector (22). For the detection of protein-bound homocysteine in plasma, laborious sample processing is often required (23).

We have recently developed a sensitive radioenzymic assay for the determination of homocysteine in tissues (11,12) and plasma (19). This assay is based on the enzymic conversion of homocysteine to radioactive AdoHcy, and can be carried out in solutions containing native proteins, and therefore allows the determination of both free (acid soluble) and protein-bound homocysteine in biological extracts and plasma.

The radioenzymic assay has been adapted for urine analysis (19). In addition, urinary homocysteine has also been determined with HPLC and electrochemical detector equipped with a mercury electrode (24).

Accurate determination requires rapid processing of tissue or plasma. We have recently observed that rapidly prepared plasma contains somewhat less homocysteine (free plus bound) than serum. This can be explained by a release of homocysteine from blood cells in whole blood left at room temperature. In contrast, when whole blood is kept on ice, there is no change in either free or protein-bound homocysteine within 0.5 hours, and total homocysteine remains stable for 12 hours under these conditions.

There is a redistribution between free and protein-bound homocysteine in plasma at room temperature. Total homocysteine remains constant whereas free homocysteine declines. Repeated freezing and thawing have similar effect.

AGENTS AFFECTING HOMOCYSTEINE METABOLISM AND DISPOSITION

Nucleoside Analogues.

Numerous adenosine analogues function as inhibitors of AdoHcy hydrolase (25). Since this enzyme is the only known source of homocysteine, one might expect that these agents induce depletion of intracellular homocysteine.

This possibility was first investigated in whole mice injected with the drug combination 9-ß-D-arabinofuranosyladenine plus 2'-deoxy-coformycin. Although AdoHcy catabolism was profoundly inhibited, depletion of homocysteine in tissues was not observed (11). The effect on homocysteine in extracellular media like plasma and urine was not investigated.

Studies with isolated and cultured cells have enlightened this enigma. Cells in suspension export large amounts of homocysteine, and the homocysteine egress is profoundly inhibited by 3-deaza-adenosine or 3-deazaaristeromycin in proportion to their inhibitory effect on AdoHcy catabolism(13,14). Homocysteine associated with the cells is either decreased, as in fibroblasts, or is even increased , as in liver cells, under these conditions. It is conceivable that homocysteine egress may be important as a cellular adjustment to imbalance in homocysteine supply relative to the metabolic need. Such a mechanism may be important for some cell types, but may be of less importance in liver cells where the turnover of AdoMet and related compounds is high (3) .

Cantoni et al. (26) pointed out some metabolic consequences of severe depression of the activity of AdoHcy hydrolase. They suggested that compounds inhibiting this enzyme, like 9-ß-D-arabino-furanosyladenine, may inhibit the regeneration of tetrahydrofolate from 5-methyltetrahydrofolate because of lack of homocysteine. In addition, inhibition of *de novo* methionine synthesis, which supplements dietary methionine, may cause methionine deficiency.

Boss and Pilz (27) have provided some data in favour of these suggestions. They recently demonstrated that the methionine synthesis was inhibited in T-lymphoblasts and to a lesser extent in B-lymphoblasts in the presence of 2'-deoxyadenosine, 9-ß-D-arabinofurano-syladenine or 2'-deoxyguanosine, and the inhibition was reversed by homocysteine (27). The pronounced inhibition of methionine synthesis in T-lymphoblasts correlates with the cytotoxic effects of these nucleosides on these cells. The authors conclude that purine nucleoside toxicity may partly be mediated through inhibition of methionine synthesis, and by trapping reduced folates as 5'-methyltetrahydrofolate. The latter possibility gains support from the observation that some adenosine deaminase and nucleoside phosphorylase deficient patients have megaloblastic anemia (27).

Two reports provide direct evidence that lack of homocysteine plays a role in the cytostatic action of nucleoside analogues inhibiting AdoHcy catabolism. Kim et al. (28) have shown that addition of homocysteine counteracts the cytostatic effect of 3-deaza-aristeromycin in mouse macrophages. Likewise, Wolfson et al. (29) have reported that the cytostatic action of neplanocin A was inhibited by homocysteine in rat pituitary cells. These observations contrast to no effect of homocysteine on the cytostatic action of 3-deaza-aristeromycin in HL-60 cells (Aarbakke, J., personal communication).

Methotrexate

The primary target for methotrexate is the enzyme dihydrofolate reductase, the enzyme responsible for the regeneration of tetrahydrofolate from dihydrofolate (30). Inhibition of this enzyme is expected to cause cellular depletion of reduced folates, including 5-methyltetrahydrofolate. Since quantitation of intracellular folates has met with technical obstacles, the effect of methotrexate on the cellular folate pools has not been evaluated until recently. In the spring of 1986 two papers were published which describe the differential effect of methotrexate on reduced folates in various cell types in culture, including human breast cancer cells. Notably, both reports independently show that, among the reduced folates, 5-methyltetrahydrofolate is particularly sensitive towards the inhibitory effects of methotrexate. The cellular content of this particular folate was profoundly reduced within minutes under conditions where the amount of other reduced folates was slightly (18) or not affected (31). Similar results were obtained with cells grown i.p. in mice injected with methotrexate (31). These findings are important in relation to the possible effects of methotrexate on homocysteine metabolism.

We have recently demonstrated that methotrexate increases homocysteine export several-fold in chemically transformed murine fibroblasts. Larger concentrations were required for the enhancement of homocysteine egress from the non-transformed counterpart, which was essentially methotrexate resistant. The increase in homocysteine egress may be explained by lack of 5-methyltetrahydrofolate relative to the metabolic demand (15).

The results with cells in culture prompted us to investigate the effect of high-dose methotrexate on homocysteine in plasma and urine from cancer patients. There was a marked increase in plasma homocysteine and urinary excretion of homocysteine within 12 hours after drug infusion (32). The homocysteine response was extinguished after a few infusions. The acute response is in accordance with the *in vitro* data (15), whereas the mechanism behind the gradual appearance of a refractory state remains an enigma.

In psoriatics receiving low dose (10-25 mg) methotrexate treatment once a week, we observed an acute increase in plasma homocysteine, which subsided within 2-3 days. The homocysteine response regularly appeared, and no refractory state developed in patients receiving low-dose methotrexate (Refsum, H., Helland, S., and Ueland, P.M., unpublished results). Notably, Brattstrøm et al. (33) have recently reported that folic acid therapy resulted in substantial reduction in plasma homocysteine in normal men and women. These data suggest that plasma homocysteine may be a sensitive measure of intracellular folate status

Some cancer patients and most patients with extensive psoriatic lesions have remarkable high plasma homocysteine levels. Plasma homocysteine decreased a few days after high-dose methotrexate treatment, but not in psoriatics receiving low-dose treatment (Refsum, H., Helland, S., and Ueland, P.M., unpublished results). One may speculate whether homocysteine in plasma and urine may, partly at least, originate from rapidly proliferating cells, including cancer cells or basal cells in psoriasis. Exposure to cytostatic concentrations of methotrexate may reduce the number of proliferating cells, which in turn may account for reduction in plasma homocysteine. The possibility that homocysteine egress may be dependent on the proliferation rate is supported by *in vitro* experiments (16), cited in a preceding paragraph.

The clinical consequences of altered homocysteine metabolism during methotrexate therapy have not been settled. Long-term treatment of psoriatics with methotrexate induces liver cirrhosis and fibrosis in 20-25 % of the patients (34). Based on experimental evidence, Barak et al. (35) have suggested that liver hepatotoxicity is caused by inhibition of the 5-methyltetrahydrofolate dependent synthesis of methionine from homocysteine, which in turn impose lipotrope deficiency. The possible consequences of altered plasma homocysteine, a possible risk factor for arteriosclerotic disease, is an open but intriguing question.

Nitrous Oxide

The anaesthetic agent, nitrous oxide, once considered to be chemically inert, reacts with transition metal complexes in solution, including the cobalt-containing vitamin B12. Oxidation of cobalamin in the enzyme, 5-methyltetrahydrofolate-homocysteine methyltransferase, irreversibly inactivates this enzyme (36). The enzyme is rapidly inactivated in rodents, but biopsi data suggest that the onset of inhibition is slower in man. Plasma methionine is decreased in rat and in man during prolonged (>12 hours) nitrous oxide exposure whereas short exposure does not affect plasma methionine in man (37 and references herein). It is conceivable that plasma homocysteine is a more responsive biochemical parameter during nitrous oxide exposure, but to our knowledge, this has not been evaluated to date.

The data cited above show that methotrexate and nitrous oxide has a common biochemical target, namely the enzymatic conversion of homocysteine to methionine (Fig. 2). In addition, nitrous oxide may affect the cellular content of reduced folates according to the methyl trap mechanism. The clinical data on homocysteine in plasma of patients treated with methotrexate (32) show that this drug in clinical use affects homocysteine metabolism. Therefore, it is conceivable that the drug combination of nitrous oxide plus methotrexate, which is used in some pediatric oncology units, may have some unforeseen clinical effects (38). This possibility is supported by experimental data showing that nitrous oxide enhances the antileukemic effect of methotrexate in rats (39)

Steroids

An experimental study has recently been initiated by Thomson et al. to investigate whether constituents of the oral contraceptives may affect urinary homocysteine excretion (24, 40, 41). Such a study is motivated by the fact that oral contraceptives increase the incidence of thromboembolic disease. In addition, it has been reported that premenopausal women have a more efficient methionine metabolism than men and postmenopausal women (42).

These authors found that injection of the synthetic estrogen, ethynyl estradiol (40) as well as ethynyl estradiol disulfate (41), increased the urinary homocysteine excretion several fold. Progesteron was without effect.

Further experimental and clinical studies of the possible effect of natural and synthetic estrogens and drugs affecting estrogen metabolism on homocysteine metabolism, are warranted.

REFERENCES

1. DuVigneaud, V.E. (1952) *A Trail of Research in Sulfur Chemistry*. Cornell University Press, Ithaca.
2. Carson, N.A.J., and Neill, D.W. (1962) *Arch. Dis. Child.* **37**, 505-513.
3. Mudd, S.H., and Levy, H.J. (1983) in *Metabolic Basis of Inherited Diseases* (Standbury, J.B., ed) Ed. 5, pp. 522-559, McGraw-Hill Publications, New York.
4. McCully, K.S. (1983) *Atherosclerosis Reviews* **11**, 157-246.
5. Mudd, S.H. (1985) *N. Engl. J. Med.* **313**, 751-753.
6. Hoffman, R.M. (1984) *Biochim. Biophys. Acta* **738**, 49-87.
7. Christa, L., Kersual, J., Auge, J. and Perignon, J-L. (1986) *Biochem. Biophys. Res. Commun.* **135**, 131-138.
8. Cantoni, G.L. (1986) in *Biological Methylation and Drug Design. Experimental and Clinical Roles of S-Adenosylmethionine* (Borchardt, R.T., Creveling, C.R., and Ueland, P.M., eds.) pp. 227-238, Humana Press, Clifton, NJ.
9. Noronha, J.M., and Silverman, M. (1962) *In Vitamin B12 and Intrinsic Factor, 2nd Eur. Symp.* (Heinrich, H.C.,ed.) pp. 728-736, Ferdinand Enke, Stuttgart.
10. Herbert, V., and Zalusky, R. (1962) *J. Clin. Invest.* **41**, 1263-1276
11. Ueland, P.M., Helland, S., Broch, O.J., and Schanche, J.-S. (1984) *J. Biol. Chem.* **259**, 2360-2364
12. Svardal, A., Refsum, H., and Ueland, P.M. (1986) *J. Biol. Chem.* **261**, 3156-3163
13. Svardal, A. M., Djurhuus, R., and Ueland, P.M. (1986) *Mol. Pharmacol.* , in press.
14. Svardal, A. M., Djurhuus, R., Refsum, H., and Ueland, P.M. (1986) *Cancer Res.* , in press.
15. Ueland, P.M., Refsum, H., Male, R., and Lillehaug, J.R. (1986) *J. Natl. Cancer Inst.* **77**, 283-289
16. Iizasa, T., and Carson, D.A. (1985) *Biochim. Biophys. Acta* **844**, 280-287
17. German, D.C., Bloch, C. A., and Kredich, N.M: (1983) *J. Biol. Chem.* **258**, 10997-11003
18. Allegra, C.J., Fine, R.L., Drake, J.C., and Chabner, B.A. (1986) *J. Biol. Chem.* **261**, 6478-6485
19. Refsum, H., Helland, S., and Ueland, P.M. (1985) *Clin. Chem.* **31**, 624-628
20. Finkelstein, J.D., and Martin, J.J. (1984) *J. Biol. Chem.* **259**, 9508-9513
21. Gupta, V.J., and Wilcken, D.E.L. (1978) *Eur. J. Clin. Invest.* **8**, 205-207.

22. Saetre, R., and Rabenstein, D.L. (1978) *Anal. Chem.* **90**, 684-692
23. Kang, S.-S., Wong, P.W.K., Cook, H.Y., Norusis, M., and Messer, J.V. (1986) *J. Clin. Invest.* **77**, 1482-1486
24. Bond, A.M., Thomson, S.B., and Tucker, D.J. (1984) *Anal. Chim. Acta.* **156**, 33-42
25. Ueland, P.M. (1982) *Pharmacol. Rev.* **34**, 223-253
26. Cantoni, G.L., Aksamit, R.R., and Kim, I-K. (1981) *N. Engl. J. Med.* **307**, 1079
27. Boss, G.R., and Pilz, R.B. (1984) *J. Clin. Invest.* **74**, 1262-1268.
28. Kim, I-K., Aksamit, R.R., and Cantoni, G.L. (1982) *J. Biol. Chem.* **257**, 14726-14729
29. Wolfson, G., Chisholm, J., Tashjian, A.H.jr., Fish, S., and Abeles, R.H. (1986) *J. Biol. Chem.* **261**, 4492-4498
30. Jackson, R.C. (1984) *Pharmac. Ther.* **25**, 61-82
31. Kesavan, V., Sur, P., Doig, M.T., Scanlon, K.J., and Priest, D.G. (1986) *Cancer Lett.* **30**, 55-59
32. Refsum, H., Ueland, P.M., and Kvinnsland, S. (1986) *Cancer Res.*, in press.
33. Brattstrøm, L.E., Hultberg, B.L., and Hardebo, J.E. (1985) *Metabolism* **34**, 1073-1077
34. Nyfors, A. (1986) *Rheumatology* **9**, 192-212
35. Barak, A.J., Tuma, D.J., and Beckenhauer, H.C. (1984) *J. Am. Coll. Nutr.* **3**, 93-96.
36. Nunn, J.F. (1984) *Trends Pharmacol. Sci.* **5**, 225-227
37. Nunn, J.F., Sharer, N.M., Bottiglieri, T., and Rossiter, J. (1986) *Br. J. Anaesth.* **58**, 1-10.
38. Ueland, P.M., Refsum, H., Wesenberg, F., and Kvinnsland, S. (1986) *N. Engl. J. Med.* **314**, 1514
39. Kroes, A.C.M., Lindemans, J., Schoester, M., and Abels, J. (1986) *Cancer Chemother. Pharmacol.* **17**, 114-120.
40. Thomson, S.B., Tucker, D.J., and Briggs, M.H. (1984) *Steroids* **44**, 531-538
41. Thomson, S.B., and Tucker, D.J. (1986) *IRCS Med. Sci.* **14**, 237
42. Boers, G.H., Smals, A.G., Trijbels, F.J., Leermakers, A.I., and Kloppenborg, P.W. (1983) *J. Clin. Invest.* **72**, 1971-1976

C-8-SUBSTITUTED GUANOSINE ANALOGUES ARE NOVEL IMMUNOSTIMULANTS AND DIFFERENTIATING AGENTS FOR NEONATAL, NORMAL AND X-LINKED IMMUNE DEFECTIVE (xid) B LYMPHOCYTES

Ateeq Ahmad

Department of Applied Biochemistry
Division of Biochemistry
Walter Reed Army Institute of Research
Washington, DC 20307-5100

ABSTRACT

It was recently demonstrated that bromination or thiolation of guanosine at the C-8 position endowed it with potent biological activities, including the capacity to induce blast transformation of murine B lymphocytes and to enhance the secretion of specific antibody when administered with antigen. The guanosine, which is itself inhibitory to murine B cells, can also be converted to an immunostimulatory molecule after substitution at its C-8 position with methoxy or hydroxy groups. The present paper demonstrates that 8-hydroxyguanosine and 8-methoxyguanosine can also act as potent in vitro immunoadjuvants and the bromo or thio group is not essential for conferring biological activity to this nucleoside. Substitution of guanosine at C-8 position with $-NH_2$, $-OH$ and $-OCH_3$ groups has differential effects in influencing B-cell activation and differentiation.

In vitro responses of B lymphocytes or spleen cells from neonatal mice and from xid immune defective (CBA/N x DBA/2) F_1 male mice to TNP-Ficoll were investigated. B cells from these mice are immunologically immature and unresponsive to antigen challenge with polysaccharide antigens including haptenated Ficoll. In the presence of 8-mercaptoguanosine, TNP-Ficoll induced TNP-specific

responses in <u>xid</u> B cells and neonatal B cells equal in
magnitude to those generated in cells from control
mice.   It is suggested that C-8 substituted guanosine
analogues may function as differentiating factors for B
lymphocytes.   The use of these analogues should prove to
be powerful probes for investigating the triggering
mechanisms underlying the proliferation and
differentiation pathways of B lymphocyte at the molecular
level.

INTRODUCTION

Bromination or thiolation of guanosine at the C-8
position endowed it with potent <u>in vitro</u> immunoadjuvant
activity (Fig 1).   These analogues enhance the secretion
of specific antibody when administered with antigen
(1-3).

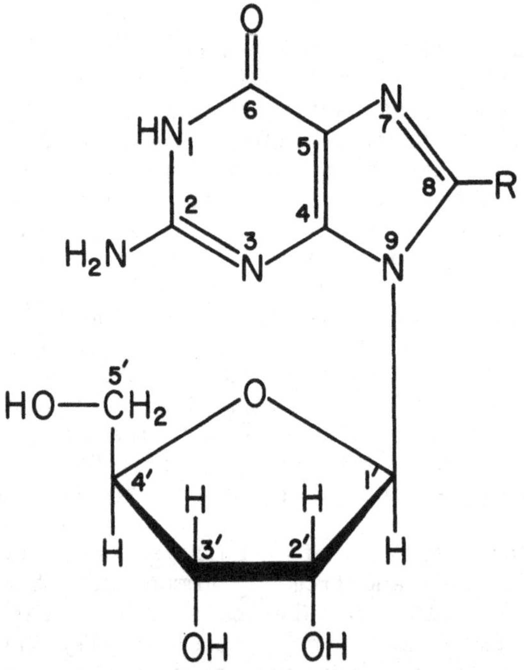

FIG. 1. Molecular structure of C-8-substituted guanosine
analogs: guanosine, R = H; 8-mercaptoguanosine, R = SH;
8-hydroxyguanosine, R = OH; 8-aminoguanosine, R = NH$_2$;
8-bromoguanosine, R = Br; 8-methoxyguanosine; R = -OCH$_3$.

This study investigated, the ability of C-8-substituted guanosine analogues to enhance primary antibody response in vitro.

CBA/N mice carry an x-linked immune defect which precludes them from responding to polysaccharide antigens (4). In this regard they resemble the immune system of newborn mice which are also hyporesponsive to this group of antigens. To test whether 8sGuo could correct a "non-responder" cell into a "responder" cell, cells from CBA/N mice and neonatal mice were cultured with TNP-Ficoll and 8sGuo. The results presented in this report indicate that C-8 substituted guanosine analogue, 8sGuo can restore the anti-TNP-Ficoll responses in B cells from these mice to a level which was comparable to that seen in control B cells from responder mice.

MATERIALS & METHODS

Mice. CBA/N mice and (CBA/N X DBA/2)F_1 male or female mice 8 to 12 week of age were obtained from the Division of Research Services, National Institutes of Health; all F_1 male mice resulting from a cross with CBA/N (xid/xid) females carry the xid gene and are phenotypically immune defective.

B cell purification. Splenocytes were teased and were washed in Hank's balanced salt solution. T cells were removed by treatment with a mixture of monoclonal antibodies at 4°C for 45 min (5). The mixture of monoclonal antibodies was comprised of a monoclonal rat anti-Thy 1.2 antibody and HO 13-4.9, a noncytotoxic monoclonal rat anti-Lyt-1 combined with a cytotoxic monoclonal mouse anti-rat k-chain antibody (MAR 18.5)(American Type Culture Collection; ATCC, Rockville, MD). Cells were then washed one time in medium and were resuspended in baby rabbit complement (Pel-Freeze Biologicals) at a 1/10 dilution.

Antigen. TNP-AECM-Ficoll was prepared as described (6) and used at a concentration of 1.0 to 10.0 ng/ml. 8sGuo (Sigma) was dissolved in a small volume of 0.1 N NaOH, then was brought to pH 7.0 with 1.0 N HCl, and was finally diluted in Mishell Dutton medium.

Cell cultures. B cells were cultured in modified

Mishell-Dutton medium containing 10% endotoxin free fetal calf serum (FCS) and 5×10^{-5} M 2-mercaptoethanol in flat-bottom microtiter plates (No. 3040; Falcon Plastics, Oxnard, CA) at 0.2 ml medium per well. Plates were incubated in a humidified 6% CO_2-94% air atmosphere at 37°C.

Assay of plaque forming cells (PFC). Cells were collected after culture, and the number of PFC that secreted antibodies against TNP were evaluated by using a modification of the hemolytic plaque assay of Jerne and Nordin(7).

RESULTS AND DISCUSSION

To investigate the efficacy of C-8 substituted analogues to enhance antibody response in vitro, purified B cells from DBA/2 mice were cultured together with antigen and adjuvant. B lymphocytes were incubated with 0.25 or 1.0 mM concentrations of guanosine analogues in the presence or absence of the type 2 antigen TNP-Ficoll, and after 3 days the cells were processed, collected, and evaluated for number of antibody forming cells. The results of these studies demonstrate that 8sGuo, 8-OHGuo, 8-BrGuo, and 8-OMeGuo could stimulate polyclonal immunoglobulin secretion (Table I) and in the presence of antigen enhance the magnitude of the anti-TNP plaque-forming-cell antibody response to TNP-Ficoll. Maximum stimulation of anti-TNP antibody secretion was achieved by the 8-substituted guanosine at 1.0 mM concentrations and their relative potencies in enhancing antibody secretion was in the following order:
8sGuo > 8-OHGuo > 8-BrGuo > 8-OMeGuo.

Addition of 8-aminoguanosine at all concentrations was suppressive to in vitro antibody formation, probably by its inhibition of purine nucleoside phosphorylase (8).

8sGuo Restores the Ability of (CBA/N x DBA/2)F_1 Male Splenic B Cells to Respond to TNP-Ficoll.

Spleen cells from immune defective (CBA/N X DBA/2)F_1 male mice were cultured in vitro with TNP-Ficoll in the presence or absence of 8sGuo (Table 2). In all of the experiments, 8sGuo stimulated a significant increase in the number of "background" anti-TNP PFC in cultures of

TABLE 1

Derivatization of Guanosine at C-8 Position
Enhances antibody responses of B lymphocytes.

PFC/culture Guanosine analog added (molarity)	Medium	Antigens: Anti-TNP TNP-Ficoll
1. Medium (0.0)	14 (1)	8 (2.4)
2. Guo (0.25)	5 (1.22)*	8 (1.07)
Guo (1.0)	1	6 (1)
3. 8-OMeGuo (0.25)	16 (1.65)	28 (1.95)*
8-OMeGuo (1.0)	41 (1.19)*	85 (1.15)**
4. 8-OHGuo (0.25)	40 (1.25)*	130 (1.13)*
8-OHGuo (1.0)	118 (1.47)**	200 (1.25)**
5. 8-BrGuo (0.25)	37 (1.16)*	120 (1.16)**
8-BrGuo (1.0)	78 (1.03)**	198 (1.07)**
6. 8sGuo (0.25)	42 (1.25)*	134 (1.18)**
8sGuo (1.0)	80 (1.09)**	296 (1.03)**
7. 8-NH$_2$Guo (0.25)	0	0
8-NH$_2$Guo (1.0)	0	0

Note: B Cells were prepared as described under Materials and Methods, and cultured in flat-bottom microtiter culture dishes at 5×10^5/well in modified Mishell-Dutton medium containing 10% FCS. C-8-substituted guanosine analogs were added at a final concentration of 0.25 or 1.0 mM. Anti-TNP PFC were enumerated on Day 3 of culture. TNP-Ficoll was used at 10 ng/ml and was added to cultures on day zero. The results for anti-TNP PFC represent geometric mean (log of SE) of triplicate cultures. Significance compared to control was calculated by Student's t test.
   * P<0.05
  ** P<0.01

TABLE 2

Restoration of in vitro responsiveness of
spleen cells from mice with the xid defective
mice to TNP-Ficoll with 8sGuo[a]

	Anti-TNP PFC response to (Anti-TNP PFC/Culture)
Medium	0
TNP-Ficoll	0
8sGuo	31 (1.60)
TNP-Ficoll + 8sGuo	200 (1.06)

[a]Spleen cells from (CBA/N x DBA/2)F_1 male mice were cultered at 1×10^6 cells/well, in modified Mishell-Dutton medium. The concentration of 8sGuo used was 1.0 mM. TNP-Ficoll was used at 2.5 ng/ml. After 3 days, cells were harvested and anti-TNP PFC were determined. The results represent geometric mean (X/÷SE) of triplicate cultures.

cultures of xid cells as might be expected of such a potent polyclonal B cell activator. Addition of TNP-Ficoll, which by itself was unable to stimulate anti-TNP responses in xid spleen cells, induced a significant increase in the number of anti-TNP PFC in the presence of 8sGuo.

To determine whether the observed enhancement induced by 8sGuo in responses to TNP-Ficoll reflected a direct stimulatory effect on B cells, xid or normal cells were cultured with TNP-Ficoll in the presence or absence of the adjuvant (Table 3). It is known that in vitro responses to TNP-Ficoll are T cell dependent, and thus purified populations of normal B cells are unable to respond to this antigen. However, in the presence of 8sGuo, TNP-Ficoll stimulated equivalent increases in the number of anti-TNP PFC in both xid (F_1 male) and normal (F_1 female) B cells.

TABLE 3

Restoration of in vitro responsiveness of B cells
from xid mice to TNP-Ficoll with 8sGuo[a]

Source of B Cells			Anti-TNP PFC Response to (Anti-TNP-PFC/Culture)	
	Medium	TNP-Ficoll	(8sGuo)	TNP-Ficoll +8sGuo
(CBA/N X DBA/2)F_1 male	0	0	91 (1.16)	181 (1.38)
(CBA/N X DBA/2)F_1 female	0	3 (1.7)	83 (1.32)	222 (1.17)

[a]B cells from F_1 male and F_1 female mice were cultured at 1.5 X 10^6 cells/well and 1 x 10^6 cells/well, respectively, for evaluation of in vitro anti-TNP PFC responses to TNP-Ficoll, and were harvested 3 days later. The concentration of 8sGuo used was 0.25 nM. The concentration of TNP-Ficoll used was 2.5 ng/ml. The results for anti-TNP PFC represent geometric mean (X/÷ SE).

8sGuo is an Effective Adjuvant for Neonatal B Lymphocytes.

Spleen cells from 3, 6 and 11 day old mice were cultured with TNP-Ficoll and 8sGuo (Table 4) and anti-TNP plaque forming cell responses enumerated 3 days later. B cells from these young mice are unresponsive to this antigen in the absence of 8sGuo and they are responsive in its presence. Thus it appears that TNP-Ficoll could initiate the early steps of B cell activation even in the immature B cells of neonatal mice and 8sGuo could exert its immuno-stimulatory effects on these activated B cells.

TABLE 4

8sGuo[a] Restores In Vitro Responsiveness
of Neonatal Spleen Cells To TNP-Ficoll

Age of Mice	8sGuo	TNP-Ficoll	TNP- Ficoll + 8sGuo
3 days	30 (1.58)	3 (1.80)	114 (1.32)
6 days	76 (1.38)	0	222 (1.14)
11 days	73 (1.43)	3 (1.25)	190 (1.15)

[a]Spleen cells from CBA/J mice were cultured at 1 X 10^6 cells/well in modified Mishell-Dutton medium. The concentration of 8sGuo used was 1.0 mM. TNP-Ficoll was used at 2.5 ng/ml. After 3 days, cells were harvested and anti-TNP PFC were determined. The results represent geometric mean (X/÷SE) of triplicate cultures.

CONCLUSIONS

1.   Differences do exist in the structural requirements   needed   for   C-8-substituted   guanosine analogues to activate B lymphocytes and more specifically that substitution of the thio and bromo group at the C-8 position of guanosine is not absolutely critical for enhancing B-cell immune responses, since 8-OHGuo and 8-OMeGuo exhibited immunostimulatory activity.

2.   The mechanism whereby the substituted guanosine

analogues exert their adjuvant effect is unclear at the present time.   Their stimulatory activity is exerted rather rapidly after culture with B cells and within 3 hr after in vitro incubation with B cells they induce a significant increase in expression of B-cell surface I-region-associated antigens (Data not shown).

3.   The ability of 8sGuo to induce responsiveness of xid B cells to TNP-Ficoll may result from its ability to enhance clonal expansion of TNP-Ficoll-specific precursor B cells, or from its ability to function as a differentiation factor.

4. The use of these new immunostimulants should prove to be powerful probes for investigating the triggering mechanisms underlying the proliferation and differentiation pathways of B lymphocyte at the molecular level.

REFERENCES

1. Goodman, M.G. and Weigle, W.O. (1982) J. Immunol. **128**, 2399-2404.

2. Goodman, M.G. and Weigle, W.O. (1983) J. Immunol **130**, 551-557.

3. Goodman, M.G. and Weigle, W.O. (1983) J. Immunol. **130**, 2580-2585.

4. Scher, I. (1982) Adv. Immunol. **33**, 1-71.

5. Mond, J.J. (1982) Immunol. Rev. **64**, 99-115.

6. Inman, J.K. (1975) J. Immunol. **114**, 704-709.

7. Jerne, N.K. and Nordin, A.A. (1963) Science (Washington, DC) **140**, 405.

8. Stoeckler, J.D. Cambor, C., C., Kuhns, V., Chu, S.H. and Parks, R.E. (1982) Biochem. Pharmacol. **31**, 163-171.

Cell Interactions and Differentiation

DIFFERENTIATION AS A MECHANISM FOR CONTROL OF

MALIGNANCY IN HUMAN CELL HYBRIDS

Eric J. Stanbridge

Microbiology and Molecular Genetics
University of California, Irvine
Irvine, California
U.S.A.

INTRODUCTION

The notion that aberrant cell differentiation is a consistent and important characteristic of malignant cells has been a popular theme in cancer research for many years. Theories concerning phenomena such as dedifferentiation, misprogramming of differentiated lineages, and inappropriate or ectopic expression of genes associated with embryonic development have often been linked to the progression of malignancy (1,2).

This regulation of differentiation has been documented in a number of experimental systems, and includes situations where malignant cells appear to be frozen in maturation arrest at some point in a given lineage. This is particularly the case with hematopoetic malignancies, and there are also documented cases of being able to reinstitute the program of terminal differentiation in malignant leukemia cells by treatment with appropriate drugs (3,4). These phenomena have been referred to as "blocked ontogeny," (5) and neoplasms have also been referred to as caricatures of tissue renewal (6).

The technique of somatic cell hybridization has been extremely useful in studies of gene mapping and control of expression of differentiated functions (7,8). This technique has also been applied to the study of the genetic analysis of malignancy (9). It is now well established that when malignant cells are fused with normal diploid cells of the same species the resulting hybrid cells retain their transformed phenotype in culture, but are completely suppressed with respect to their tumorigenic behavior. Rare tumorigenic variants arise which have fully regained their tumorigenic potential. Extensive analyses of these hybrid populations have revealed that they express many of the phenotypic traits of the malignant parent in culture; however, most of the differentiated functions of the normal parental cell are extinguished (10,11). However, when the nontumorigenic hybrid cells are inoculated into immune-deficient animals, they fail to form tumors and the reason that they fail to do so is because the hybrid cells are induced to terminally differentiate in the host animal (12,13). The following article is a brief discussion of these phenomena and how they may be used to investigate the differentiation process and control of malignancy in human cells. Because of the limited space of this article, I will confine my remarks to those dealing with intraspecies human cell hybrids; although the reader should be aware that a great deal of work has also been undertaken with rodent cell hybrids and inter-species rodent cell hybrids (for reviews see references 9 and 14).

A BRIEF OVERVIEW OF HUMAN CELL HYBRIDS

The early studies with intraspecies human cell hybrids were undertaken using HeLa as the tumorigenic parental cell and diploid fibroblasts as the normal parental cell (15). HeLa was fused with a number of different fibroblast cell strains. In all cases, the hybrid cells behaved as transformed cells in culture and shared many phenotypic properties in common with the HeLa parental cells. However, these same cells failed to form tumors in nude athymic mice, even when as many as 1×10^8 cells were inoculated (approximately 1×10^5 HeLa cells under similar conditions will give 100% tumor incidence). Rare tumorigenic segregants were obtained from the nontumorigenic hybrid population, often after only prolonged periods of time in culture (11). Similar results were found when hybrids were generated from the fusion of HeLa with human foreskin keratinocytes (12).

The availability of paired combinations of hybrid cells (one transformed but nontumorigenic; the other transformed and tumorigenic) prompted the comparative analysis of their phenotypic characteristics in culture. Comparative studies of such hybrid cells quickly identified that many so-called markers of malignancy that had been claimed in a variety of other studies were phenotypes expressed by both nontumorigenic and tumorigenic segregant cell hybrids. Surprisingly, this also included the trait of anchorage independence, a phenotype that has been repeatedly claimed as a correlate of tumorigenicity. In this human hybrid cell system, both nontumorigenic and tumorigenic segregant hybrid cells grow equally as well in suspension in soft agar or methyl cellulose (16). These results clearly demonstrated that the transformed and tumorigenic phenotypes are under separate genetic control, a finding which has been shown by other investigators in other hybrid cell systems (9,14).

In addition to comparing phenotypic characteristics of the nontumorigenic hybrid cells and their tumorigenic segregants, it was also possible to do comparative cytogenetic analyses to determine if specific chromosome loss is associated with re-expression of tumorigenicity. These studies were carried out by Klinger's group and also our own. Stanbridge and colleagues described loss of one copy each of two chromosomes, 11 and 14, associated with re-expression of tumor-forming ability in HeLa x fibroblast hybrids (17). Klinger and associates, in a similar exten-sive study, also provided evidence supporting a role for human chromosome 11 in suppression of the tumorigenic phenotype. In their case, however, they also indicated that other human chro-mosomes, namely 2, 13, 17 and 20 may contain genetic information capable of suppressing the tumorigenic phenotype (18). The cytogenetic analyses performed on the intraspecies human hybrid cells could, however, be only described as tentative. Owing to the lack of morphologic markers identified by chromosome banding techniques, it is impossible to determine the parental origin of those specific chromosomes that are absent in the tumorigenic segregants. The availability of chromosome-specific restriction fragment length polymorphism (RFLP) probes has now made it possible to identify specific chromosomes from different individuals, and thereby to ascertain the presence or absence of such chromosomes in somatic cell hybrids. When this analysis was applied to the HeLa x fibroblast human hybrid cells using RFLP probes specific for chromosome 11, the loss of a single copy of normal chromosome 11 from the hybrids was confirmed (19,20). However, no such correlation with loss of normal chromosome 14 was found (19).

Further confirmation of the role of chromosome 11 in control of tumorigenic expression in HeLa cells was obtained by the technique of microcell transfer. In this technique single chromosomes are transferred from donor to recipient cell in interphase micronuclei via cell fusion (21,22). This method has the distinct advantage that the transferred chromosome is retained in the recipient cell in a heritable fashion, and maintains its chromosome structural integrity. It has now been shown that if a normal human chromosome 11 is transferred into tumorigenic segregant HeLa x fibroblast hybrids, complete suppression of the tumorigenic phenotype results (23). It is as yet unknown whether other single human chromosomes are capable of effecting sup-pression of the tumorigenic phenotype.

DIFFERENTIATION AS A MECHANISM OF SUPPRESSION OF TUMORIGENICITY

One of the general features of nontumorigenic malignant x normal hybrid cell populations is that they behave as transformed cells in culture (10,11,24). An important question, therefore, is why the nontumorigenic hybrids fail to form tumors in immuno-suppressed mice when the growth behavior in culture is almost identical with that seen with the tumorigenic segregant hybrid populations. Answers to this question were obtained by examining the growth behavior of the hybrid cells in the intact animal (24). When nontumorigenic HeLa x fibroblast hybrid cells were inoculated subcutaneously into athymic mice the cells initially proliferated as if they would form tumors. However, approximately four days post-inoculation there was a dramatic decrease in mitotic activity. By day seven virtually all mitotic activity had ceased and the cells underwent a morphological alteration to a more fibroblastoid morphology. There was no evidence of lymphoid cell infiltration and the tissue nodules remained well vascularized. The histopathology of the nodules also indicated that the HeLa x fibroblast hybrids may have undergone differentiation into fibroblastoid tissue. Further evidence for differentiation came when nontumorigenic HeLa x keratinocyte hybrids were examined (12). Once again, the cells initially proliferated and then gradual cessation of mitosis occurred. In the case of these hybrid cells, however, a very dramatic histological change was seen. The cells were rather rapidly induced to terminally differentiate and, most interestingly, the nature of this terminal differentiation was that of keratinizing epithelium. Considerable evidence has now accumulated to suggest that the nontumorigenic hybrid cells are induced to differentiate terminally in the athymic mouse and that the hybrid cell takes on the phenotypic "signature" of the normal parental cell regardless of the origin of the malignant parental cell. For example, HeLa x keratinocyte hybrids differentiate into keratinizing tissue, and HeLa x fibroblast differentiate into fibroblastoid tissue in the intact animal. In all cases the tumorigenic segregants of these hybrids form tumors that are undifferentiated anaplastic carcinomas, indistinguishable from those formed by the parental HeLa cells. A similar induction of differentiation has been noted by Harris in intraspecies rodent cell hybrids (13).

GENERATION OF MONOCLONAL ANTIBODIES AGAINST DIFFERENTIATION-SPECIFIC ANTIGENS

Given the fact that the nontumorigenic phenotype of the hybrid cells appears to be intrinsically linked to the process of differentiation it obviously becomes of interest to determine whether the induction of the differentiated phenotype follows the normal program of differentiation or whether some aberrant program is activated. It should be noted at this juncture that when normal human diploid fibroblasts or keratinocytes are inoculated into nude athymic mice they are induced to terminally differentiate extremely rapidly, and features of terminal differentiation are seen within 24 hours post-implantation. During our comparative analysis of the nontumorigenic and tumorigenic segregant hybrid cells we initiated a program of study to determine whether antigenic differences between the two cell types could be identified. To accomplish this antisera were raised in rabbits to the two hybrid cell types using live cells as immunogens. These initial studies were undertaken with HeLa x fibroblast hybrids. As expected, when the antisera were tested against a panel of cells consisting of parental HeLa and fibroblast cell lines and the paired nontumorigenic and tumorigenic segregant hybrid populations, both antisera reacted against all four cell types. Each antiserum was then extensively cross-absorbed with the other cell type; that is, antiserum against the nontumorigenic hybrid cell population was absorbed with tumorigenic segregant cells and vice versa. When these absorbed antisera were then tested against the same panel of cells several interesting results were noted (see Table I). The antiserum against the tumorigenic segregant (TS) HeLa x fibroblast hybrid cells, which had been absorbed extensively against the nontumorigenic (NT) hybrid cells, reacted only against the TS hybrid cells and parental HeLa. Further analysis of this absorbed antiserum showed that it reacted with a single 75 kD polypeptide that is a membrane glycophosphoprotein and a candidate tumor-associated antigen (25,26).

The absorbed anti-NT antiserum had an even more interesting pattern of reactivity. When the absorbed antiserum was tested by immunofluorescence against the NT hybrid cells (the immunogen), no reactivity was seen. This result indicated that the TS cells had absorbed out all of the antibodies directed against the NT cells, and suggested that all antigenic determinants (as recognized by the rabbit) expressed by NT cells are also expressed by TS cells. The absorbed anti-NT antiserum, as expected, also failed to react with the TS or parental HeLa cells (Table I). However, when this absorbed antiserum was tested against parental fibroblasts, strong positive staining was seen. This result seems somewhat paradoxical because the absorbed anti-NT antiserum did not react with the NT cells, which were the immunogen, but did react with human fibroblasts

Table I. Identification of Differentiation-Specific Products Using Absorbed Antisera and Immunofluorescent Staining[a]

		Parental cells		Hybrid cell populations	
Antiserum[b]	Absorption with	HeLa	Fibroblast	NT HeLa/fibroblast	TS HeLa/fibroblast
Anti-TS	—	+	+	+	+
Anti-NT	—	+	+	+	+
Anti-TS	NT cells	+[c]	—	—	+[c]
Anti-NT	TS cells	—	+	—	—
Anti-NT	NT cells	—	+	—	—

[a]See text for details.
[b]NT, Nontumorigenic HeLa/fibroblast hybrid cells; TS, tumorigenic segregant HeLa/fibroblast hybrid cells.
[c]75-kD phosphoglycoprotein. (Adapted from reference 27.)

to which the rabbit had never been exposed. Furthermore, even when the anti-NT antiserum was extensively absorbed with NT cells, the reactivity toward the human fibroblasts persisted.

The key to this paradox lies in the nature of the immunogen. Viable NT hybrid cells were used in the immunization protocol. It is our contention that these live cells were induced to differentiate rapidly in the rabbit—in a fashion analogous to that seen in the nude mouse—and that certain differentiation-specific (DS) products were rapidly expressed before the rabbit mounted its immune response against the foreign NT antigens. Antibodies were then synthesized against the spectrum of NT antigens, including the DS products. Because these DS products are not expressed by the NT hybrid cells in culture, extensive absorption of the anti-NT antiserum with NT cells did not remove antibodies directed against the DS products. It was shown by immunoprecipitation of solubilized, metabolically labeled fibroblast cell antigens with the absorbed anti-NT antiserum that several fibroblast DS antigens were recognized by this absorbed antiserum (27).

Advantage was taken of this property of differentiation induction in the host animal to develop a general method to produce monoclonal antibodies (MAbs) against differentiation-specific antigens. Viable nontumorigenic hybrid cells were used as the immunogen to immunize conventional mice. At the end of the immunization regimen spleens were removed and then hybridomas produced by fusion of the splenocytes with a nonproducing mouse myeloma cell line. Growth medium supernatants from wells containing hybridoma cells were then screened by ELISA or immunofluorescence for reactivity against a restricted panel of parental and hybrid cells. The novel feature of this approach is to use as immunogens viable nontumorigenic hybrid cells that are undifferentiated in culture but which terminally differentiate in the host animal. The desired reactivity is the hybridoma supernatant that fails to react with the cultured hybrid cells that constitute the immunogen, but which do react against the normal parental cells in culture which are expected to express certain differentiated functions. A test to investigate the validity of this hypothesis was done using nontumorigenic HeLa x keratinocyte hybrid cells as immunogen (28). As illustrated in Table II, a variety of patterns of reactivity were seen as would be expected, but most importantly, the predicted pattern of reactivity against only the normal keratinocyte parental cell was seen with 5 of approximately 90 hybridoma supernatants tested. Further evidence that these reactivities were indeed against DS antigens was obtained by testing the MAbs against frozen sections of

Table II. ELISA reactions of hybridoma supernatants against parental and hybrid cells[a].

Number of hybridoma supernatants	HeLa (H)	Keratinocyte (K)	Nontumorigenic H x K hybrid (Immunogen)	Tumorigenic H x K hybrid
12	+	+	+	+
6	+	−	+	+
3	−	+	+	+
5	−	+	−	−
63	−	−	−	−

[a]See text for details.
ELISA was performed on cell monolayers in 20-well dishes. Cells were fixed with 2% paraformaldehyde and 0.1% glutaraldehyde prior to testing. (Adapted from reference 28.)

human skin. The MAbs reacted with a number of epidermal antigens, including basement membrane and stratum corneum, thereby proving the validity of the experimental system (28). These MAbs and others which have been generated against fibroblast DS antigens (27) and human breast epithelial antigens (Casey and Stanbridge, unpublished observations) will provide extremely useful reagents to begin to probe the nature of the process of differentiation of the nontumorigenic hybrids in nude athymic mice.

IS DIFFERENTIATION-INDUCTION THE SOLE CONTROLLING MECHANISM OF TUMORIGENIC EXPRESSION OF HUMAN HYBRID CELLS?

The studies described above clearly implicate the induction of differentiation as a mechanism to control the tumorigenic expression of the human hybrid cells. Indeed, there has been no exception to this induction of differentiation when hybrid cells derived from whole cell fusions have been examined; however, it is important to appreciate that the fusion of a malignant cell with a normal cell means that an entire genome of a normal cell is introduced into the cancer cell. The pattern of differentiation in vivo is that of the normal parental cell, and therefore it would seem reasonable to assume that the genes which are activated during this differentiation process are those of the normal parental cell. A schematic consideration of this is shown in Figure 1, where we assume that HeLa arose from a progenitor stem cell, which if it had undergone its orderly lineage of differentiation, would have terminated as an ectocervical epithelial cell. This hypothetical situation is based upon the original reports which identified the probable source of HeLa as a cervical carcinoma (29). The malignant HeLa, again using hypothetical license in this example, is assumed to have arisen as a consequence of a block in this normal differentiation lineage, also probably accompanied by other genetic changes. Now, when the HeLa cell is fused with a fibroblast the resulting nontumorigenic hybrid population differentiates into fibroblastoid tissue in the nude mouse. If fused with a keratinocyte, the nontumorigenic hybrid differentiates into keratinizing tissue in the nude mouse. In both cases, one must assume that the program of differentiation is driven by activation of the genes of the normal parental cell, which in some fashion override the neoplastic behavior of the cancerous HeLa cells.

As described above, however, we are now able to accomplish suppression of the tumorigenic phenotype by transfer of a single normal human chromosome. This has been accomplished in two experimental systems where the same normal human chromosome 11 when transferred either into HeLa cells or Wilms tumor cells results in complete suppression of the tumorigenic phenotype (23,30).

Epithelial stem cell → → Hela // → → Ectocervical Epthelial Cell

HeLa x fibroblast hybrid $\underset{\text{environment}}{\xrightarrow{\text{in vivo}}}$ fibroblast

HeLa x keratinocyte hybrid $\underset{\text{environment}}{\xrightarrow{\text{in vivo}}}$ keratinocyte

Figure 1. Schematic representation of induction of differentiation in whole cell hybrids. In the upper line is the hypothetical lineage of differentiation that the progenitor of HeLa would have undergone. Blockage of this lineage and other genetic changes result in the neoplastic HeLa cell. The lower two lines indicate that HeLa x normal cell hybrids express the differentiated phenotype of the normal parental cell in the in vivo environment of the nude mouse. See text for further explanatory details.

Continuing with the HeLa paradigm, possible reasons for the suppression of tumorigenicity in HeLa following the introduction of a normal human chromosome 11 derived from a fibroblast cell line are outlined in Figure 2. One possibility is that HeLa cells containing the fibroblast chromosome 11 differentiate into fibroblastoid tissue in the nude mouse. This would indicate the switch-on of the entire program of fibroblast differentiation in these cells. It is of course ridiculous to assume that the genes responsible for the program of fibroblast differentiation all reside on chromosome 11; therefore one would have to postulate that some genetic information on the fibroblast chromosome 11 in some way activates HeLa genes which then participate in the fibroblast differentiation process. This would be somewhat akin to a master genetic switch capable of activating genes which presumably have never been switched on, even during HeLa's early pre-neoplastic history when its ancestral cell was committed to the differentiated lineage of ectocervical epithelium. An alternative possibility could be that the fibroblast chromosome 11 provides genetic information which allows the

HeLa cell in some way to overcome the original hypothetical block in the differentiation process of its progenitor cell and, thereby, in some fashion allow the HeLa cell to now once again proceed down the pathway to the differentiated state of ectocervical epithelium. This would be somewhat akin to the switching-on of normal developmental programs that have been seen in certain myeloid leukemia cell lines, most notably that of HL-60, where treatment of the leukemia cells with a variety of compounds (for example, dimethylsulfoxide) leads to their differentiation into macrophages and granulocytes (2,4).

(1) HeLa + fibroblast chromosome 11 ⟶ Fibroblast cell

(2) HeLa + fibroblast chromosome 11 ⟶ Ectocervical epithelial cell

(3) HeLa + fibroblast chromosome 11 ⟶ Inhibition of proliferation No differentiation

Figure 2. Theoretical consequences of the introduction of a normal fibroblast chromosome (FC) 11 into HeLa via microcell transfer. Three possible states exist following implantation of the cells into nude mice. In (1) a master gene switch on FC 11 activates genes of the HeLa genome to produce a differentiated fibroblast. In (2) gene(s) on FC 11 provide the means for HeLa to overcome the block in its original lineage pathway resulting in completion of development into an ectocervical epithelial cell. In (3) failure to form a tumor occurs because of an inhibition of proliferation of the HeLa cell without induction of differentiation.

Finally, it is possible that the suppression of tumorigenicity effected by the introduction of the normal chromosome 11 occurs by some mechanism other than induction of differentiation, for example, merely by inhibiting proliferation. This result would effectively dissociate the induction of differentiation from the control of tumorigenic behavior. We are currently investigating these possibilities.

CONCLUSIONS AND PROSPECTS FOR FUTURE STUDY

Somatic cell hybrids have provided a valuable means of investigating the genetic control of transformation and tumorigenicity in human cells. Conclusions that have been obtained from these studies include the fact that the transformed and tumorigenic phenotypes are under separate genetic control; that specific chromosomes are implicated in the control of malignant expression; and that, at least with whole cell hybrids, the induction of differentiation appears to be an important mechanism in controlling tumorigenicity. The hybrid cells have also allowed us to generate valuable reagents such as monoclonal antibodies against differentiation-specific antigens that will allow researchers to probe more specifically into the program of differentiation. These studies, particularly those dealing with the transfer of single chromosomes, will now make the cloning and characterization of tumor-suppressor genes a feasible goal. It is also hoped that when the tumor-suppressor genes are finally isolated and functional studies are able to be undertaken, that it will then be possible to determine whether neoplasia is indeed a disease of cell differentiation (1).

REFERENCES

1. Markert, C. L. (1968) Cancer Res. **28**, 1908-1914.

2. Greaves, M. F. (1986) Science **234**, 697-704.

3. Metcalf, D. (1985) Science **229**, 16-22.

4. Sachs, L. (1984) Cancer Surveys **3**, 219-228.

5. Potter, V. R. (1978) Brit. J. Cancer **38**, 1-23.

6. Pierce, G. B. (1974) Am. J. Pathol. **77**, 103-118.

7. McKusick, V. A. and Ruddle, F. H. (1977) Science **196**, 390-405.

8. Davidson, R. L. (1974) <u>Somatic Cell Hybridization</u>. Raven Press, New York.

9. Harris, H. (1986) J. Cell Sci. **4**, 431-444.

10. Straus, D. S., Jonasson, J. and Harris, H. (1976) J. Cell Sci. **25**, 73-86.

11. Stanbridge, E. J. et al. (1982) Science **215**, 252-259.

12. Peehl, D. M. and Stanbridge, E. J. (1982) Intl. J. Cancer **30**, 113-120.

13. Harris, H. (1985) J. Cell Sci. **79**, 83-94.

14. Sager, R. (1985) Adv. Cancer Res. **44**, 43-68.

15. Stanbridge, E. J. (1976) Nature **260**, 17-20.

16. Stanbridge, E. J. and Wilkinson, J. (1980) Intl. J. Cancer **26**, 1-8.

17. Stanbridge, E. J. et al. (1982) Somatic Cell Genet. **7**, 699-712.

18. Klinger, H. P. (1982) Cytogenet. Cell Genet. **32**, 68-84.

19. Srivatsan, E. S., Benedict, W. F. and Stanbridge, E. J. (1986) Cancer Res. **46**, 6174-6179.

20. Kaelbling, M. and Klinger, H. P. (1986) Cytogenet. Cell Genet. **41**, 65-70.

21. Ege, T. et al. (1977) Methods Cell Biol. **15**, 339-357.

22. Fournier, R. E. K. and Ruddle, F. H. (1977) Proc. Natl. Acad. Sci. **74**, 319-323.

23. Saxon, P. J., Srivatsan, E. S. and Stanbridge, E. J. (1986) EMBO J. **5**, 3461-3466.

24. Stanbridge, E. J. and Ceredig, R. (1981) Cancer Res. **41**, 573-580.

25. Der, C. J. and Stanbridge, E. J. (1981) Cell **26**, 429-439.

26. Sutherland, D. R. et al. (1986) J. Biol. Chem. **261**, 2418-2424.

27. Stanbridge, E. J., Fagg, B. A. and Der, C. J. (1983) In: Human Carcinogenesis (C. Harris and H. Autrup, eds.) pp. 97-122. Academic Press, New York.

28. Stanbridge, E. J. et al. (1986) Cancer Res. **46**, 4759-4764.

29. Jones, H. W. et al. (1971) Obstet. Gynecol. **38**, 945-949.

30. Weissman, B. E. et al. Science (in press).

INTERACTION BETWEEN BRAIN TISSUE AND MALIGNANT GLIOMA CELLS IN ORGAN CULTURE

O.D. LAERUM, R. BJERKVIG AND S.K. STEINSVÅG

DEPARTMENT OF PATHOLOGY, THE GADE INSTITUTE,

UNIVERSITY OF BERGEN, N-5016 HAUKELAND HOSPITAL, NORWAY

The direct spread of malignant cells from a primary tumour into the surrounding tissues is considered as one of the most important properties that govern malignant behaviour. At the same time such invasiveness is a necessary condition for the occurrence of metastases. Despite intensive research the general knowledge of this process is still limited. One of the reasons for this is the complexity of cellular reactions that take place in the borderzone between a malignant tumour and the surrounding normal tissue (Fig.1).

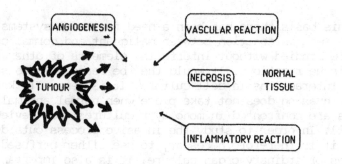

Fig. 1. Schematic diagram of tissue reactions near a malignant tumour.

INVASIVENESS:

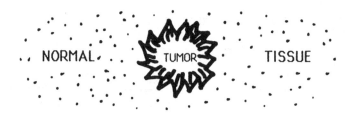

1. CELLS OCCUPY ANOTHER TISSUE

2. PROGRESSIVE PROCESS,
   i.e will continue and increase with time

3. DESTRUCTION OF NORMAL TISSUE

Fig. 2. Definition of invasiveness.

On this basis there has been a need for model systems where
the direct interaction between malignant and normal cells
can be studied without interfering elements of other types
of tissue reactions. It would then be reasonable to study
such interactions in cell culture. It is generally known
that invasion does not take place when normal and malignant
cells are confronted in monolayer cultures (for review
see 1). In order to study the invasive process outside the
body it is, therefore, necessary to use either perfused
organs or ordinary organ culture. It is also important to
state that invasiveness is a complex property which rests
on several cellular functions. The strict definition is as
shown in (Fig. 2).

MALIGNANT DEVELOPMENT IN THE NERVOUS SYSTEM

From a clinical point of view it is   generally known that
malignant brain tumours may exhibit a rather short time
period from the onset of clinical symptoms until the

terminal phase. At the same time the preclinical stages of
these neoplasms may go over several years. From animal
systems it is known that even after the administration of
a strong, specific neurocarcinogenic agent, it may take a
great part of the lifespan of the animal before a tumour
is evident (see e.g. 2).

When a tumour is evident in the nervous system, it is often
outside the reach of surgically intervention, due to the
local spread into the surrounding brain tissue. It has,
therefore, been a need for research in this area, both
applying to how malignancy develops and how the malignant
cells may infiltrate. On this background our research group
has for several years been studying malignant transformation in the nervous system by transplacental administration
of the alkylating carcinogen ethylnitrosourea to 18-day-old
rat fetuses (3,4). This process could also be studied outside the body by explanting cells from the treated brains
shortly afterwards to longterm cell culture. Under these
conditions, malignant transformation would take place in a
similar way as in the intact brains in vivo, and during the
same time period, i.e. 7 months (3). Thus, the different
stages of malignant transformation could be observed
directly. It was found that the transformation occurred as
a stepwise process, where the cells acquired one and one
property characteristic of malignant cells. The sequence
was as follows: Growth of hyperplastic nodules/microtumours→
rapid proliferation of morphologically altered cells→loss
of anchorage dependence→tumourigenicity by reimplantation
into isogeneic host animals.

However, it could not be established at what period the
cells acquired invasive properties. On this background a
collaboration project with the University of Gent was
initiated, where several organ culture systems were employed in order to study directly the interactions between
malignant and normal cells. The final goal was to obtain a
system where the glioma cells could use their natural
target tissue in organ culture, i.e. rat brain tissue (5).

EXPLANTS OF SOLID BRAIN TISSUE AS TARGET

A system has been especially developed for this purpose,
where pieces of hemisphere tissue from the brains of
18-day-old BD-IX rat fetuses were explanted to microwell

dishes where the bottom had been covered with an agar base
on beforehand. By this procedure the tissue would not
attach to the substratum and remained free in suspension
in the medium. Within a few days the explants would round
up and form spheroids with preservation of the organoid
structures. At the same time, a cell proliferation and
migration mimicking the layer formation and differentiation
process taking place in the intact brains was observed (6).
When these explants were confronted with aggregates of
malignant rat glioma cells, the tumour cells first migrated
around the explant to varying extents. Then tumour cell
invasion and replacement of one and one layer of the brain
tissue was observed (7). The tumour cell invasion occurred
as a massive replacement process ending with a small central
core of remaining brain tissue surrounded by a large mass
of malignant cells.

INVASION INTO REAGGREGATING BRAIN CELL CULTURES

The experiments described above were hampered by the great
difference between the loose tumour cell aggregate,
enabling more or less free movement of the malignant cells,
and the solid matrix and limited possibilities for movement
of the normal cells. It could, therefore, not be excluded
that some of the phenomena were due to this difference.
To test this possibility, another system was developed,
where cell suspensions were made by mechanical dispersion
of 18-day fetal rat brains which were transferred to
culture dishes coated with an agar base. After a few days
the cells would reaggregate and form organoid nodules in a
similar way as has been known from other systems. However,
the main difference from other types of reaggregating brain
cell cultures was that this was done in a stationary
system in order to avoid interference due to mechanical
forces when cultures were shaken continuously(8,9).

Also in this system, malignant glioma cells would surround
and thereafter invade the normal brain tissue that had
formed. Depending on the cell lines studied, tumour cell
invasion was characterized by a massive solid cell replacement, or single cell invasion was observed (8-10).

Firstly, two normal brain cell aggregates were placed
together. Within a few days they fused and made one large
aggregate. When two glioma cell aggregates were placed

together, they also fused rapidly and formed one single aggregate. However, when one normal brain cell aggregate was confronted with a glioma cell aggregate or to glioma cells in suspension, the malignant cells progressively invaded the brain tissue (10; Fig. 3 and 4).

In both these confrontation systems it was possible to identify single malignant cells within the brain tissue with several methods. One was to prelabel the glioma cells with ^{3}H-thymidine and perform autoradiography (7). The other was to study differentiation markers such as glial fibrillary acidic protein, S-100 protein and neuron specific enolase. For these three markers fetal brain tissue and glioma cells had different patterns depending on the stage of brain development in culture and on the type of glioma line (8).

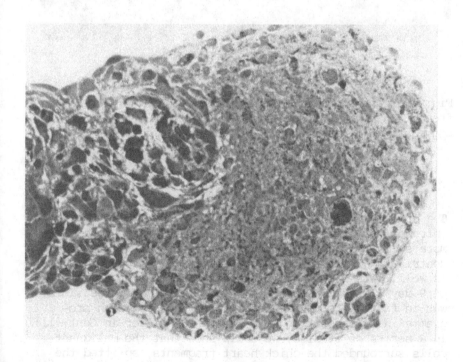

Fig. 3. After 144 hrs of confrontation, the tumour cells have partly penetrated and replaced the normal brain tissue. Semithin toluidine stained section. Magnification x 380.

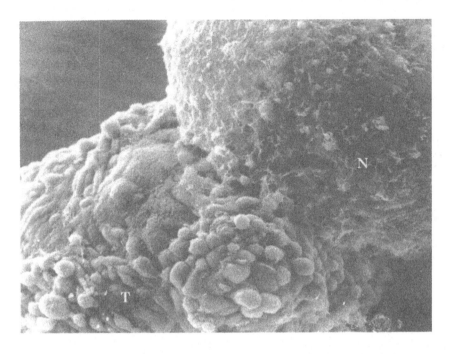

Fig. 4. Scanning electron micrograph after 24 hrs of confrontation between a tumour spheroid (T) and a normal brain
aggregate (N). Magnification x 1150.

FETAL HEART SYSTEM

The brain is known as a rather soft tissue, where the
entrance of malignant cells might be far easier than in
more solid tissues. In order to exclude that this was a
contributing factor, it was necessary to test other organs
as well. This was done by confronting precultured fragments
of 9-day-old chick hearts to glioma cell aggregates. This
was in fact the study that initiated this research pro-
gramme in collaboration with Dr. Leo De Ridder in Gent (11).
In a series of studies, we could show that the malignant
cells surrounded the chick heart fragments, splitted the
heart cell junctions and invaded the tissue. The pattern of
invasion was dependent on the type of glioma line, and glioma
and neurinoma lines had different histological appearence

(12). By electron microscopy it was also observed that cytoplasmic processes of the malignant cells were extended into the heart tissue between muscle cells and thereafter splitting their junctions at a short distance (13). It was also found a high endo/exocytotic activity both on the surface of the malignant and the normal cells.

An important finding was that the acquisition of invasiveness was a rather late phenomenon during the carcinogenic process. With the chick heart system, we found that invasiveness occurred at the same culture passage as when carcinogen treated brain cells had become tumourigenic (11). We could also show that a revertant cell line that was no longer tumourigenic was also no longer invasive. This could indicate that the acquisition of invasiveness is a rather late event during the process of carcinogenesis, although it can not be excluded that the culture system can interfere.

PROPERTIES RELATED TO INVASIVENESS

As documented in the presented data and in accordance with earlier investigations, several cell properties are associated with tumour cell invasion (Fig. 5). It has been shown that cell locomotion is a necessary condition for the occurrence of invasion (1). In the brain-glioma co-culture system this appears as a directional migration of the malignant cells after they have extended cytoplasmic processes towards the surface of the normal tissue (14). Thereafter, cytoplasmic extensions are extruded between normal cells, a phenomenon that is also observed in the chick heart system (13).

Surprisingly, cell proliferation does not appear to be a necessary condition for invasive behaviour (15).

The importance of phagocytic properties of the invasive cells has been debated for a long time (see e.g. 15). Using a new flow cytometric method for automated quantitation of phagocytic activity in malignant cells, we could show that the phagocytic capacity of some invasive cell lines was of the same magnitude as in normal fetal brain cells, i.e. about 30-40% of the cells would take up foreign particles such as bacteria, zymosan particles, erythrocytes and fluorescent cell debris (16). However, when divided

LYSIS OF NORMAL CELLS AND BREAKDOWN OF CELL BOUNDARIES

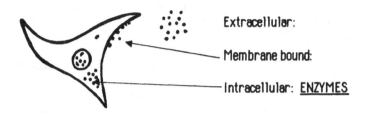

Extracellular:

Membrane bound:

Intracellular: <u>ENZYMES</u>

PHAGOCYTOSIS
(Property of all cells)

CELL LOCOMOTION
(Cytoskeleton - microtubules)

Fig. 5. Some phenomena associated with invasiveness.

into glioma cell lines with high and low phagocytic capacity, respectively, it turned out that those with high activity also had a strong lytic effect on the normal brain tissue. This could even occur at some distance from the invaded cells (16). At present it can not be established whether this is a direct relation or indirect, e.g. that cells with a high endocytic activity also have a high exocytic activity with excretion of lysosomal enzymes and toxic cell products. We are now investigating the excretion of different types of proteases from these cell lines in order to identify the active lytic agents (17).

It has often been claimed that highly differentiated tumours are less malignant than those with a low differentiation. However, we could not establish a direct relationship between differentiation pattern and the pattern of invasion. When looking at the presence of brain specific proteins, such as glial fibrillary acidic protein (GFAP), S-100 protein, neuron specific enolase and the nCAM adhesion protein (18), both positive and negative cell lines were invasive (11). To what extent subpopulations within the

same cell lines have different invasive properties according to the differentiation pattern has not yet been
established.

It should also be noted that there do not seem to be
species differences according to invasiveness i organ
culture, since also human glioma cells invade in the same
way as rat gliomas (19).

GENERAL COMMENTS AND CONCLUSIONS

From the presented data it is evident that the property of
invasiveness by glioma cells can now be selectively studied
in organ culture, using their natural target organ outside
the body. The histological pattern of invasion turned out
to be identical in vitro and after intracranial transplantation in vivo (10). Hence, the presented co-culture
systems may be used for further elucidating one of the most
critical properties for biological malignancy. It should
also be noted that the co-culture system allows the study
of both malignant and normal cells under exactly the same
conditions, including properties as cell proliferation,
cell attachment and migration, invasion and tissue destruction. At the same time the direct interactions between
normal and malignant cells of the same tissue origin can be
studied at the membrane level and with high magnification
(see e.g. 20; Fig. 4 and 5).

According to observations with malignant brain tumours in
CNS, one could postulate that invasion is partly the result
of lack of space following uncontrolled and progressive
cell proliferation in a tumour. However, this occurs not
to be the case, since there is certainly no lack of space
in the co-culture system.

Since the invasion process also can be quantitated and
followed in time, the dynamics of this process can also be
elucidated. Apart from the generally known phenomenon of
lysosomal enzyme secretion, phagocytic properties seem to
be related to the lytic effects of tumour cells, while
differentiation protein markers did not show such
correlation (16).

We conclude that invasiveness is one of the most important
biological properties for malignancy in the nervous system.
This property can now be studied specifically outside the
body using organ co-culture systems which enable selective
investigations of different cell functions related to this
property. Our systems are now available for large scale
use in the search for alternative cancer treatment
modalities as well as for the study of mechanisms underlying invasive behaviour.

REFERENCES

1. Mareel, M.M. (1984) in *Invasion: Experimental and Clinical Implications* (Mareel, M.M., and Calman, K.C., eds) pp.275-300, Oxford University Press, Oxford

2. Kleihues, P., Rajewsky, M.F. (1984) in *Progress in Experimental Tumor Research* (Rosenblum, M.L., and Wilson, C.B., eds) Vol. 27, pp.1-16, S. Karger, Basel

3. Laerum, O.D., and Rajewsky, M.F. (1975) *J. Natl. Cancer Inst.* **55**, 1177-1187

4. Laerum, O.D., Mørk, S.J., and De Ridder, L. (1984) in *Progress in Experimental Tumor Research* (Rosenblum, M.L., and Wilson, C.B., eds) Vol. 27, pp 17-31, S. Karger, Basel

5. Laerum, O.D., Steinsvåg, S.K., and Bjerkvig, R. (1985) *Acta Neurol. Scand.* **72**, 529-549

6. Steinsvåg, S.K., and Laerum, O.D. (1985) *Experientia* **41**, 1517-1524

7. Steinsvåg, S.K., Laerum, O.D., and Bjerkvig, R (1985) *J. Natl. Cancer Inst.* **74**, 1095-1104

8. Bjerkvig, R., Steinsvåg, S.K., and Laerum, O.D. (1986) *In Vitro* **22**, 180-192

9. Bjerkvig, R. (1986) *In Vitro* **22**, 193-200

10. Bjerkvig, R., Laerum, O.D., and Mella, O. (1986) *Cancer Res.* **46**, 4071-4079

11. De Ridder, L., and Laerum, O.D. (1981) *J. Natl. Cancer Inst.* **66**, 723-728

12. Mørk, S., De Ridder, L., and Laerum, O.D. (1982) *Anticancer Res.* **2**, 1-10

13. Mørk, S., Laerum, O.D., and De Ridder, L. (1983) *Anticancer Res.* **3**, 373-384

14. Steinsvåg, S.K. (1985) *Invasion Metastasis* **5**, 255-269

15. Mareel, M.M. (1980) *Int. Rev. Exp. Pathol.* **22**, 65-129

16. Bjerknes, R., Bjerkvig, R., and Laerum, O.D. (1986) *J. Natl. Cancer Inst.* In press

17. Andersen, K.-J., Bjerkvig, R., and Laerum, O.D., (1987) in *Investigation o, Cellular Dearrangements* (Reid, E., and Andersen, K.-J., eds) Plenum Press, New York. In press

18. Laerum, O.D., Mørk, S.J., Haugen, Å., Bock, E., Rosengren, L., and Haglid, K. (1985) *J. Neuro-Oncol.* **3**, 137-146

19. De Ridder, L., Laerum, O.D., Mørk, S.J., and Bigner, D.D. (1986) *Acta Neuropathol.* In press

20. Steinsvåg, S.K., and Laerum, O.D. (1985) *Anticancer Res.* **5**, 137-146

TUMOR PROMOTER-MEDIATED MODULATION OF CELL DIFFERENTIATION AND COMMUNICATION:THE PHORBOL ESTER - ONCOGENE CONNECTION

Monica HOLLSTEIN and Hiroshi YAMASAKI

International Agency for Research on Cancer

150 cours A.Thomas 69372 Lyon cedex 08 France

INTRODUCTION

Proto-oncogenes, when expressed inappropriately or in altered form have the potential to cause cancer. Cancer is usually accompanied by a loss of cellular differentiation and by enhanced proliferation. As the normal function of proto-oncogenes appears to include control of cell differentiation and proliferation, aberrant function of these oncogenes is probably involved in the various molecular events that contribute to the development of malignancy.

The tumor promoter phorbol esters which can enhance the transformed phenotype _in vitro_ and the appearance of tumors in experimental animal systems, also have the capacity to modulate cell differentiation and proliferation. The biological effects of tumor promoters on differentiation are worthy of analysis because the transformed cell phenotype is usually associated with loss of differentiation-associated characteristics such as disappearance of biochemical markers and specific cell functions. Since proto-oncogenes can be involved in the development of neoplasia when they are deflected from their proposed normal role of controlling differentiation processes, there is a theoretical basis for the hypothesis that tumor promoters affect differentiation and encourage malignant growth by perturbing some members of this set of control switches: the cellular oncogenes.

At the cellular level cell-cell interaction appears to play an important role in the control of differentiation and proliferation. Cells in almost all tissues, with the exception of blood cells, acquire specific structures through which they communicate by direct exchange of physiological molecules and ions. This specific communication pathway, gap-junctional intercellular communication, is considered to be of fundamental importance in the maintenance of tissue homeostasis. Phorbol ester tumor promoters were the first class of chemical agents shown to inhibit junctional intercellular communication. It is postulated that phorbol ester-mediated inhibition of cell communication may lead to modulation of cell differentiation.

Phorbol ester tumor promoters may exert many, if not all of their effects by activating protein kinase C. Recent studies from different laboratories suggested to us that the "phosphatidyl inositol cycle - protein kinase C" pathway may be one of the key signal traducing systems for many growth factors.

It is the aim of this article to discuss cellular and molecular mechanisms of phorbol ester-mediated modulation of cell differentiation and intercellular communication with special emphasis on the relationship between phorbol ester tumor promoters, protooncogene expression and protein kinase C.

PHORBOL ESTER-INDUCED MODULATION OF CELL DIFFERENTIATION IN VITRO IS ACCOMPANIED BY ALTERATIONS IN PROTO-ONCOGENE EXPRESSION (Table I and references therein)

Tumor promoting phorbol esters modulate cell differentiation in a variety of cell types, and the nature of this effect depends on the cell system (1): both inhibition and stimulation of differentiation can occur. For example, treatment of mouse Friend erythroleukemic cells (FELC), neuroblastoma cells, and epidermoid cultures with TPA blocks the appearance of the differentiated phenotypes; this same compound induces terminal differentiation of human medullary thyroid carcinoma TT cells, promyelocytic HL60 cells, and U937 human monocytes. While at first glance such contradictory effects might appear to lead to unnecessary complications, it is clear that these experimental systems can be extremely useful tools for studying the parameters involved in cell differentiation and growth control: with each of these classic model systems and their TPA resistant variants, it should be possible to separate association and causation, and to select among the pleiotropic effects of TPA those biochemical events specifically linked to induction, or prevention as the case may be, of the differentiated phenotype.

Exposure to TPA ultimately results in the appearance or disappearance of a wide variety of gene products (depending on the cell type), some of which serve as markers characteristic of differentiation, such as beta-globin in Friend erythroleukemia cells (FELC). This phenomenon argues for a mechanism involving some ubiquitous and fundamental gene regulation control system, triggerred by external cellular signals (e.g., TPA) and the particular internal environment (determined by the cell type), that governs stage-tissue-specific patterns of gene expression.

As is the case for TPA, the products of certain proto-oncogenes apparently are able to induce, and some are able to block cellular differentiation (2); it is likely that the normal function of certain proto-oncogenes is the proper control of cell differentiation. As expression of this family of genes is programmed developmentally and modulates tissue differentiation, there is a strong argument for the supposition that aberrant proto-oncogene function causes aberrations in differentiation programmes and consequently, neoplastic-like phenotypic changes. From the aspect of cancer as cell proliferation gone out of balance, it is also relevant to note that a) certain proto-oncogene products appear to be tightly linked to control of cell division processes (e.g., fos, myc); b) some proto-oncogene products are growth factors/receptors (erbB, sis, fms), and c) certain programs of cell differentiation may be induced by specific oncogene products (e.g., src and neuronal differentiation). In addition, viral oncogenes, which can be viewed as modified proto-oncogenes, malignantly transform cells. Since both phorbol ester tumor promoters and proto-oncogenes affect cell growth, differentiation, and malignant transformation, it is tempting to suggest that these entirely separate entities, i.e., an external chemical stimulus (TPA), and cellular proto-oncogene products, either interact at some level or affect the same biochemical pathway at some point. Evidence that there is at least an indirect interplay

between proto-oncogenes and tumor promoters is provided by
the numerous examples showing that expression of certain
proto-oncogenes can undergo dramatic shifts when cells are
exposed to TPA (Table I).

Since, phorbol ester exposure may elicit differentiation, block differentiation, or have no apparent phenotypic
effect depending on the cell system, several hypotheses can
be tested as to which proto-oncogene expression alterations
are particularly relevant to differentiation control, and
how, at a molecular level, tumor promoters may be affecting
a cell's malignant potential. For example, experiments
with the U937 and HL60 leukemia cell lines have shown that
a rapid increase in c-fos mRNA occurs following phorbol
ester stimulation of terminal differentiation into macrophages; however, DMSO induced HL60 differentiation to
granulocytes is not accompanied by an increase in c-fos
mRNA, suggesting either that c-fos induction during differentiation is lineage-dependent and/or that TPA might
elicit c-fos mRNA independent of whether differentiation
ensues, and is thus an indiscriminate c-fos mRNA inducer.
This second interpretation is supported by the observation
that TPA induces fos expression in a wide variety of other
cells, e.g., erythroleukemia cells, bladder epithelial
cells, pheochromocytoma cells and fibroblasts (Table I), in
some instances independent of whether differentiation-like
phenotypic changes follow exposure to the tumor promoter.
In addition, two chemical stimuli can elicit enhanced c-fos
expression in pheochromacytoma cells (3), yet only one of
the two treatments induces these cells to differentiate.
At present, these results are consistent with the interpretation that a burst in c-fos mRNA, though perhaps a necessary component in the pathway to differentiation of some
lineages, is not a universal requirement of cell differentiation, and when necessary, is nevertheless insufficient.

A powerful approach to determine precisely the role of
proto-oncogene   expression   alterations   essential   in
differentiation control is the use of cell systems in which
a given oncogene is constitutively expressed. With this
approach it has been shown that Friend erythroleukemia
cells transfected with a c-myc containing plasmid and
constitutively expressing c-myc mRNA are unable to
differentiate (4, 5, 6). In this way, it is possible to
distinguish between whether chemical induction of a

Table I - Phorbol ester tumor promoter modulation of cell growth and differentiation: Concommittant alterations in proto-oncogene expression*

DESCRIPTION OF CELL SYSTEM	TREATMENT	EFFECT on phenotype	EFFECT on proto-oncogene mRNA		REFERENCES
Human myeloblast leukemia cell line (HL60)	TPA	macrophage differentiation	fos	+	34, 35
			myc	-	36, 39, 74
			fms	+	7
			src	+	42
			N-ras	0	36
	DMSO	granulocyte differentiation	fos	0	34
			myc	-	36, 37, 74
			fms	0	7
			N-ras	0	36
Variant clone (HL60[R])	TPA or DMSO	No differentiation	fms	0	7
Human myeloblast leukemia cell line (ML-1)	TPA	differentiation	myb	-	38
Human monocytic hematopoietic cell line (U937)	TPA	macrophage differentiation	src[1]	+	42
			myc	-	39
			fms	+	28
			fos	+	34

*Differentiation induction by other chemicals besides TPA are included[1] for comparison.
Symbols: (+), increase; (-), decrease; (0), no change observed.   [1] pp60src

DESCRIPTION OF CELL SYSTEM	TREATMENT	EFFECT on phenotype	on proto-oncogene mRNA		REFERENCES
Friend erythroleukemia mouse cell line (FELC 19-101)	HMBA or DMSO	differentiation	myc	−	10,40,31,39,41,74
	HMBA + TPA	No differentiation	myc fos	− +	10
Variant clone (FELC 19-9)	HMBA + TPA	differentiation	myc fos	− +	10
Myeloid human (TT) medullary thyroid carcinoma cell line	TPA	differentiation	myc	−	43
Human embryonic mega-karyocitic cell line (K562)	TPA	differentiation	sis	+	44
Human epidermal carcinoma cell line (A431)	TPA	(not reported)	fos myc	+ +	46
	EGF	Growth inhibition	fos myc	+ +	46
Variant clone (A431R)	EGF	No growth inhibition	fos myc	+ +	

DESCRIPTION OF CELL SYSTEM	TREATMENT	EFFECT on phenotype	on proto-oncogene mRNA		REFERENCES
Human epidermoid carcinoma cell line (KB)	TPA	(not reported)	erbB	+	47
	EGF		erbB	+	
Human bladder epithelial cell line (HCV 29)	TPA	cell-contact morphology	fos	+	45
			myc	0	
			H,Kras	0	
Rat pheochromocytoma cell line (PC12)	TPA	No differentiation	fos	+	3
			myc	+	
	EGF	No differentiation	fos	+	3
			myc	+	
	NGF	neuronal differentiation	fos	+	3
			myc	+	
Mouse fibroblast cell lines BALB/c or NIH/3T3[1]	TPA	mitogenic	myc	+	32, 48
			fos	+	48, 49
			fms	0	49
	PDGF	mitogenic	myc	+	32
			fos	+	49
Mouse skin, normal and and cancerous (in vivo)	TPA	skin tumor promoter	H, Kras	0	50
			fos,myc,raf		

[1]Chemical treatment of quiescent cultures

proto-oncogene has a functional role in differentiation control, or whether the chemical simply induces the alterations without evident phenotypic consequences. Clarification of this sort is also feasible with the use of tumor promoter-resistant variants. For example, the use of a HL60 cell variant resistant to TPA-induced differentiation (7) has permitted the tentative conclusion that TPA is not a general inducer of c-fms expression unlike the situation for c-fos, and that increased c-fms mRNA in HL60 cells sensitive to TPA-induced differentiation has a function in the differentiation process. Murine erythroleukemic cells offer a particularly interesting model system for this type of approach since variants with all possible differentiation responses to TPA are available and expression of certain proto-oncogenes has been studied in detail.

We have isolated TPA-resistant variants of murine Friend erythroleukemic cells (8) which we use to analyse TPA-induced proto-oncogene expression alterations in erythrocyte differentiation. This system is attractive from the point of view of tumor promoter mechanisms because in the prototypic FELC TS 19-101 cell line TPA blocks rather than stimulates differentiation, and thus serves as a model of the in vivo observation that tumor promoters cause phenotypic effects consistent with a loss of differentiated functions in cell tissues. The proto-oncogenes, c-fos, intensively studied in HL60 cell system (2), c-abl, the viral analog of which induces embryonic beta-globin production (9), and myc, constitutive expression of which blocks FELC differentiation (see above), are of particular interest. Using this cell line and its variant we have shown that in FELC TPA appears to be a general inducer of c-fos, which is consistent with findings in other in vitro model systems, and that increased c-fos expression does not necessarily result in differentiation (10). Since expression of some gene families is influenced by the degree of cytosine methylation at certain sequences, and since TPA exposure, as well as FELC differentiation, affect methylation of FELC cell DNA, we also examined the methylation pattern of c-fos sequences in these variants using HpaII, the CCGG methylation sensitive restriction enzyme isoschizomer of MspI. We found that the methylation of c-fos sequences is different in these variants, and has remained stable over time (1 year continuous culture). We have seen no alteration in c-fos methylation after 48 hours differentiation induction, and c-fos methylation does not appear to correlate with TPA's induction of c-fos mRNA. Since overall methylation of DNA in the TPA resistant cell variant is considerably greater than the parent TS 19-101 TPA-sensitive cell line (as seen by ethidium bromide staining following gel electrophoresis of total HpaII digested DNA), we are continuing to test the possibility that the TPA-resistant phenotype may be in part a consequence of methylated sequences, indicating a silenced gene, perhaps a proto-oncogene.

From an empirical basis, TPA effects on proto-oncogene expression and cell differentiation permit the following tentative generalisations: 1) TPA affects expression of a wide variety of proto-oncogenes, 2) this alteration in proto-oncogene expression is frequently associated with changes in differentiation and growth, and 3) changes in proto-oncogene mRNA levels following TPA exposure often parallel those elicited by growth factors, some of which are products (or ligands) of proto-oncogene proteins.

TPA-INDUCED AND ONCOGENE-INDUCED CHANGES IN INTERCELLULAR COMMUNICATION AND CELLULAR TRANSFORMATION: SIMILARITIES

Homeostasis of an organ appears to be assured *in vivo* by communication of cells with each other, permitting signal transduction, and thereby perhaps controlling metabolism and cell proliferation. Various facets of cell-cell contact may be important: interaction of CAM proteins, gap junction structures, and other surface structures may function in this type of communication. Numerous reports demonstrate that a perturbation of intercellular communication is linked to re-stimulation of the potential for cellular multiplication. Also, it is well known that partial hepatectomy results in a sharp decrease in the number of gap junctions and simultaneously, stimulation of hepatocyte proliferation. *In vitro* cell communication studies using the techniques of electric coupling, metabolic cooperation, and microinjection of fluorescent dye suggest that growth control is associated with the capacity of cells to communicate with each other.

Phorbol Esters Block Intercellular Communication and
Promote Expression of the Transformed Phenotype
(Table II and references therein)

One can consider carcinogenesis as a process involving
several stages that fall into two fairly distinct phases:
an initiation phase in which the carcinogen damages the DNA
by a mutation, and a promotion phase, in which there is a
clonal expansion of initiated cells which proliferate more
rapidly than neighboring normal cells, and form a tumor
under conditions favorable to neoplastic growth. Although
this model of initiation and promotion stems primarily from
animal experiments, in particular mouse skin carcinogenesis
experiments (11), it is likely that a similar process can
occur in human cancers (12).   Tumor promoting chemicals
such as phorbol esters which act at this second phase of
the carcinogenesis process presumably have the capacity to
stimulate clonal outgrowth of altered cells, but the
mechanisms by which this effect is elicited have not been
defined.

In the last several years, the interesting observation
was made that phorbol esters could inhibit the intercellular communication typically present among normal cells, and
this phenomenon has been confirmed by several different
methods and in numerous cell systems (Table II).   The
mechanism by which TPA could promote tumor growth may be
this metabolic isolation of aberrant cells from normal
cells, permitting clonal growth of initiated cells.

The precise action of phorbol esters at the intracellular level is not yet well understood, but it is known
that the most potent of this class of chemicals, TPA, is
not only a tumor promoter as discussed above, but also, an
activator of the calcium and phospholipid dependent enzyme
protein kinase C (13). The relevant feature of TPA exposure
and oncogene induced transformation as modulators of intercellular communication could be phosphorylation of a specific target protein involved in the communication machinery
at the cell membrane, since protein kinase phosphorylation
is the common event at the molecular level of TPA exposure
and the presence of active proto-oncogene protein kinases.
Although the action of oncogenes on communication has not
been the topic yet of many studies, it would be interesting
to compare the effect of various oncogene products with
that of phorbol esters on intercellular communication.

Table II. Inhibition of gap junctional intercellular communication by tumour promoting stimuli

Method of junctional communication measurement	Promoting stimulus	Target cells or tissue	Reference
Metabolic cooperation			
HGPRT$^+$/HGPRT$^-$(a)	Phorbol esters and many other tumor promoting agents	Chinese hamster V79	51
		Human fibroblasts	55
		Rat hepatocytes/rat liver epithelial cells	56
^{3}H-uridine metabolites transfer	Phorbol esters	Mouse epidermal cell line /Swiss 3T3 cells	22
ASS$^-$/ASL$^-$(b)	Phorbol esters, DDT	Human fibroblasts	57
Electrical coupling	Phorbol esters	Human amniotic membrane epithelial cells	53
		BALB/c 3T3 cells	54
Dye transfer			
Microinjection	Phorbol esters and certain other tumour promoting agents	Human colon epithelial	58
		Mouse epidermal cell line	59
		BALB/c 3T3 cells	60
		Chinese hamster V79	61
Photobleaching	Partial hepatectomy	Rat liver	62
	TPA and dieldrin	Human teratocarcinoma cells	63

Method of junctional communication measurement	Promoting stimulus	Target cells or tissue	Reference
Gap junction structure analysis			
Electron microscope	Phorbol esters	Chinese hamster V79	64
	Phorbol esters	Mouse skin in vivo	65
	Skin wounding	Urodele skin	66
	Phenobarbital or DDT administration	Rat liver in vivo	67
Gel electrophoresis analysis	Phorbol esters	Chinese hamster V79	68
Analysis with gap junction antibody	Partial hepatectomy	Rat liver in vivo	69

(a) HGPRT, hypoxanthine guanine phosphoribosyltransferase
(b) ASS⁻, angininosuccinate synthetase-deficient; ASL⁻, argininosuccinate lyase-deficient

Cellular Transformation by Oncogenes Causes
Intercellular Communication Block

Viewing cellular transformation in part as a perturbation of growth control, several research groups have shown that cellular transformation is accompanied by a block in intercellular communication (14,15,16). BALB/c 3T3 cells, frequently used in transformation experiments, form foci upon treatment with carcinogens, e.g., MCA, or following pEJras oncogene transfection. These transformed cells are incapable of communicating with surrounding normal cells (17, Figure 1). Communication inhibition, leading to increased cell growth, would then be one mechanism in the multi-step process ultimately permitting the appearance of foci, or clonal outgrowth of initiated cells. The relevance of this phenotypic change is supported by the observations discussed above showing that tumor promoting phorbol esters are potent inhibitors of intercellular communication (18). This, in conjunction with the finding that rat kidney cells infected with a temperature sensitive mutant of the oncogenic avian sarcoma virus become less permeable (19) make reasonable the supposition that reduced communication capacity allows expression of the transformed phenotype which otherwise would be blocked by the presence of surrounding cells. To analyse the temporal and mechanistic requirements of cell-cell contact effects on transformation, one can compare the effect of oncogene transfection with that of TPA exposure upon expression of transformation. For example, in cultures of 3T3 cells immortalised by plT, E1A or myc transfection in which no foci appear ordinarily, foci are induced by TPA treatment. Thus, here TPA acts in a manner analogous to pEJras which, when co-transfected with these so-called "immortalising" genes also results in the appearance of transformed foci (20). Rat embryo fibroblasts (21) and C3H10T1/2 (22) transfected with pEJras alone also form foci only if also exposed to TPA, and the presence of untransformed cells apparently has no effect on this stimulation of initiated cells (21). The capacity of TPA treatment to increase the appearance of foci in carcinogen or oncogene treated cultures may be quite specific for cell type. Intercellular communication studies in these cultures will indicate whether and when cell interaction is linked to TPA development of foci.

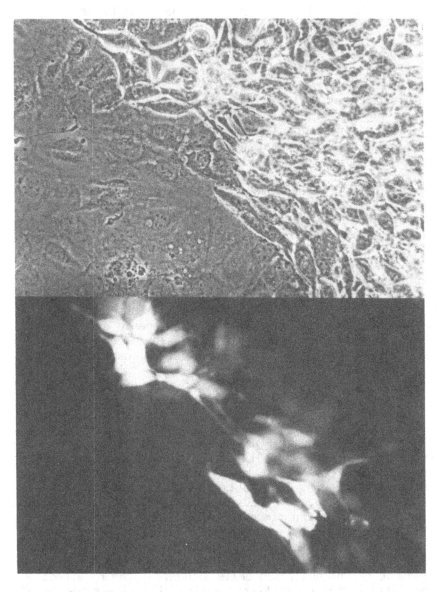

Figure 1. Intercellular communication block between normal
BALB/c 3T3 cells and cells transformed by pEJras
oncogene DNA transfection. A, pEJras transformed
cell at the periphery of a transformed focus was
microinjected with fluorescent dye. Upper panel:
phase contrast micrograph; lower panel: fluorescent micrograph of the same area.

RELATIONSHIPS BETWEEN TUMOR PROMOTING PHORBOL ESTERS, PROTO-ONCOGENES AND PROTEIN KINASE C
(Table III and references therein)

From a theoretical standpoint, a mechanistic link between oncogenes and TPA is provided by the demonstration that protein kinase C is the specific binding receptor of TPA and that many oncogenes code for protein kinases. Since tumor promoting phorbol esters directly activate protein kinase C (13) and since diacylglycerols also activate this enzyme, it is probable that most if not all pleiotropic effects of TPA, including its effects on cell differentiation and oncogene expression, occur through protein kinase C activation, subsequent modulation of cellular protein phosphorylation events, and the consequences of this phosphorylation. In evaluating this deduction, it would be useful to know 1) whether TPA treatment results in phosphorylation of oncogene products; 2) whether protein kinase C activation by diacylglycerol affects oncogene expression in the same way that TPA exposure does; 3) whether oncogene kinases and protein kinase C have substrates in common, or 4) whether cell variants resistant to the phenotypic effects of TPA have either some alterations in protein kinase C activity or localisation, or some functional change in a target protein phosphorylated by protein kinase C. In this way, one can probe for the biochemical intersections of protein kinase C activation and proto-oncogene activity.

Theoretically, one may envisage several possibilities including the hypotheses a) that among the protein kinase C substrates, there is a key protein kinase C phosphorylation of a proto-oncogene product, which then alters the proto-oncogene's capacity to function; b) that protein kinase C and proto- oncogene tyrosine kinases share a common substrate that in turn controls expression of other oncogenes governing cell growth, proliferation or differentiation (candidates for this class of substrate could include transcription regulatory factors controlling expression of oncogenes that are implicated, for example, in cell division control); or c) that protein kinase C activity and oncogene-ligand binding, by separate pathways, cause the accumulation of common intracellular messengers, e.g., products of the arachidonic acid cascade, and these messengers have essential effects on gene transcription

Table III – Information which suggests functional relationship between phorbol esters, diacylglycerols, protein kinase C and oncogene products

Oncogene/ growth factor	Observations	Ref.
src	TPA-induced HL-60 leukemial cell differentiation is accompanied by activation of pp60[src]	27
EGF	TPA and DAG reduce EGF binding in rat tracheal epithelial cells by changing affinity	24
EGF-R	TPA treatment of embryonic carcinoma cells causes phosphorylation of EGFR thr-654, and this may regulate EGF binding and EGFR tyrosine kinase activity	23
EGF-R	Purified protein kinase C modulates EGFR affinity, possibly by receptor phosphorylation	25
EGF-R	pp60[src] and EGFR substrates inhibit phospholipase A2: these substrates are also phosphorylated by protein kinase C. Phospholipid breakdown products may be a trigger for differentiation and transformation	26, 29
EGF	PD and OAG treated cells phosphorylate tyrosine residues of a 42kd protein which has been shown to be phosphorylated by EGF, PDGF-stimulated, and avian sarcoma virus-transformed cells	30

Oncogene/ growth factor	Observations	Ref.
src	Proteins that bind to actin cytoskeleton are phosphorylated by src and protein kinase C	28, 29
src	v-src transformed NIH/3T3 cells showed enhanced protein kinase C activity and reduced intercellular communication. TPA also blocks NIH/3T3 cell communication	73
myc	There is a drop in cellular DAG within two hours of chemically induced FELC differentiation and this precedes the decrease in c-myc mRNA	31
myc	Protein kinase C binds to upstream c-myc enhancer sequences; agents that activate protein kinase C stimulate c-myc expression	28, 71
PDGF	PDGF addition to quiescent 3T3 fibroblasts causes an increase in protein kinase C activity and in c-myc mRNA. TPA also has these effects	33
NGF	NGF, EGF, PMA all increase fos mRNA in rat pheochromocytoma cells and all phosphorylate tyrosine hydroxylase at a specific site	70
FSH	FSH stimulates granulosa cell differentiation. TPA blocks this differentiation, as do DAGs 37	72

control, transformation and differentiation. Experiments providing examples of each of these possibilities are cited in Table III: TPA phosphorylates the EGF receptor (encoded by the proto-oncogene erbB) (23) which may affect receptor ligand binding affinity (24,25). Protein kinase C phosphorylates pp60^{src} (26), and cell exposure to TPA enhances tyrosine kinase activity (27). Various inducers of fos transcription other than TPA, such as EGF, PDGF and NGF, can activate protein kinase C. Several proteins that bind to the actin cytoskeleton, for example calpactin, may be phosphorylated via either protein kinase C activation or the src oncogene product (28,29). Which phosphorylation events if any are essential features in expression of malignant phenotypes is the subject of intensive study. To determine which protein kinase C substrates are particularly relevant in the context of cell transformation, overlap can be sought between the transforming protein pp60^{src} and protein kinase C substrates (26,30); there is evidence that alteration in phospholipid metabolism is an important consequence of activity of these two kinases (29).

There are also several reports suggesting that protein kinase C is closely linked to control of c-myc expression: TPA and DAG cause a decrease in c-myc prior to FELC differentiation (31) and PDGF effects on c-myc mRNA in fibroblasts, which are similar to those of TPA exposure (32), are accompanied by an increase in protein kinase C activity (33). Whether protein kinase C binding to c-myc upstream enhancer sequences (28), phosphorylation of some trans-acting regulatory protein, or indirect control of regulatory molecules through other intermediates generated by protein kinase C activity is responsible for reported effects on c-myc expression is unclear.

CONCLUSIONS

In the past several years evidence has accumulated showing that molecular mechanisms by which phorbol esters enhance tumor formation include modulation of oncogene function, thereby de-regulating "healthy" differentiation and proliferation control. This link has been established by three avenues of inquiry.

1) Exposure to phorbol esters in various cell systems can affect cell differentiation. These changes in

differentiation are tightly linked to changes in proto-oncogene expression. Secondly, many growth factors (some are oncogene products or oncogene product ligands) mimic the pattern of proto-oncogene expression alterations induced by phorbol ester treatment.

2) Phorbol esters and transfected oncogenes can have similar or co-ordinating effects on transforming or differentiating cells in culture. Examples have been shown in which either an oncogene or phorbol esters can inhibit (or in some cell systems, induce) the differentiated phenotype. Oncogene transfection, viral transformation and phorbol ester treatment, have been shown to affect inter-cellular communication, a proposed control factor in co--ordinate cell growth, clonal outgrowth of initiated cells, and foci formation.

3) Protein kinase C is the membrane acceptor for phorbol esters, and ligand binding activates this enzyme. In the biochemical pathways of the cell, there are numerous points of intersection with regard to oncogenes, growth factors, and protein kinase C activation by phorbol esters.

Taken together, these observations support the working hypothesis that phorbol esters exert their tumor promoting effects by activating protein kinase C and that it is this activation, perhaps through a series of steps or signal intermediates, which has an important effect on oncogene functions, causing the appearance of transformed cell characteristics. One model of this "phorbol ester-protein kinase C activation-oncogene" connection would be one in which both protein kinase C activation, activation of oncogene kinases and growth factor ligand binding share a common biochemical consequence. This could be either phosphorylation of a shared substrate or the triggering of a second (later) messenger which alters cell metabolism and gene control. Another model of this connection would be one in which protein kinase C, perhaps indirectly, affects the expression of pivotal proto-oncogenes. It is also feasible that protein kinase C when altered in structure, function, or localisation would be capable of transforming cells, and would then itself fall into a functional definition of a proto-oncogene.

ACKNOWLEDGEMENTS

The contributions of M. Mesnil, and the secretarial assistance of C. Fuchez are gratefully acknowledged.

REFERENCES

1. Yamasaki, H. and Weinstein, I.B. (1985) In: Vouk, V.B., Butler, G.C., Hoel, D.G. and Peakall, D.B., eds., Methods for Estimating Risk of Chemical Injury, 155-180
2. Muller, R. (1986) TIBS 11, 129-132
3. Greenberg, M.E., Greene, L.A. and Ziff, E.B. (1985) J. Biol. Chem. 26, 14101-14110
4. Coppola, J.A. and Cole, M.D. (1986) Nature 320, 760-763
5. Dmitrovsky, E., Kuehl, W.M., Hollis, G.F., Kirsch, I.-R., Bender, T.P. and Segal, S. (1986) Nature 322, 748-750
6. Prochownik, E.V. and Kukowska, J. (1986) Nature 322, 848-850
7. Sariban, E., Mitchell, T. and Kufe, D. (1985) Nature 316, 64-66
8. Yamasaki, H., Drevon, C. and Martel, N. (1982) In: Hecker, E., Fusenig, N.E., Kunz, W., Marks, F. and Theilmann, H.W., eds., Cocarcinogenesis and Biological Effects of Tumor Promoters, 359-377
9. Lopez, A.R., Barker, J., Deisseroth, A.B. (1986) Proc. Natl. Acad. Sci. USA 83, 2042-2046
10. Giroldi, L., Hollstein, M. and Yamasaki, H. Manuscript in preparation
11. Berenblum, I. (1975) In: Becker, F.F., ed., Cancer: A Comprehensive treatise, vol. 1, pp. 323-344
12. Day, N.E. (1982) In: Hecker, E., Fusenig, N.E., Kunz, W., Marks, F. and Thielmann, H.W., eds., Cocarcinogenesis and Biological Effects of Tumor Promoters, pp. 183-199
13. Nishizuka, Y. (1984) Nature 308, 693-698
14. Loewenstein, W.R. (1979) Biochim. Biophys. Acta 560, 1-65
15. Mehta, P.P., Bertram, J.S. and Loewenstein, W.R. (1986) Cell 44, 187-196
16. Atkinson, M.M., Menko, A.S., Johnson, R.G., Sheppard, J.R. and Sheridan, J.D. (1981) J. Cell. Biol. 91, 573-758
17. Yamasaki, H., Hollstein, M., Mesnil, M., Martel, N., Aguelon, A-M. and Piccoli, C. (submit. for publication)

18. Yamasaki, H. (1986) In: Genetic Toxicology of Environmental Chemicals, Part A, 285-294
19. Goldberg, A.R., Delclos, K.B. and Blumberg, P.M. (1980) Science 208, 191-192
20. Connan, G., Rassoulzadegan, M.and Cuzin, F. (1985) Nature 314, 277-279
21. Dotto, G.P., Parada, L.F. and Weinberg, R.A. (1985) Nature 318, 472-475
22. Hsiao, W.L.W., Gattoni-Celli, S. and Weinstein, I.B. (1984) Science 226, 552-554
23. Davis, R.J. and Czech, M.P. (1985) Proc. Natl. Acad. Sci. US, 82, 1974-1978
24. Jetten, A.M., Ganong, B.R., Vandenbark, G.R., Shirley, J.E., and Bell, R.M. (1985) Proc. Natl. Acad. Sci. USA 82, 1941-1945
25. Fearn, J.C. and King, A.C. (1985) Cell 40, 991-1000
26. Huang, K.S., Wallner, B.P., Mattahano, R.J., Tixard, R., Burne, C., Frey, A., Hession, C., McGray, P., Sinclair, L.K., Chow, E.P., Browning, J.L., Ramachandran, K.L., Tang, J., Smart, J.E. and Pepinsky, R.B. (1986) Cell 46, 191-199
27. Barnekow, A. and Gessler, M. (1986) EMBO J. 5, 701-705
28. Abstracts. UCLA Symposium Steamboat Springs, Colo., April 1986. J. Cell. Biochem. (in press)
29. Brugge, J.S. (1986) Cell 46, 149-150
30. Gilmore, T. and Martin, G.S. (1983) Nature 306, 487-490
31. Faletto, D.L., Arrow, A.S. and Macara, I.G. (1985) Cell 43, 315-325
32. Kelly, K., Cochran, B.H., Stites, C.D. and Leder, P. (1983) Cell 35, 603-610
33. Kaibuchi, K., Tsuda, T., Kikuchi, A., Tanimoto, T., Yamashita, T. and Takai, Y. (1986) J. Biol. Chem. 261, 1187-1192
34. Mitchell, R.L., Zokas, L., Schreiber, R.D., Verma, I.M. (1985) Cell 40, 209-217
35. Muller, R., Curran, T., Muller, D. and Guilbert, L. (1985) Nature 314, 546-548
36. Watanabe, T., Sariban, E., Mitchell, T. and Kufe, D. (1985) Biochem. Biophys. Res. Comm. 126, 999-1005
37. Filmus, J. and Buick, R.N. (1985) Cancer Res. 45, 822-825
38. Craig, R.W. and Bloch, A. (1984) Cancer Res. 44, 442-446
39. Einat, M., Resnitzky, D. and Kimchi, A. (1985) Nature 313, 597-600

40. Watanabe, T., Sherman, M., Shafman, T., Iwata, T. and Kufe, D. (1986) J. Cell. Physiol. 127, 480-484
41. Lachman, H.M. and Skoultchi, A.I. (1984) Nature 310, 592-594
42. Gee, C.E., Griffin, J., Sastre, L., Miller, L.J., Springer, T.A., Piwnica-Worms, H.J. and Roberts, T.M. (1986) Proc. Natl. Acad. Sci. USA 83, 5131-5135
43. de Bustros, A., Baylin, S.B., Berger, C.L., Roos, B.A., Leong, S.S., and Nelkin, B.D. (1985) J. Biol. Chem. 260, 98-104
44. Colamonici, O.R., Trepel, J.B., Vidal, C.A., Neckers, L.M. (1986) Mol. Cell. Biol. 6, 1847-1850
45. Skouv, J., Christensen, B., Skibshøj, I. and Autrup, H. (1986) Carcinogenesis 7, 331-333
46. Bravo, R., Burckhardt, J., Curran, T. and Muller, R. (1985) EMBO J. 4, 1193-1197
47. Clark, A.J.L., Ishii, S., Richert, N., Merlino, G.T. and Pastan, I. (1985) Proc. Natl. Acad. Sci. USA 82, 8374-8378
48. Rabin, M.S., Doherty, P.J. and Gottesman, M.M. (1986) Proc. Natl. Acad. Sci. USA 83, 357-360
49. Greenberg, M.W. and Ziff, E.B. (1984) Nature 311, 433-438
50. Toftgard, R., Roop, D.R. and Yuspa, S.H. (1985) Carcinogenesis 6, 655-657
51. Yotti, L.P., Chang, C.C. and Trosko, J.E. (1979) Science 206, 1089-1091
52. Murray, A.W. and Fitzgerald, D.J. (1979) Bioch. Biophsy. Res. Comm. 91, 395-401
53. Enomoto, T., Sasaki, Y., Shiba, Y., Kanno, Y. and Yamasaki, H. (1981) Proc. Natl. Acad. Sci. USA 78, 5628-5632
54. Yamasaki, H., Enomoto, T., Shiba, Y., Kanno, Y. and Kakunaga, T. (1985) Cancer Res. 45, 637-641
55. Mosser, D.D. and Bols, N.C. (1982) Carcinogenesis 3, 1207-1212
56. Williams, G.M., Telang, S. and Tong, C. (1981) Cancer Letters 11, 339-344
57. Davidson, J.S., Baumgarten I. and Harley, E.H. (1985) Cancer Res. 45, 515-519
58. Friedman, E.A. and Steinberg, M. (1982) Cancer Res. 42, 5096-5105
59. Fitzgerald, D.J., Knowles, S.E., Balland, J. and Murray, A.W. (1983) Cancer Res. 43, 3614-3618
59. Mascioli, D.W. and Estensen, R.D. (1984) Cancer Res. 44, 3280-3285

60. Enomoto, T., Martel, N., Kanno, Y. and Yamasaki, H. (1984) J. Cell. Physiol. 121, 323-333
61. Zeilmaker, M.J. and Yamasaki, H. (1986) Cancer Res. (in press)
62. Meyer, D.J., Yancey, S.B. and Revel, J.P. (1981) J. Cell Biol. 91, 505-523
63. Wade, M.H., Trosko, J.E. and Schindler, M. (1986) Science 232, 525-528
64. Yancey, S.B., Edens, J.E., Trosko, J.E., Chang, C.C. and Revel, J.P. (1982) Exp. Cell Res. 19, 329-340
65. Kalimi, G.H. and Sirsat, S.M. (1984) Cancer Letters 22, 343-350
66. Loewenstein, W.R. and Penn, R.D. (1967) J. Cell Biol. 33, 235-242
67. Sugie, S., Mori, H. and Takahashi, M. (1984) Int. Cell Biol. p. 316 (abstract)
68. Finbow, M.E., Shuttleworth, J., Hamilton, A.E. and Pitts, J.D. (1983) EMBO J. 2, 1479-1486
69. Traub, O., Druge, P.M. and Willecke, K. (1983) Proc. Natl. Acad. Sci. USA 80, 755-759
70. Kruijer, W., Schubert, D. and Verma, I.M. (1985) Proc. Natl. Acad. Sci. USA 82, 7330-7334
71. Coughlin, S.R., Lee, W.M.F., Williams, P.W., Giels, G.M., Williams, L.T. (1985) Cell 43, 243-251
72. Shinohara, O., Knecht, M., Catt, K.J. (1985) Proc. Natl. Acad. Sci. USA 82, 8518-8522
73. Chang, C.C., Trosko, J.E., Kung, H.J., Bombick, D. and Matsumura, F. (1985) Proc. Natl. Acad. Sci. USA 82, 5360-5364
74. Grosso, L.E. and Pitot, H.C. (1985) Cancer Res., 45, 847-850.

Subject Index